THE
JUICE LADY'S™
GUIDE TO
JUICING
FOR
HEALTH

CHERIE CALBOM

a member

The information and procedures contained in this book are based upon the research and the personal and professional experiences of the author. They are not intended as a substitute for consulting with your physician or other health care provider. The publisher and author are not responsible for any adverse effects or consequences resulting from the use of any of the suggestions, preparations, or procedures discussed in this book. All matters pertaining to your physical health should be supervised by a health care professional. It is a sign of wisdom, not cowardice, to seek a second or third opinion.

Cover design: Doug Brooks
and Oscar Maldonado
Typesetter: Gary A. Rosenberg
In-house editor: Lisa James

Avery
a member of
Penguin Putnam Inc.
375 Hudson Street
New York, NY 10014
www.penguinputnam.com

The material on BMI in Appendix B is adapted from D. Heber, *The Resolution Diet* (1999), pages 28–29 and S. Woodruff, *Secrets of Cooking for Long Life* (1999), page 41; both books by Avery Publishing Group, Garden City Park NY.

THE JUICE LADY is a trademark of Salton-Maxim Housewares, Inc.

Cataloging-in-Publication Data
Calbom, Cherie.
    The juice lady's guide to juicing for health :
unleashing the healing power of whole fruits and
vegetables / by Cherie Calbom. — 1st ed.
      p. cm.
      Includes index.
      ISBN: 0-89529-999-2

      1. Fruit juices—Health aspects. 2. Vegetable
juices—Health aspects. I. Title.

RA784.C23 1999   613.2'6
                                   QBI99-871

Printed in the United States of America

20 19 18 17

Contents

To Norman Walker,
the great pioneer of juicing.

Acknowledgments

I wish to express my deep and lasting appreciation to the people who have assisted me with this book, especially the Nutrition Department at Bastyr University; the help of Dr. Mark Kestin and Alia Calender was invaluable in coordinating the research. A special thanks to the following Bastyr University students who did a superb job researching various topics: Cathy Mourey, Artemis Morris, Terry Monaghan, Pushpa Larsen-Giacalone, Carolyn Bell, Trina Fykerud, Kelly Morrow, Nicole Jensen, Beth DiDomenico, Norlinda Ghazali, Patti Pritchard, and Laura Behenna.

A very special thanks to Wendy Keller, my agent, for her expert help and guidance.

Much thanks to my editor, Lisa James, for her superb input to make this book a success.

Finally, my deep gratitude and continued appreciation to John, my husband, who has been my official "taste tester" for all my juice recipes and "the wind beneath my wings."

Introduction

People often ask me where I get the energy to keep the schedule I have of writing, traveling worldwide, and appearing on television. That question always causes me to pause. The energy I enjoy today is something I didn't experience for most of my life, but the fatigue and ill health that stalked me for so long have disappeared like mist before the sun.

I can't remember ever being particularly healthy and energetic, even as a child. My grandmother told me that I was sick a great deal of the time in childhood, sidelined because of colds and flus. I'm convinced that my problems began before I was born. My maternal heritage was not one of good health; my mother had never been well and died of cancer when I was six years old.

The surprising part of my health history was that not one doctor ever figured out why I was so tired and why I kept getting sick so much. Once a doctor suggested that I might have an allergy to dairy products and when I stopped eating them, my health improved slightly. Maybe I should have seen a veterinarian instead—growing up in Iowa and with relatives that farmed in Minnesota, I often heard people question what the cattle or other farmyard animals had been eating when they got sick. No one ever asked me what I had been eating.

What I was eating might have killed a healthy, strong gorilla! I loved junk food, candy, soft drinks, ice cream—anything sweet or salty and saturated with fat. Never having considered the connection between a healthy diet and a healthy body, I rarely thought twice about what I put in my mouth. I can't ever remember eating fresh green vegetables in the winter. Though I lived with my maternal grandmother, who grew a bountiful organic garden each year and prepared lots of vegetables for summertime meals, I didn't think most vegetables were particularly appealing. I liked eating sweet peas and baby carrots right out of the garden, corn off the cob

1

with lots of butter, and berries picked fresh off the vine—but that was about it. For the most part, my interest centered on my grandmother's homemade bread with plenty of butter plus her mouth-watering pies and cookies.

Through junior high I continued to catch nearly every cold and flu bug that circulated in school and was often home due to illness and fatigue. There were many mornings when I was so exhausted I could barely drag myself from bed. Feeling tired and unwell became a natural state of being for me, one I accepted without question for many years.

My health fluctuated through high school and my twenties. In order to stay thin, I started avoiding sweets, which helped my health to a degree, but I also put myself on a number of crash or starvation diets. Lacking the nutrients it needed, my body was crying for help. Once an aunt convinced me to take vitamin and mineral supplements. I noticed an increase in energy almost immediately when I took them, but I still suffered from bouts of fatigue and flu. Whatever good I was doing by taking nutritional supplements was nearly canceled out by my poor diet and occasional binges on sweets.

My real health crisis came when I turned 30 and developed a devastating case of chronic fatigue syndrome. I felt as though I had a never-ending flu and was perennially lethargic. In constant pain, I also had what is now diagnosed as fibromyalgia. That, coupled with hypoglycemia and infection with *Candida albicans* (a systemic yeast infection), meant I had never felt worse. I visited a holistic doctor who tested me for food allergies, and I left his office with a list of allergens longer than my arm. It was one of the most discouraging times of my life.

Not finding any clear answers from the medical profession as to how to correct my physical condition, I finally went to a health food store. I talked with employees and browsed the bookshelves. There I found answers. Clearly, I was eating poorly, not providing my body with the nutrients it needed to heal and gain energy. Most importantly, I learned about the energizing benefits of juicing fresh vegetables and fruits and the healing, restorative power of juice fasting. My body was toxic; an iridologist and a reflexologist both pointed this out. I was in great need of a cleansing program. The information I'd gathered offered me the first rays of hope—there *was* something I could do to restore my health.

Too tired to work, but armed with a juicer, I moved to my father's home and made it a full-time job to get healthy. I started a self-designed program with a five-day juice fast of mostly vegetable juices. I then turned to vegetarian eating, along with drinking lots of vegetable juices, for the next three months. The results were astounding. At the end of my program, I was completely well. I felt vibrant, healthy, and strong—three words I had never used to describe myself.

Praising this program as the best cure on earth, I still did not connect the fact that this way of eating was what would give my body the energizing fuel it needed to stay healthy. I returned slowly to some former eating habits. Little by little, old symptoms came back, and I had to admit that my healthy style of eating and juicing needed to be a way of life. Though I did not remain vegetarian, I stuck closely, most of the time, to my healthy diet—lots of fresh organically grown vegetables, juices, salads, whole grains, fish, and naturally raised chickens and eggs, with no sweets and little fat.

I became so passionate about what had brought about my newfound health and vitality that I finally decided to attend graduate school and pursue a master's degree in nutrition. This way I could be a credible source of information when I told people what juicing and eating right could do for them. Bastyr University in Seattle was my choice—a school dedicated to teaching natural medicine. It was there, before I had graduated, that I met the owners of the Juiceman company. They were looking for a couple of graduate students to write a little booklet containing juice recipes and nutrition information to accompany the juicer. I was one of the people chosen for the project.

One thing leads to another. I started lecturing for the Juiceman seminars before I had graduated. I was passionate about juicing; it had saved my life as far as I was concerned, and I considered it a privilege to help other people find nutritional answers for their needs. By the time I had graduated with my master's degree, I was the company's Juice Lady. I traveled the country almost weekly teaching people about health and nutrition, and about what juicing could do for them. I was so caught up in this mission and felt so healthy and strong that I neglected my own health. Getting little exercise, eating on the run, drinking fruit juices that I made on stage (fruit sugars are not good for my body), and not getting enough sleep all contributed to the return of chronic fatigue syndrome and fibromyalgia along with *Candida albicans* and parasites in 1993.

I took most of that year off and worked to restore my health with a strict diet and vegetable juices, a dedicated workout program, and homeopathic remedies prescribed by my naturopathic physician. By the end of the year, I was completely well again. I then wrote my first cookbook, *The Healthy Gourmet*, which is filled with my favorite healthy, tasty recipes. That same year the Juiceman juicer was bought by Salton-Maxim Housewares, Inc. It was through this new relationship that I met heavyweight boxer George Foreman at a trade show, where he was introducing his new

Lean, Mean, Fat-Reducing Grilling Machine. I became George's nutritionist, appeared in all the grill infomercials with him, and cowrote *George
Foreman's Knock Out the Fat Barbecue & Grilling Cookbook*. I have made
numerous appearances on QVC and The Shopping Channel of Canada,
and at the time of this writing, I have sold about 1.5 million books.

I want you to find juicing as easy and fun as possible, and to look forward to drinking the juices you make so you can experience their life-giving benefits. I am thrilled to pass on to you the knowledge about juicing
and dietary choices that I've learned, both on my own journey toward
health and through the dedicated scientific research of others. One of the
greatest gifts I can give you is the knowledge of the healing power of a
good diet, and of juicing in particular, along with an understanding of the
cause and prevention of disease.

To that end, I've written a book that gives you everything you need to
know about juicing in a simple, easy-to-understand format. First, I'll give
you some basic information about juicing, including the nutritional
advantages of juice, how to choose a juicer, and tips on how to get the
most out of your juicer. Then, I will provide diet and nutrition recommendations for a number of common health problems, including juice recipes.
Finally, I'll tell you about how to complement fresh juice with a healthy
diet and with cleansing programs that will allow you to naturally and
safely eliminate toxins from your body.

I wish you the best of health, which is one of the most precious gifts
you'll ever have.

Cherie Calbom
The Juice Lady

All About Juice

Do you eat between five and nine servings of fruits and vegetables every day, the number of servings recommended by the federal government to maintain good health? If you are like most Americans, your answer to this question is "No." Surveys show that only one in eleven people eats even the minimum of five servings each day. Fresh produce can require a lot of preparation and cooking time, and many people find the dinner hour to be the most rushed hour of the day. Juicing is the only way I know to easily and quickly supplement your diet with fruits and vegetables given the fast-paced lives most of us lead.

It is very easy to incorporate juicing into your life. Fresh juice is a great way to start the day, and it's far more energizing than a cup of coffee. Make some extra juice, and take it to work in an insulated container for a midmorning pick-me-up. Before dinner, start with a "salad in a glass" instead of a cocktail—all the nutrients fresh juice offers are far more calming, and you'll sleep better at night. Once you start experiencing the benefits of fresh juice, juicing will become a habit.

If you have a health problem, it is even more important to juice fresh vegetables and fruits. Fresh juice offers increased energy and strengthened immunity, plus the raw materials that help your body heal more quickly and completely. If you want to prevent disease, the surest path to a disease-free life begins with a diet rich in plant foods. Juicing provides the nutritional advantages of plant foods in a concentrated form that is easy to absorb. It is a delicious, simple way to increase your consumption of these life-giving foods.

In this section, I'll first explain why juicing is good for you. I'll then answer several commonly asked questions about juicing before telling you how to find the juicer that best meets your needs and how to most productively use the juicer you buy. Finally, I will explain why you should use organic produce to get the best possible juice.

LOOK AT WHAT FRESH JUICE OFFERS!

If you want a vitamin-mineral cocktail with all the nutrients you need, fresh juice is your answer. Juice provides your body with an abundance of water, along with easily absorbed protein, carbohydrates, essential fatty acids, vitamins, minerals, enzymes, and phytonutrients. And researchers are continuing to explore how the nutrients found in juice can ease specific disorders; see "The Science-Based Juice Pharmacy" below.

The Science-Based Juice Pharmacy

Scientific research supports the idea that fresh juice is good for you. Many studies have been published in some of the most prestigious medical journals on the benefits of the various nutrients found in fruits and vegetables, and a number of studies attest to the health benefits of specific juices.

❥ **Cabbage juice.** Dr. Garnet Chaney from Stanford University's School of Medicine performed several studies with cabbage juice, and found it was extremely effective in treating peptic ulcers. (Cheney, G, et al. "Anti-Peptic Ulcer Dietary Factor (Vitamin "U") in the Treatment of Peptic Ulcers," *Journal of the American Dietetic Association* 25:668–672, 1950.)

❥ **Cherry juice.** Cherry juice has been shown to be effective in easing attacks of gout and gouty arthritis, with patients reporting greater freedom of movement in their fingers and toes. Keracyanin, the pigment found in cherries, is believed to be the beneficial agent. (Blau, LW. "Cherry Diet Control for Gout and Arthritis," *Texas Report on Biology and Medicine* 8:309–312, 1950.)

❥ **Citrus juice.** One study showed that drinking citrus juices regularly, along with reducing dietary sodium, helped prevent kidney stones. ("Keeping Kidneys Stone-Free: Hold the Salt and Pass the OJ," *Modern Medicine* 63:15, January 1995.)

❥ **Cranberry juice.** Cranberry juice has been shown effective in the treatment and prevention of urinary tract infections. (Kuzminskik, LN. "Cranberry Juice and Urinary Tract Infections: Is There a Beneficial Relationship?" *Nutrition News* II:S87–S90, November 1996.)

❥ **Grape juice.** Grape juice, and specifically a compound called trans-resveratol, is likely to reduce the risk of atherosclerosis.

Water. Juice provides an abundance of water, which accounts for about 75 percent of the body's composition. About two-thirds of the body's water supply is in the cells, while the rest is used to transport nutrients. Water lubricates joints, assists in maintaining a constant body temperature, creates chemical reactions in a process called hydrolysis, generates energy, helps form the structure of cell membranes, and regulates all bodily func-

(Pace-Aselak, CR, et al. "Wines and Grape Juice as Modulators of Platelet Aggregation in Healthy Human Subjects," *Clinical Chimica Acta* 246:163–182, 1996.) Other studies found that drinking three glasses of purple grape juice a day reduced platelet aggregation, an important part of the clotting process, by 40 percent. According to the researchers, this suggests that grape juice provides as much protection against heart attack as a daily aspirin for patients with heart disease. (Mann, Denisek. "Purple Grape Juice, Wine and Beer All Cardioprotective," *Medical Tribune* 26, 1 May 1997.) Grape seed contains antioxidants known as proanthocyanidins that are more potent destroyers of free radicals than vitamin C or E. Juicing grapes with the seeds provides these antioxidants. (Bagchi, D, et al. "Oxygen Free Radical Scavenging Abilities of Vitamins C and E, and a Grape Seed Proanthocyanidin Extract *In Vitro*," *Research Communication in Molecular Pathology and Pharmacology* 95(2): 179–189, February 1997.)

❢ **Tomato juice.** A Harvard study showed that men who eat at least ten servings a week of tomato-based foods are up to 45 percent less likely to develop prostate cancer, while men who eat four to seven servings a week show a 20 percent reduction in prostate cancer rates. Tomatoes and tomato juice contain large amounts of lycopene, which is a powerful antioxidant. ("Cancer and Tomatoes," *Nutrition Week* 7, 15 December 1995; taken from 6 December 1995 issue of *Journal of the National Cancer Institute.*)

❢ **Vegetable juices.** In a study conducted at Norway's Oslo Rheumatism Hospital, rheumatoid arthritis patients drank fresh carrot, celery, and beet juices as part of a special dietary program. Doctors found a substantial reduction in disease activity among these patients. (Kjeldsen-Kragh, J, et al. "Controlled Trial of Fasting and One Year Vegetarian Diet in Rheumatoid Arthritis," *The Lancet* 338:899–902, 12 October 1991.)

tions. Fresh juice, especially if it is made from organic produce, provides pure water—the body's most important requirement.

Protein. Protein is the next most plentiful bodily component. The body uses various proteins to form muscles, ligaments, tendons, hair, nails, and skin. Proteins are needed to create enzymes, which direct chemical reactions, and hormones, which direct bodily processes. Fruits and vegetables contain lower quantities of protein than such high-protein foods as meat and dairy products, and are therefore thought of as poor protein sources. However, juices are concentrated forms of fruits and vegetables, and so provide an abundance of easily absorbed amino acids, the building blocks that make up protein. For example, sixteen ounces of carrot juice (two to three pounds of carrots) provides about five grams of protein (the equivalent of one hot dog or two ounces of tofu). Vegetable protein does not provide all the amino acids your body needs. You will need to add other protein sources, such as legumes (beans, lentils, and split peas) and whole grains, and/or low-fat animal proteins, to your daily diet (see Basic Guidelines for the Juice Lady's Health and Healing Diet, page 313). But juice is an excellent protein supplement, especially for vegetarians.

Carbohydrates. The third most plentiful substance in the body, carbohydrate is the fuel that provides the body with the energy needed for movement, heat production, and chemical reactions. The chemical bonds of carbohydrates lock in the energy a plant receives from the sun, and this energy is released when the body burns plant food as fuel. There are three categories of carbohydrates: simple (sugars), complex (starches), and fiber. There are more simple sugars in fruit juice than vegetable juice, which is why you should juice more vegetables than fruits if you have a sugar-metabolism problem. Soluble fiber is found in juice, and both soluble and insoluble fiber is found in whole fruits and vegetables. While both types are needed, remember that soluble fiber is proven effective in helping to control cholesterol levels.

Essential Fatty Acids. There is very little fat in fruit and vegetable juices, but the fats juice does contain are essential to your health. The essential fatty acids (EFAs)—linoleic and alpha-linolenic acids in particular—found in fresh juice function as components of nerve cells, cellular membranes, and hormonelike substances called prostaglandins. They are also required for energy production.

Vitamins. There are more than a dozen major vitamins—vitamins A, C, D, E, and K, along with the B complex—and they are all essential to your good health. Vitamins take part, along with minerals and enzymes, in chemical reactions. For example, vitamin C participates in the production of collagen, one of the main types of protein found in the body. Fresh fruit and vegetable juices are excellent sources of water-soluble vitamins (the B complex and vitamin C) and some fat-soluble vitamins (the carotenes, known as provitamin A, and vitamin K).

Minerals. There are about two dozen minerals that your body needs to function normally. Minerals—along with vitamins—are components of enzymes. Minerals also make up part of bone and blood tissue, and help maintain normal cell function. The major minerals include calcium, chloride, magnesium, phosphorus, potassium, sodium, and sulfur. Trace minerals—those needed in very small amounts—include boron, chromium, cobalt, copper, fluoride, manganese, nickel, selenium, vanadium, and zinc. Plants incorporate minerals, which occur in inorganic forms in the soil, into their tissues. As a part of this process, the minerals are combined with organic molecules into easily absorbable forms, which makes plant food an excellent dietary source of minerals. Juicing is believed to provide even better mineral absorption than whole fruits and vegetables because the process of juicing liberates minerals into a highly absorbable form.

Enzymes. Fresh juices are chock full of enzymes—those "living" molecules that work, often with vitamins and minerals, to speed up reactions necessary for the human body to function. Without enzymes, we would not have life in our cells. Enzymes are prevalent in raw foods, but heat, such as cooking or pasteurization, destroys them. Fresh juice contains enzymes that help break down food in the digestive tract, thereby sparing the body's digestive system from overwork. This sparing action is known as the "law of adaptive secretion of digestive enzymes." According to this law, if some of the food you eat is digested by enzymes from the food itself, the body will secrete less of its own enzymes. This allows the body's energy to be shifted from digestion to other functions such as repair and rejuvenation. Fresh juices require very little energy expenditure to digest. And that is one reason why people who start drinking fresh juice regularly often report that their energy levels increase.

Phytochemicals. Plants contain substances that protect them from disease, injury, and pollution. These substances are known as *phytochemicals;* "phyto" means plant and "chemical" in this context means nutrient. There are tens of thousands of phytochemicals in the foods we eat. For example, the average tomato may contain up to 10,000 different types of phytochemicals. Phytochemicals give plants their color, odor, and flavor. (Unlike vitamins and enzymes, they are heat stable and can withstand cooking.)

Researchers have found that people who eat the most fruits and vegetables, which are the best sources of phytochemicals, have the lowest incidence of cancer and other diseases. Drinking fruit and vegetable juices gives you these vital substances in a concentrated form. Here are just a few of these plant heroes and what they do for us:

- *Allyl sulfides,* in garlic and onions, have been found to lower the risk of stomach cancer.

- *Curcumins,* present in ginger and the spice turmeric, stimulate the activity of chemicals called glutathione S-transferases, which are thought to be cancer inhibitors.

- *Ellagic acid,* found in grapes and strawberries, neutralizes cancer-causing agents and prevents these agents from altering the DNA in cells (the first step in the process by which cancer develops).

- *Gingerol,* found in ginger, has been shown to help reduce inflammation, lower cholesterol levels, and heal ulcers.

- *Indoles, isothiocyanates,* and *sulforaphanes,* which are found in the cruciferous (broccoli, cabbage, and cauliflower) vegetable family, are thought to lower the risk of breast, lung, and stomach cancer.

- *Limonene,* found in citrus fruits, stimulates enzymes that break down carcinogens.

- *Lycopene,* abundant in tomatoes, has been shown to lower the risk of stomach and prostate cancer.

- *Monoterpenes,* found in cherries, has been shown to lower the risk of breast, skin, liver, lung, stomach, and pancreatic cancer.

SOME COMMONLY ASKED QUESTIONS ABOUT JUICING

Now that you know why juice is so good for your health, you may have some questions about juicing.

Isn't It Better to Eat Whole Fruits and Vegetables for the Fiber?

Good question. Of course we need whole vegetables and fruits for fiber. But while fiber is very important for colon health, it is the juice of fruits and vegetables that nourishes our bodies. Some people have thought that a significant amount of nutrients remained in the fiber after juicing, but that theory has been disproved. The Department of Agriculture analyzed twelve fruits and found that 90 percent of the antioxidant activity was in the juice rather than the fiber. That is why juice makes such a great supplement to a high-fiber diet (see Basic Guidelines for the Juice Lady's Health and Healing Diet, page 313).

Is Fresh Juice Better Than Commercially Processed Juice?

Fresh juice is much healthier than canned, bottled, frozen, or packaged juice because it contains far more nutrients at the peak of their effectiveness. It also contains enzymes, phytochemicals, and other "living" ingredients. In contrast, commercially processed juices have been pasteurized, which means the juice has been heated to high temperatures, and many of the vitamins, minerals, enzymes, and other live ingredients have been killed or removed. This means the juice will have longer shelf life, but it won't give you more life. Making your own juice also allows you to use a wider variety of fruits and vegetables. For example, some of the recipes in this book include Jerusalem artichokes and jicamas. These sweet, crisp tubers are not found in processed juices.

How Long Can Fresh Juice Be Stored?

The sooner you drink juice after you make it, the more nutrients you will get. However, you can store juice and not lose too many nutrients by keeping it cold, such as in an insulated container, or covered in the refrigerator. (For more advice on storage and other things you should know about juicing, see page 12.) *On a personal note:* When I had chronic fatigue syndrome, I would juice in the afternoons, when I had the most energy, and store the juice covered in refrigerator and drink it for the next twenty-four hours until I juiced my next batch.

How Much Produce Do You Need to Make a Glass of Juice?

People often ask me if it takes a bushel basket of produce to make a glass of juice. Actually, if you're using a good juicer, it takes a surprisingly small amount of produce. For example, all of the following items, each weighing roughly a pound, yield about one 8-ounce cup of juice: three medium apples, five to seven carrots, two medium oranges. The following yield about a half-cup: three large (thirteen-inch) stalks of celery, one large (about eight ounces) cucumber. These yields make juicing economical as well as nutritious.

CHOOSING THE RIGHT JUICER

To gain the greatest benefits of juicing, choose a juicer that is right for you. It can make the difference between juicing daily and never juicing again.

Before I go on, I need to distinguish between a blender and a juicer. A juicer separates the liquid from the pulp. A blender liquefies everything that is placed in it; it doesn't separate the pulp from the juice. If you think it might be a good idea to have carrot, beet, or celery pulp in your juice for added fiber, I can tell you from experience that it tastes like juicy sawdust. For the most flavorful juice, I recommend using a juicer. Look for the following features:

- Choose a machine with adequate horsepower (hp). I recommend one with 0.5 hp. Weak machines with low horsepower ratings must run at extremely high rpm (revolutions per minute). A machine's rpm does not accurately reflect its ability to perform effectively because rpm is calculated when the juicer is running idle, not while it is juicing. When you feed produce into a low-power machine, the rpm will be reduced dramatically, and sometimes the juicer will come to a full stop. I have "killed" some machines on the first carrot I juiced.

- Look for a machine that has electronic circuitry that sustains blade speed during juicing.

- Make sure the machine can juice tough, hard vegetables and fruits, such as pineapple skins, watermelon rinds, carrots, and beets, as well as delicate greens, such as parsley, lettuce, and herbs. Make sure it does not need a special citrus attachment.

- Look for a large feed tube so that you don't have to cut your produce into very small pieces before juicing.

- Choose a juicer that ejects pulp into a receptacle. This design is far better than one in which all the pulp stays inside the machine, and so has to be scooped out frequently. Juicers that keep the pulp in the center basket rather than ejecting it cannot juice continuously. You will need to stop the machine often to wash it out.

- Look for a juicer with only a few parts to clean. The more parts a juicer has, and the more complicated the parts are to wash, the longer it will take to clean your juicer and put it back together. That makes it less likely you will use your machine daily. Also, make sure the parts are dishwasher safe.

GETTING THE MOST FROM YOUR JUICER

Juicing is a very simple process. Simple as the procedure is, though, it helps to keep a few guidelines in mind to get the best possible results:

- Wash all produce before juicing; fruit and vegetable washes are available at many grocery and health food stores. Cut away all moldy, bruised, or damaged areas.

- Always peel oranges, tangerines, and grapefruits before juicing because the skins of these items contain bitter-tasting oils that can cause digestive problems. (Lemon and lime peels can be juiced, if organic.) Leave as much of the white pithy part on the citrus fruit as possible, since it contains the most vitamin C and bioflavonoids. Always peel mangoes and papayas, since their skins contain an irritant that is harmful when eaten in quantity. Also, I recommend that you peel all produce that is not labeled organic, even though the largest concentration of nutrients is in and next to the skin. The peels and skins of sprayed fruits and vegetables also contain the largest concentration of pesticides.

- Remove pits, stones, and hard seeds from such fruits as peaches, plums, apricots, cherries, and mangoes. Softer seeds from oranges, lemons, watermelons, cantaloupes, grapes, and apples can be juiced without a problem. Because of their chemical composition, large quantities of apple seeds should not be juiced for young children, but should not cause problems for adults.

- Do not remove the stems and leaves of most produce—for example, beet stems and leaves, strawberry caps, and small grape stems—since they offer valuable nutrients. Discard larger grape stems, as they can dull the juicer blade. Also remove carrot and rhubarb greens because they contain toxic substances.

- Cut most fruits and vegetables into sections or strips that will fit your juicer's feed tube. You will learn from experience what size works best for your machine.

- Place a plastic bag—the kind you find in the produce section of a grocery store—in the pulp receptacle of your juicer. When you are done juicing, you can either toss the pulp or use it in cooking or composting, but you won't need to wash the receptacle.

- Keep in mind that some fruits and vegetables don't juice well. Most produce items contain a lot of water, which makes them ideal for juicing. Those vegetables and fruits that contain much less water, such as bananas, mangoes, papayas, and avocados, will not juice well. They can be used in smoothies and cold soups by first juicing any other produce, and then placing the juice and the drier produce in a blender for the final processing.

- Drink your juice as soon as it's made, if you can. If you can't, store it in an insulated container or an airtight, opaque container in the refrigerator for up to twenty-four hours—light, heat, and air will destroy nutrients quickly. Be aware that the longer juice sits before you drink it, the more nutrients it loses. If juice turns brown, it has oxidized and lost a large amount of its nutritional value. After twenty-four hours, it may become spoiled. Melon and cabbage juices do not store well at all.

CHOOSE ORGANIC PRODUCE

The best way to get the healthiest juice possible is to use organic produce whenever you can. The popularity of organic foods has increased dramatically in recent years, and continues to grow. Sales of organic foods reach into the billions of dollars each year and have been growing 20 percent annually. It appears that more and more people want to avoid the 1.2 billion pounds of pesticides and herbicides sprayed onto or added to our crops yearly. And for good reason: it is estimated that only about 2 percent of this amount actually fights insects and weeds, while the rest is absorbed into our air, soil, and water. These pesticide residues pose long-term health risks, such as cancer and birth defects, and immediate health risks from acute intoxication, such as vomiting, diarrhea, blurred vision, tremors, convulsions, and nerve damage. If pesticides and herbicides do not, as we are told, pose a risk to our health, then why is there is a greater incidence of cancer—lymphoma, leukemia, and cancer of the brain, skin, stomach, and prostate—among farmers and their families when compared with cancer rates among the general public?

I'm often asked if organic produce is more nutritious as well as more healthful. At least one study indicates that it is. Organically grown tomatoes were found to have higher concentrations of vitamin C and calcium than tomatoes cultivated inorganically. Couple that with fewer chemical residues, and you can see that buying organically grown food is well worth the effort and additional pennies.

When choosing organically grown foods, look for labels marked "certified" organic. This means the produce has been cultivated according to strict uniform standards that are verified by independent state or private organizations. Certification includes inspection of farms and processing facilities, detailed record keeping, and pesticide testing of soil and water to ensure that growers and handlers are meeting government standards. You may occasionally see a label that says "transitional organic." This means the food was grown on a farm that recently converted—or is in the process of converting—from chemical to organic farming.

When organic vegetables or fruits that you want are not available, ask your grocer to get them. Certain items are especially prone to pesticide contamination, and should always be purchased as organic produce (see page 19): apples, apricots, bell peppers, celery, cherries, Chilean grapes, cucumbers, green beans, Mexican cantaloupes, peaches, spinach, and strawberries. You also can look for small-operation farmers in your area. A number of them can't afford to use many chemicals in farming. Another option is to order organic produce by mail (see Appendix A).

While you are looking for organic produce, stay away from irradiated fruits and vegetables. Some food producers use gamma-ray radiation to kill pests and germs in stored food, and to increase the food's shelf life. Although the Food and Drug Administration has approved the practice, eating irradiated food is not something I recommend. The average dose of radiation used to decontaminate most foods can be up to 5 million times that of a typical chest X ray. This practice destroys vitamins and minerals. It also generates harmful byproducts such as free radicals, toxins that can damage cells, and harmful chemicals known as radiolytic products, including formaldehyde and benzene. Irradiation of fruits and vegetables poses an even greater problem than irradiation of other foods because the large quantities of water found in produce allows for greater free-radical production. The answer to foodborne diseases is not irradiation, but stopping the overuse of pesticides and ensuring more sanitary conditions in food-processing plants.

Juicing is an easy, delicious way to add the goodness of fruits and vegetables to your daily diet. A good juicer and clean produce will allow you to enjoy a wealth of nutrients every day, which is important even if your health is good. If your health is not good, proper nutrition is even more vital. In the next section, I'll show you how to use juicing in the treatment of various disorders.

Using Juices for Healing

*Diseases are crises of purification, of toxic elimination.
Symptoms are natural defenses of the body. We call
them diseases, but in fact they are the cure of diseases.*

Hippocrates

People all over the world have found healing from ailments such as chronic fatigue syndrome, high blood pressure, heart disease, arthritis, and many other conditions by juicing and making dietary changes. The body was made to heal itself. When you provide it with the materials it needs for repair and rejuvenation, and remove irritating substances, the healing process begins. Therefore, make sure you add fresh juice (and a healthy diet) to whatever treatment plan your health care provider recommends.

There is a large and growing body of scientific research that shows an intimate connection between diet and the recovery process. Most of the diet and juice recommendations for the disorders covered in this section are based on such research, much of it done in the past few years. I want you to benefit from the most up-to-date information. In addition, I have included remedies that are time-honored traditions; people have used them for years and passed them down for generations because they worked. I have included herb recommendations. And finally, I have made some lifestyle recommendations because I want you to have a well-rounded health plan. My desire is that this book can be your resource guide. I don't want you to have to search, as I did for such a long time, to find answers to your health questions. I want you to find what you need in an easily accessible format.

There are a few things you should be aware of before using this section. While using organic produce is always a good idea, it is especially important for some fruits and vegetables (see "Avoid the 'Dirty Dozen'" on page 19). If you have more than one ailment, you may find some conflicting advice, such as the recommendation to add fruit juice under one disorder and the caution to omit all fruit under another. In this case, always *omit* the items as advised. You should also note that wherever I have recommended you undertake one of the cleansing programs (pages 323 to 339), you should use the Kidney Cleanse before moving on to the recommended program. That is because the kidneys must filter the toxins released via any cleansing program, and it will make their job easier if they are functioning as efficiently as possible.

Be aware that getting well can be like unraveling a tangled ball of yarn; sometimes the situation gets worse before it gets better. Such "healing crises" are often a sign that the body is ridding itself of toxins. If your symptoms are a source of concern, talk to your health care provider. Actually, if you have a chronic disorder, you should talk to a professional anyway before making wholesale changes in diet, or before starting to use herbal or other alternative therapies. This allows you and your health care provider to better plan your course of treatment. The important point is for you not to give up on your recovery efforts. (It helps to work with a health care provider who understands the importance of nutrition in healing. Look for either a naturopathic doctor or a medical doctor who specializes in nutrition or wholistic medicine.)

Finally, if your health professional has prescribed nutritional supplements for your condition, note that such supplements work best when taken with juices that are high in those nutrients. Nature has combined vitamins, minerals, enzymes, phytochemicals, and many other compounds that act as cofactors, or helpers, to make your vitamins and minerals more effectively absorbed and utilized. You will get the maximum healing potential when you incorporate freshly made juices, especially vegetable juices, into your health and healing recovery plan.

Allergies

Airborne allergens, such as pollen, dander, and dust mites, can cause what is popularly called hay fever. Hay fever (known medically as allergic rhinitis) is marked by watery nasal discharge, sneezing, and itchy eyes and nose. It occurs when the immune system overreacts to the allergen(s), causing the release of an inflammatory chemical called histamine.

Food allergy is a negative reaction that occurs after eating an offend-

Avoid the "Dirty Dozen"

Though I recommend that you buy all organically grown produce, I have specified "organic" in my recipes for the fruits and vegetables on the "dirty dozen" list. The nonprofit research organization Environmental Working Group reports periodically on health risks posed by pesticides in produce. The group says you can cut your pesticide exposure in half simply by avoiding twelve conventionally grown fruits and vegetables that have been found to be the most contaminated. At the time of this writing, the items on this list are: apples, apricots, bell peppers, celery, cherries, Chilean grapes, cucumbers, green beans, Mexican cantaloupes, peaches, spinach, and strawberries.

ing food or substance. Symptoms include dark circles or puffiness under the eyes, chronic fluid retention, and swollen glands, in addition to such digestive complaints as gas, nausea, and diarrhea. Immune function is also impaired. Some people are sensitive to naturally occurring substances found in a variety of foods, including dairy, wheat, corn, eggs, chocolate, peanuts, and shellfish. The number of people suffering from food allergies and other adverse reactions to food has gone up dramatically in recent years, and now includes between 10 and 15 percent of the American population. The primary cause of this increase appears to be an increase in the frequent consumption of such food additives as dyes, stabilizers, preservatives, and flavorings (items often found in commercially prepared foods), and overconsumption of such foods as wheat and dairy products. Other causes of food allergies are linked to heredity, stress, infection, nutritional status, early weaning, and impaired digestion.

Lifestyle Recommendations

❥ **For airborne allergies, eliminate allergens to the extent possible.** Clean often and well carpets, rugs, upholstered furniture, and other surfaces where allergens can collect. Allergy-proof your bedroom. Encase the mattress, box spring, and pillows in allergen-proof covers, and wash bedding, towels, curtains, and clothing in additive-free, fragrance-free detergent. Install an air purifier with a HEPA filter, a special filter that can trap tiny particles. Use a vacuum cleaner that has a HEPA filter. And have your furnace and air ducts cleaned yearly. Dust can build up in these places and make your allergy symptoms worse.

❥ **Reduce stress levels as much as possible.** Stress weakens the immune system, which increases susceptibility to, and magnitude of, an allergic response. To learn more about stress, *see* **Stress.**

Diet Recommendations

❥ **For food allergies, identify the offending food(s).** The Elimination Diet (page 321) can help you pinpoint the offenders. Keep in mind a food allergy may be something you like and eat often, since people frequently develop cravings for foods to which they are allergic (*see* **Cravings**). Once allergenic foods are identified, the next step is to rotate foods, both to control preexisting allergies and to prevent the formation of new allergies. As much as possible, continue to avoid all foods to which you are especially sensitive.

❥ **Consume more raw fruits, vegetables, and fresh juices.** Strengthening the immune system is at the root of improving the body's response to all allergens, and this requires high-level nutrition. At least 50 percent of your diet should consist of raw fruits, vegetables, juices, sprouts, nuts, and seeds. Eating junk foods, along with too many cooked and commercially prepared foods, strains the digestive system. The organs that produce digestive juices are then overburdened because enzymes are missing in these "empty" foods. This leads to deficiencies in important enzymes that are needed to break down foods properly and provide nutrients for the cells. In addition, constant stimulation of the digestive organs can result in excess acidity within the body and an overstressed enzymatic system, which leads to allergies. Raw foods and freshly made juices alkalinize the body and provide an abundance of enzymes that help the digestive system return to balance. After one eats raw foods freely for a period of time, many allergies subside, as confirmed by Dr. John Douglas, who has worked with allergy patients at the Kaiser-Permanente Medical Center in Los Angeles. For more information, see Basic Guidelines for the Juice Lady's Health and Healing Diet (page 313).

❥ **Avoid sugar and alcohol.** Sugar produces an acidic condition in the body that can accentuate allergic reactions, especially those to airborne allergens. Alcohol acts like sugar in the body.

Nutrient Recommendations

❥ **Bioflavonoids,** especially quercetin, have been shown to both reduce histamine levels and relieve allergy symptoms. Quercetin acts by inhibiting the release within the body of an inflammatory chemical called arachidonic acid. Yellow onions and shallots are particularly rich sources of quercetin. In addition, bioflavonoids enhance the actions of vitamin C (see the vitamin C entry on this list). Best juice sources of bioflavonoids: apricots, bell peppers, berries (blueberry, blackberry, and cranberry), broccoli, cabbage, cantaloupes, cherries, citrus fruit, grapes, parsley, plums, prunes, and tomatoes.

❧ **Gamma-linolenic acid (GLA)** is a fatty acid the body uses to make inflammation-inhibiting substances called prostaglandins. GLA is found in evening primrose oil, which is best taken in supplement form.

❧ **Vitamin C** benefits allergy sufferers by providing an important cellular defense against oxidizing agents, tissue-damaging substances that are produced in increased amounts during allergic reactions. Best juice sources of vitamin C (in order of effectiveness): kale, parsley, broccoli, Brussels sprouts, watercress, cauliflower, cabbage, strawberries, papaya, spinach, citrus fruit, turnips, mangoes, asparagus, and cantaloupes. Carotenes enhance vitamin C's effectiveness, and are found abundantly in most fruits and vegetables that are high in vitamin C.

Herb Recommendations

❧ **Angelica** is useful in the prevention and treatment of allergic symptoms involving the digestive tract. Make sure you use *Angelica archangelica*, not *Angelica dahurica* (wild angelica).

❧ **Ginkgo biloba** inhibits a substance called platelet activating factor, a chemical activated during an allergic response that starts inflammatory reactions.

❧ **Licorice** inhibits phospholipase A, an enzyme that, like platelet activating factor, starts inflammatory reactions. Use a medicinal form of the herb, not licorice candy. Avoid licorice if you have high blood pressure, and do not use for prolonged periods of time.

Juice Ingredient Recommendations

❧ **Alfalfa sprout** and **celery** juices raise blood alkalinity, which helps reduce allergic reactions.

❧ **Parsley** juice helps stop hay fever attacks, and ounce for ounce has more than three times the vitamin C of oranges. A safe, therapeutic dose is $1/2$ to 1 cup of parsley juice per day. Parsley can be toxic in overdose, and should be especially avoided by pregnant women.

Juice Recipes

ALFALFA SPROUT DRINK

1 organic cucumber, scrubbed well

1 handful sunflower sprouts, rinsed

1 small handful alfalfa sprouts, rinsed

½ organic tart apple, such as Pippin, washed

½ small or medium lemon, washed, or peeled if not organic

Cut the cucumber in half lengthwise. Bunch up the sprouts, and push through the feed tube with the cucumber, apple, and lemon. Stir to combine, pour into a glass, and serve chilled or at room temperature.

ALLERGY RELIEF

1 small bunch parsley, rinsed

2 stalks organic celery with leaves, washed

2–3 large carrots, scrubbed well, green tops removed, ends trimmed

½ small or medium lemon, washed, or peeled if not organic

Bunch up the parsley and push it through the feed tube with the celery, carrots, and lemon. Stir the juice, and pour it into a glass. Serve at room temperature or chilled, as desired.

WALDORF TWIST

1 organic Red or Golden Delicious apple, washed

3 stalks organic celery with leaves, washed

¼ small or medium lemon, washed, or peeled if not organic

Cut the apple into sections that will fit your juicer's feed tube, and juice along with the celery and lemon. Stir the juice, and pour into a glass. Serve at room temperature or chilled, as desired.

GINGER TWIST

1 organic Red or Golden Delicious apple, washed

1 handful parsley, rinsed

4 carrots, scrubbed well, green tops removed, ends trimmed

1-inch piece fresh ginger root, washed

¼ small or medium lemon, washed, or peeled if not organic

Cut the apple into sections that fit your juicer's feed tube. Bunch up the parsley and push it through the feed tube with the apple, carrots, ginger, and lemon. Stir the juice, and pour into a glass. Serve at room temperature or chilled, as desired.

The Morning Energizer

½ organic Red or Golden Delicious apple, washed

5 medium carrots, scrubbed well, green tops removed, ends trimmed

½ small beet with leaves and stems, scrubbed well

½ small or medium lemon, washed, or peeled if not organic

½- to 1-inch piece fresh ginger root, washed

Cut the apple into sections that will fit your juicer's feed tube. Juice the apple along with the carrots, beet, lemon, and ginger. Stir the juice, and pour into a glass. Serve at room temperature or chilled, as desired.

Antiaging Cocktail

1 small bunch organic purple grapes (about 1 cup) with small stems* and seeds, washed

½ cup blueberries, blackberries, or raspberries, washed

½ small or medium lemon, washed, or peeled if not organic

½-inch piece fresh ginger root, washed

*Large stems can dull your juicer's blade.

Juice the grapes, berries, lemon, and ginger. Stir the juice, and pour into a glass. Serve at room temperature or chilled, as desired.

Alzheimer's Disease

Alzheimer's disease (AD) is marked by tissue atrophy within the frontal and temporal parts of the brain, resulting in the loss of mental capacity. AD typically affects people over age seventy, although it can strike in middle age. It is estimated that 50 to 60 percent of those over age eighty-five are affected by dementia, most of which is caused by AD. In the United States, approximately 250,000 people are diagnosed with Alzheimer's each year.

AD is characterized by a loss of cognitive function and memory, and typically interferes more and more with daily activities until the person loses all ability to care for himself or herself. Symptoms can include depression, incontinence, delusions, hallucinations, aggression, wandering, binge-eating, and lack of sexual constraint. Symptoms usually worsen with time.

AD occurs when protein-based plaques are deposited in the brain. Doctors believe that the plaques and tangles seen in this disease cause the brain damage. While family history is an important risk factor, environmental factors play a significant role in AD, such as chronic exposure to aluminum and/or silicon, exposure to toxins, and free-radical damage. In particular, considerable circumstantial evidence points to aluminum concentrations in the brain, which are considerably higher than normal in people with AD, as a key factor.

Diet Recommendations

❥ **Eat only fresh, whole foods.** Since AD is thought to be caused by an accumulation of toxins in the brain, it very important to avoid all packaged and processed foods. Prepare food yourself and choose fresh, organically grown foods as much as possible. For more information, see Basic Guidelines for the Juice Lady's Health and Healing Diet (page 313).

❥ **Drink plenty of fresh fruit and vegetable juices.** Fruits and vegetables are among the richest sources of antioxidants, and according to a recent study by the United States Department of Agriculture, 90 percent of the antioxidant activity is in the juice, not in the fiber. Antioxidants bind with toxins called free radicals and prevent further cell damage. They also help to cleanse the body of toxins. *On a personal note:* One woman who contacted me was caring for an AD patient. She started giving the lady fresh vegetable juice every day, and noticed a striking improvement in the lady's health and cognitive abilities. She said that even the neighbors began commenting on the improvement in the patient's condition. For more information on the healing power of raw foods and juices, see the appropriate section in Basic Guidelines for the Juice Lady's Health and Healing Diet (page 313).

❥ **Eliminate aluminum from the body.** Aluminum detoxification appears to be of some help to people in the early stages of AD. It is very important that the body be able to eliminate heavy metals and other toxins. Juice fasting (see the Juice Fast, page 324) for three days several times a year can be very beneficial. The Liver Cleanse (page 333) can support the liver, which is vitally important since toxins, including heavy metals, are broken down primarily by the liver.

❥ **Avoid all substances containing aluminum.** Two studies from Norway have shown a relationship between an increased concentration of aluminum in the water supply and an increase in mortality from both Alzheimer's disease and dementia. Therefore, do not use aluminum cookware or aluminum foil as food wrapping, and avoid aluminum food packages. Also avoid antacids, many of which contain aluminum. Aluminum is added to table salt and baking powder to keep them from clumping, and to most processed cheese products. Choose only products that say "aluminum free." It is advisable to get a water purifier that removes aluminum and other heavy metals.

Nutrient Recommendations

❥ **Antioxidants** can eliminate free radicals, and an increase in free-radical damage and fat breakdown has been seen in people with AD. Antioxidants protect autonomic nerve cells (those involved in automatic bodily functions) from being destroyed. Be sure you get plenty of the following nutrients:

- *Beta-carotene* is a powerful antioxidant. Best juice sources of carotenes (in order of effectiveness): carrots, kale, parsley, spinach, chard, beet greens, watercress, mangoes, cantaloupes, apricots, broccoli, and romaine lettuce.

- *Selenium* helps activate glutathione peroxidase, an enzyme that serves as the body's own antioxidant. Best juice sources of selenium (in order of effectiveness): chard, turnips, garlic, oranges, radishes, grapes, carrots, and cabbage.

- *Vitamin C* helps protect brain cells from free-radical attack. Best juice sources of vitamin C (in order of effectiveness): kale, parsley, broccoli, Brussels sprouts, watercress, cauliflower, cabbage, strawberries, papaya, spinach, citrus fruit, turnips, mangoes, asparagus, and cantaloupes.

- *Vitamin E* helps protect cell membranes. Best juice sources of vitamin E (in order of effectiveness): spinach, watercress, asparagus, carrots, and tomatoes.

❥ **Essential fatty acids (EFAs),** which are often deficient in a typical Western diet, are essential for the creation of strong cell membranes. Faulty cell membranes play a role in degenerative diseases, such as AD. In comparing the brain cell membranes of AD patients with those of other individuals, scientists found a dramatic reduction in the EFA content and an increase in the saturated fat content. EFAs are abundant in such cold-water fish as salmon, trout, tuna, mackerel, halibut, and sardines. They are also plentiful in flaxseed and hemp oils. For more information on EFAs, see the fats and oils section in Basic Guidelines for the Juice Lady's Health and Healing Diet (page 313).

ʗ Vitamin B$_{12}$ (cobalamin) deficiency is common among AD patients. A deficiency of vitamin B$_{12}$ is associated with dementia, and prolonged B$_{12}$ deficiency may lead to irreversible changes in mental function. However, vitamin B$_{12}$ is not found in fruits and vegetables. The best food sources of this vitamin are meat, poultry, and fish; it is also available in some fermented soy-based foods, such as tofu and tempeh. One reason many older people are B$_{12}$ deficient is because they have low levels of intrinsic factor, a substance in gastric juice that increases absorption of B$_{12}$. As people age, secretion of gastric juices declines. Supplementation with HCl betaine, available at most health food stores, may aid protein digestion, thus increasing vitamin B$_{12}$ absorption. And supplements of the vitamin itself may be helpful; see your doctor to find out whether the oral or injectable form is best for you.

ʗ Zinc deficiency is a major problem in older people, and has been implicated as a factor in AD. Patients with AD who have received zinc supplementation have shown improvement in memory, understanding, socialization, and communication. Best juice sources of zinc (in order of effectiveness): ginger root, turnips, parsley, garlic, carrots, grapes, spinach, cabbage, lettuce, cucumbers, and tangerines.

Herb Recommendations

ʗ Ginkgo biloba increases blood flow to the brain, which increases cellular use of oxygen and glucose. This herb has also been shown to normalize receptors for an important brain chemical called acetylcholine and to increase transmission of nerve impulses, two functions that are decreased in Alzheimer's disease.

Juice Ingredient Recommendations

ʗ Parsley juice is rich in beta-carotene, vitamin C, and zinc. Intake should be limited to a safe, therapeutic dose of $1/2$ to 1 cup per day. Parsley can be toxic in overdose, and should be especially avoided by pregnant women.

Juice Recipes

TOMATO FLORENTINE

1 vine-ripened tomato, washed

1 handful organic spinach, washed

2–3 fresh basil leaves (optional)

$\frac{1}{2}$ small or medium lemon, washed, or peeled if not organic

Cut the tomato into sections that will fit your juicer's feed tube. Bunch up the spinach and basil leaves (if using), and push through the feed tube with the tomato and lemon. Stir the juice, and pour into a glass. Serve at room temperature or chilled, as desired.

POPEYE'S POWER

$\frac{1}{2}$ medium organic apple, washed

1 handful organic spinach, washed

1 small handful parsley, rinsed

4 medium carrots, scrubbed well, green tops removed, ends trimmed

1 stalk organic celery with leaves, washed

$\frac{1}{2}$ beet with leaves, scrubbed well

Cut the apple into sections that will fit your juicer's feed tube. Bunch up the spinach and parsley, and push them through the feed tube with the apple, carrots, celery, and beet. Stir the juice, and pour into a glass. Serve at room temperature or chilled, as desired.

WHEATGRASS LIGHT

1 organic Golden or Red Delicious apple, washed

1 small handful wheatgrass, rinsed

2–3 sprigs mint, rinsed (optional)

$\frac{1}{2}$ small or medium lemon, washed, or peeled if not organic

Cut the apple into sections that fit your juicer's feed tube. Bunch up the wheatgrass and mint (if using) and push them through the feed tube with the apple and lemon. Stir the juice, and pour into a glass. Serve at room temperature or chilled, as desired.

MEMORY MENDER

2 medium vine-ripened tomatoes, washed

$\frac{1}{4}$ small head iceberg lettuce, washed

4 cauliflower florets, washed

$\frac{1}{2}$ small or medium lemon, washed, or peeled if not organic

Cut the tomatoes and lettuce into sections that will fit your juicer's feed tube. Juice the tomatoes and lettuce along with the cauliflower and lemon. Pour into a glass and serve at room temperature or chilled, as desired.

SWEET DREAMS NIGHTCAP

2 romaine lettuce leaves, washed

1 handful parsley, rinsed

4 carrots, scrubbed well, green tops removed, ends trimmed

3 organic celery stalks with leaves, washed

Bunch up the lettuce leaves and parsley, and push through the feed tube with the carrots and celery. Stir the juice, and pour into a glass. Serve at room temperature or chilled, as desired.

ANTIAGING COCKTAIL

1 small bunch organic purple grapes (about 1 cup) with small stems* and seeds, washed

1/2 cup blueberries, blackberries, or raspberries, washed

1/4 small or medium lemon, washed, or peeled if not organic

1/2-inch piece fresh ginger root, washed

*Large stems can dull your juicer's blade.

Juice the grapes, berries, lemon, and ginger. Stir the juice, and pour into a glass. Serve at room temperature or chilled, as desired.

Anemia

Anemia is a condition marked by a deficiency either of red blood cells or of hemoglobin, the oxygen-carrying substance found in red blood cells. A nutritional deficiency often underlies anemia, and three nutrients are the most common culprits—iron, vitamin B_{12} (cobalamin), and folic acid. It is important to know which nutrient(s) is deficient in order to treat anemia effectively. General anemia symptoms include impaired intellectual performance, pale skin, light pink color (rather than red) inside the lower eyelids, canker sores, irritability, weakness, dizziness, and headaches.

Anemia caused by iron deficiency is characterized by small red blood cells and low levels of circulating hemoglobin. Iron-deficiency anemia is marked by extreme fatigue; red, even burning, tongue; inflammation of the lips; and a spoonlike deformity of the fingernails.

Vitamin B_{12} deficiency, known as pernicious anemia, is characterized by large, immature red blood cells. Symptoms include weight loss, problems with sensation and muscle control, and yellow-blue colorblindness. Vitamin B_{12} absorption requires a sufficient amount of intrinsic factor, a substance found in gastric juice. Gastrointestinal problems, such as bacterial or parasitic infection, can lead to B_{12} anemia (*see* **Parasitic Infections**). *On a personal note:* I had vitamin B_{12} deficiency anemia for years, and no amount of dietary intervention worked. It turned out that the underlying cause was a parasitic infection.

Folic acid-deficiency anemia, also called macrosydia anemia, is characterized by red blood cells that are improperly formed. This form of anemia can produce sleeping disorders and a sore, red tongue.

Diet Recommendations

◗ **If you have iron-deficiency anemia, eat an iron-rich diet.** There are two types of iron in the foods we eat: heme and nonheme. Heme iron is the type primarily found in animal foods. Nonheme iron makes up the remainder, and is the only iron present in plant foods. The absorption rate of heme iron is considerably higher than that of nonheme iron. Best food sources for heme iron include meat (especially liver), poultry, and fish. Best juice sources of nonheme iron (in order of effectiveness): parsley, dandelion greens, broccoli, cauliflower, strawberries, asparagus, chard, blackberries, cabbage, beets with greens, carrots, and pineapple. (Increase nonheme absorption by consuming extra vitamin C; see the Nutrient Recommendations.)

◗ **Limit substances that can inhibit iron absorption when eating an iron-rich meal.** Such substances can bind to iron, trapping it in insoluble complexes within the intestines so it cannot be absorbed. These substances include: phytates (in grains, legumes, and seeds), tannins (in tea and coffee), oxalates (in beets, rhubarb, and spinach), phosphates (large amounts in soft drinks), excess calcium, soybeans, antacids, and EDTA (a food preservative). For example, tannins can reduce absorption of nonheme iron by up to 50 percent.

◗ **Eat and drink dark green vegetables.** These foods contain generous amounts of nonheme iron and folic acid, as well as vitamin C and fat-soluble chlorophyll. The best green vegetables are broccoli, kale, and bok choy.

Nutrient Recommendations

◗ **Copper** in food is necessary to help your body absorb and use iron properly. Best juice sources of copper (in order of effectiveness): carrots, garlic, ginger root, and turnips.

❥ **Folic acid** can be obtained from food if you have folic acid-deficiency anemia, although you may also need to take a folic acid supplement. Best juice sources of folic acid (in order of effectiveness): asparagus, spinach, kale, broccoli, cabbage, and blackberries.

❥ **Vitamin B$_{12}$ (cobalamin)** is generally found in small amounts in animal foods, and is not available in fruits and vegetables. Strict vegans—people who eat no animal products at all—are particularly susceptible to vitamin B$_{12}$ deficiency. The best food sources of vitamin B$_{12}$ are meat, poultry, and fish; it is also available in some fermented soy-based foods, such as tofu and tempeh. You may need to take a B$_{12}$ supplement; see your doctor about whether the oral or the injectable form would be best in your case. You can also try using a digestive aid called HCl betaine, a supplement available in most health food stores. HCl betaine can help improve vitamin B$_{12}$ absorption.

❥ **Vitamin C** significantly enhances iron absorption. Best juice sources of vitamin C (in order of effectiveness): kale, parsley, broccoli, Brussels sprouts, watercress, cauliflower, cabbage, strawberries, papaya, spinach, citrus fruit, turnips, mangoes, asparagus, and cantaloupes.

Herb Recommendations

❥ **Anise** tea enhances iron absorption. Mint, caraway, cumin, and licorice teas are also effective, but anise is the best.

❥ **Gentian** is used in the treatment of anemia. It stimulates the secretion of digestive juices, thereby enhancing iron absorption.

❥ **Yellow dock** is used to raise hemoglobin levels in the blood and is a good source of iron.

Juice Ingredient Recommendations

❥ **Dandelion greens** juice is commonly used in treating anemia. It is a good source of iron and also contains significant amounts of folic acid, calcium, and potassium, as well as many trace minerals.

❥ **Parsley** juice is a good source of both iron and vitamin C. Intake should be limited to a safe, therapeutic dose of $^1/_2$ to 1 cup per day. Parsley can be toxic in overdose, and should be especially avoided by pregnant women.

❥ **Spinach, cabbage,** and **nettle** juices are used to treat anemia, as are other dark green juices, which are rich in chlorophyll.

Juice Recipes

LIVER LIFE TONIC

½ organic green apple such as Granny Smith or Pippin, washed

1 handful dandelion greens, washed

5 carrots, scrubbed well, green tops removed, ends trimmed

½ small lemon, washed, or peeled if not organic

Cut the apple into wedges that will fit your juicer's feed tube. Bunch up the dandelion greens, and push through the feed tube with the apple, carrots, and lemon. Stir the juice, and pour into a glass. Serve at room temperature or chilled, as desired.

POPEYE'S POWER

½ medium organic apple, any kind, washed

1 handful organic spinach, washed

1 small handful parsley, rinsed

4 medium carrots, scrubbed well, green tops removed, ends trimmed

1 stalk organic celery with leaves, washed

½ beet with leaves, scrubbed well

Cut the apple into sections that will fit your juicer's feed tube. Bunch up the spinach and parsley, and push them through the feed tube with the apple, carrots, celery, and beet. Stir the juice, and pour into a glass. Serve at room temperature or chilled, as desired.

TRIPLE C

¼ small head green cabbage, washed

4 carrots, scrubbed well, green tops removed, and ends trimmed

4 stalks organic celery with leaves, washed

Cut the cabbage into sections that fit your juicer's feed tube. Juice the cabbage along with the carrots and celery. Stir the juice, and pour into a glass. Serve at room temperature or chilled, as desired.

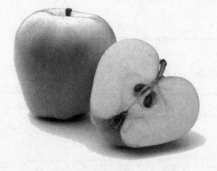

THE MORNING ENERGIZER

½ organic Red or Golden Delicious apple, washed

5 medium carrots, scrubbed well, green tops removed, ends trimmed

½ small beet with leaves and stems, scrubbed well

½ small or medium lemon, washed, or peeled if not organic

½- to 1-inch piece fresh ginger root, washed

Cut the apple into sections that will fit your juicer's feed tube. Juice the apple along with the carrots, beet, lemon, and ginger. Stir the juice, and pour into a glass. Serve at room temperature or chilled, as desired.

THE GINGER HOPPER

½ organic Red or Golden Delicious apple, washed

5 medium carrots, scrubbed well, green tops removed, ends trimmed

½- to 1-inch piece fresh ginger root, washed

Cut the apple into sections, and juice along with the carrots and ginger. Stir the juice, and pour into a glass. Serve at room temperature or chilled, as desired.

BEAUTIFUL BONE SOLUTION

1 organic Golden or Red Delicious apple, washed

1–2 kale leaves, washed

1 handful parsley, rinsed

1 stalk organic celery, washed

¼ small or medium lemon, washed, or peeled if not organic

½- to 1-inch piece fresh ginger root, washed

Cut the apple into sections that fit your juicer's feed tube. Bunch up the kale and parsley, and push through the feed tube with the apple, celery, lemon, and ginger. Stir the juice, and pour into a glass. Serve at room temperature or chilled, as desired.

Angina

See **Cardiovascular Disease.**

Ankylosing Spondylitis

See **Rheumatoid Arthritis.**

Anxiety and Panic Attacks

Anxiety is a term that describes a wide range of emotional experiences, from a general sense of internal tension to a full-blown, acute panic attack. Occasional worry or anxiety is normal. But for some people anxiety is constant, and reduces both their ability to function and their overall sense of well-being.

People with generalized anxiety often feel apprehension, uneasiness, or nervousness. They may be easily startled, and may experience a vague, nagging uncertainty about future personal or job-related matters. This constant state of tension often leads to irritability, sleeplessness, fatigue, and difficulty in concentrating. They may also suffer from depression, headaches, trembling, twitching, sweating, and muscular tension, which often results in muscle pain and soreness. People who tighten their abdominal muscles when anxious often experience constipation or diarrhea.

Acute anxiety shows itself as intense dread or terror for no objective reason, and it is often characterized by such symptoms as a pounding or racing heart, trembling, shaking, sweating, shortness of breath, smothering sensations, chest pain, and lightheadedness. Since many of these symptoms are similar to that of a heart attack, they should be taken seriously, and a heart attack should be ruled out.

Panic attacks are characterized by a sudden overwhelming fright without reasonable cause. They can be caused by environmental sensitivities, such as those to dust, molds, chemicals, and certain foods. These items can cause allergic reactions that can dramatically influence conditions such as anxiety, panic, and depression.

Lifestyle Recommendations

❥ **Eliminate respiratory allergies.** Reducing any allergic reactions you may have to airborne irritants may reduce your anxiety (*see* **Allergies**).

Diet Recommendations

❥ **Eat a high-fiber, low-fat diet.** The better your nutritional status, the better your body can cope with stressful situations that can cause anxiety. See Basic Guidelines for the Juice Lady's Health and Healing Diet (page 313).

❥ **Eat smaller meals more frequently.** Hypoglycemia, or low blood sugar, may play a role in anxiety attacks for some people. Therefore, it is important to keep your blood-sugar levels even throughout the day by eating smaller, more frequent meals that include protein, or by eating protein snacks between meals (*see* **Hypoglycemia**).

❥ **Drink fresh juices, and go on juice fasts.** Multiple chemical sensitivities have been implicated in anxiety disorder. Fresh juices and a short juice fast will help to cleanse the body of toxins. People who juice fast for short periods of time say they experience a greater sense of well-being. (See the Juice Fast, page 324.)

❥ **Identify food allergies and intolerances.** Avoid foods you are allergic to or don't tolerate well, since food allergies are known to cause anxiety and fatigue. (*See* **Allergies;** also see the Elimination Diet, page 321.)

❥ **Avoid caffeine.** Several studies have implicated caffeine as a contributing factor in anxiety disorders. Caffeine use can lead to a stress response characterized by depression, anxiety, nervousness, irritability, recurrent headaches, heart palpitations, and insomnia. Caffeine is found in coffee, black and green tea (though in much higher amounts in black), cola, chocolate, and some drugs. Even decaffeinated coffee has some caffeine.

❥ **Avoid food additives.** Food additives—such as dyes, preservatives, stabilizers, and fillers—have been implicated in hyperactivity and attention deficit disorder in children, and they should not be overlooked as contributing factors to adult anxiety. Choose fresh, whole foods, and avoid packaged and processed foods as much as possible. Choose only freshly made fruit and vegetable juices, whenever possible.

Nutrient Recommendations

❥ **B vitamins** can help reduce the effects of anxiety. In fact, B-complex vitamin deficiencies can cause anxiety. The best juice sources of B vitamins overall are green leafy vegetables. In addition, several specific B vitamins are especially beneficial:

• *Inositol* can help alleviate panic disorders. Best juice sources of inositol (in order of effectiveness): oranges, grapefruits, cantaloupes, peaches, cabbage, watermelon, strawberries, and tomatoes.

- *Pantothenic acid* is known as the antistress vitamin because it helps the body resist stress in general. Best juice sources of pantothenic acid (in order of effectiveness): broccoli, cauliflower, and kale.

- *Vitamin B_3 (niacin)* has been found to reduce anxiety because of its effect on the brain, which is similar to such benzodiazapine tranquilizers as Valium. This vitamin can also help reduce the effects of benzodiazapine withdrawal, which include anxiety, because of its calming effects. Vitamin B_3 is not found in appreciable amounts in fruits and vegetables. Best food sources of vitamin B_3 (in order of effectiveness): brewer's yeast, rice and wheat bran, peanuts, turkey, chicken, and fish.

- *Vitamin B_6 (pyridoxine)* is an important antianxiety vitamin, especially for women. Best juice sources of vitamin B_6 (in order of effectiveness): kale, spinach, turnip greens, bell peppers, and prunes.

❥ **Magnesium** deficiency has been associated with anxiety disorder. Best juice sources of magnesium (in order of effectiveness): beet greens, spinach, parsley, dandelion greens, garlic, blackberries, beets, broccoli, cauliflower, carrots, and celery.

Herb Recommendations

❥ **Ginkgo biloba** has demonstrated antistress and antianxiety activity in animal studies.

❥ **Hops** is used in a traditional remedy for insomnia caused by anxiety. To use this herb, fill a small sachet-size pillow with hops and place it near your regular pillow or within the pillowcase at night.

❥ **Kava-kava** relaxes both the central nervous system and the muscles. Studies show that kava-kava has proven long-term effectiveness in helping persons with anxiety, with none of the tolerance problems of antidepressant drugs.

Juice Ingredient Recommendations

❥ **Celery** juice has a calming effect and is helpful for insomnia.

❥ **Fennel** juice calms the mind.

❥ **Parsley** juice helps produce an overall sense of well-being. Intake should be limited to a safe, therapeutic dose of $1/2$ to 1 cup per day. Parsley can be toxic in overdose, and should be especially avoided by pregnant women.

Juice Recipes

SWEET DREAMS NIGHTCAP

2 romaine lettuce leaves, washed

1 handful parsley, rinsed

4 carrots, scrubbed well, green tops removed, ends trimmed

3 organic celery stalks with leaves, washed

Bunch up the lettuce leaves and parsley, and push through the feed tube with the carrots and celery. Stir the juice, and pour into a glass. Serve at room temperature or chilled, as desired.

THE FEEL GOOD COCKTAIL

½ pear, washed

4 medium carrots, scrubbed well, green tops removed, ends trimmed

3 fennel stalks with leaves and flowers, washed

1 stalk organic celery with leaves, washed

Cut the pear into sections that fit your juicer's feed tube, and juice along with the carrots, fennel, and celery. Stir the juice, and pour into a glass. Serve at room temperature or chilled, as desired.

WALDORF TWIST

1 organic Red or Golden Delicious apple, washed

3 stalks organic celery with leaves, washed

¼ small or medium lemon, washed, or peeled if not organic

Cut the apple into sections that will fit your juicer's feed tube, and juice along with the celery and lemon. Stir the juice, and pour into a glass. Serve at room temperature or chilled, as desired.

MAGNESIUM SPECIAL

5 medium carrots, scrubbed well, green tops removed, ends trimmed

2 stalks organic celery with leaves, washed

½ small beet with leaves and stems, scrubbed well

2 broccoli florets, washed

½ small or medium lemon, washed, or peeled if not organic

Juice the carrots, celery, beet, broccoli, and lemon. Stir the juice, and pour into a glass. Serve at room temperature or chilled, as desired.

POPEYE'S POWER

½ medium organic apple, any kind, washed

1 handful organic spinach, washed

1 small handful parsley, rinsed

4 medium carrots, scrubbed well, green tops removed, ends trimmed

1 stalk organic celery with leaves, washed

½ beet with leaves, scrubbed well

Cut the apple into sections that will fit your juicer's feed tube. Bunch up the spinach and parsley, and push them through the feed tube with the apple, carrots, celery, and beet. Stir the juice, and pour into a glass. Serve at room temperature or chilled, as desired.

MORNING EXPRESS

1 orange, peeled

4–5 carrots, well scrubbed, green tops removed, ends trimmed

Divide the orange into segments that fit your juicer's feed tube, and juice with the carrots. Stir the juice, and pour into a glass. Serve at room temperature or chilled, as desired.

LIVER LIFE TONIC

½ organic green apple such as Granny Smith or Pippin, washed

1 handful dandelion greens, washed

5 carrots, scrubbed well, green tops removed, ends trimmed

¼–½ small or medium lemon, washed, or peeled if not organic

Cut the apple into wedges that will fit your juicer's feed tube. Bunch up the dandelion greens, and push through the feed tube with the apple, carrots, and lemon. Stir the juice, and pour into a glass. Serve at room temperature or chilled, as desired.

Asthma

Asthma is a chronic disease in which the small air passages, or bronchi, in the lungs are inflamed and constricted, and there is excess mucous secretion. A variety of stimuli can provoke an asthma episode, which is marked by wheezing, coughing, and shortness of breath.

Asthma comes in two forms, extrinsic and intrinsic. Extrinsic asthma is generally considered an allergic condition. It occurs when particles to which a person has become sensitized trigger the release of an inflammatory chemical called histamine. Intrinsic asthma is set off by such nonimmune factors as exercise, emotional upset, heat or cold, stress, chemical irritants, infection, and aspirin. Increased levels of air pollution, such as those produced by cigarette smoke or a wood-burning stove, can increase the frequency and severity of asthma attacks. Wood smoke contains tiny, irritating particles, and cigarette smoke contains nitrogen oxides and toxic free radicals that are present in the tar.

The rate of asthma in the United States is rising rapidly, especially among children. The reasons include greater stress on the immune system caused by environmental pollutants, earlier weaning and introduction of solid food, and increased use of food additives. (For more information, I recommend *Asthma: Clinical Pearls in Nutrition and Complementary Therapies* by Kirk Hamilton; see Appendix A.)

Diet Recommendations

❥ **Choose a vegetarian diet supplemented by the addition of cold-water fish (unless there is an allergy to fish).** A long-term study of twenty-five asthma patients who ate a vegetarian diet showed a significant improvement in 92 percent of the participants. Adding cold-water fish, which is rich in omega-3 fatty acids—such as salmon, tuna, halibut, herring, and mackerel—provides nutrients that are beneficial for individuals with asthma (see essential fatty acids under Nutrient Recommendations).

❥ **Eliminate all food additives.** Dyes and preservatives can contribute to asthma attacks in susceptible individuals.

❥ **Eliminate mucus-forming foods.** These include dairy products, refined foods (such as white flour), and sugar (including all sweets).

❥ **Identify and eliminate all food allergens and sensitivities.** Food allergies may play a role in asthma attacks. The most common allergenic foods are dairy products, shellfish, fish, eggs, nuts, peanuts, wheat, chocolate, citrus fruit, and food colorings. (*See* **Allergies;** also see the Elimination Diet, page 321.)

Nutrient Recommendations

❥ **Essential fatty acids (EFAs),** especially eicosapentaenoic acid (EPA) and docosahexaenoic acid (DHA)—two omega-3 fatty acids found in cold-water fish—are beneficial. Studies have shown that a diet high in EPA and DHA correlates with a low incidence of asthma. You can supplement your diet daily with unrefined flaxseed or hemp oil, since the body can manufacture EPA and DHA from these plant-based oils. For more information, see the fats and oils section in Basic Guidelines for the Juice Lady's Health and Healing Diet (page 313).

❥ **Magnesium** relaxes the smooth muscles and may encourage airway dilation. Decreased levels of magnesium have been associated with an increased risk of bronchial hypersensitivity. Best juice sources of magnesium (in order of effectiveness): beet greens, spinach, parsley, dandelion greens, garlic, blackberries, beets, broccoli, cauliflower, carrots, and celery.

❥ **Vitamin B_{12} (cobalamin)** has been used as a successful asthma therapy, especially in children. It also appears to be especially helpful for individuals who are sensitive to food additives called sulfites. Vitamin B_{12} is not available in fruits and vegetables. The best food sources of vitamin B_{12} are meat, poultry, and fish; it is also available in some fermented soy-based foods, such as tofu and tempeh. See your doctor about taking B_{12} supplements in either oral or injectable form. In addition, you may want to try using a digestive aid called HCl betaine, available in most health food stores, which may improve vitamin B_{12} absorption.

❥ **Vitamin C** has been shown in studies to cause an immediate decrease in airway constriction by acting against one of the substances in the lung that induces such constriction. Patients with asthma have been shown to have lower blood concentrations of vitamin C than other individuals. Best juice sources of vitamin C (in order of effectiveness): kale, parsley, broccoli, Brussels sprouts, watercress, cauliflower, cabbage, strawberries, papaya, spinach, citrus fruit, turnips, mangoes, asparagus, and cantaloupes.

❥ **Vitamin E** deficiency has been related to the onset of asthma in adult women. Vitamin E can relax the smooth muscles of the airway by inhibiting the effects of histamine and by modifying formation of inflammation-controlling substances called prostaglandins. Best juice sources of vitamin E (in order of effectiveness): spinach, watercress, asparagus, carrots, and tomatoes.

Juice Ingredient Recommendations

❥ **Onion** juice helps eliminate mucus in the upper respiratory tract.

❥ **Parsley** juice is a traditional remedy for allergies. A safe, therapeutic dose is $1/2$ to 1 cup of parsley juice per day. Parsley can be toxic in overdose, and should be especially avoided by pregnant women.

❥ **Radish** juice is a traditional remedy for asthma.

Juice Recipes

THE PINK ONION

1 large yellow onion

1-inch piece fresh ginger root, washed

1 large pink grapefruit, peeled, or enough to make 2 cups of juice

1 small or medium lemon, washed or peeled if not organic

Cut the onion into pieces that fit your juicer's feed tube. Juice the onion and ginger, pour into a glass, then juice the grapefruit and add to the onion/ginger juice. Juice the lemon, add the lemon juice just before serving, and stir. (This is quite a strong tasting combination, and your taste buds may not be particularly fond of it. But this recipe can help if you are battling mucus in the upper respiratory tract, so hold your nose and gulp it down!)

ALLERGY RELIEF

1 small bunch parsley, rinsed

2 stalks organic celery with leaves, washed

2–3 large carrots, scrubbed well, green tops removed, ends trimmed

1/4–1/2 small or medium lemon, washed, or peeled if not organic

Bunch up the parsley and push it through the feed tube with the celery, carrots, and lemon. Stir the juice, and pour it into a glass. Serve at room temperature.

SINUS SOLUTION

2 medium vine-ripened tomatoes, washed

4 radishes with green tops, washed

1/4–1/2 small or medium lime or lemon, washed, or peeled if not organic

Cut the tomatoes into sections that fit your juicer's feed tube. Juice the tomatoes along with the radishes and lime or lemon. Stir the juice, and pour into a glass. Serve at room temperature.

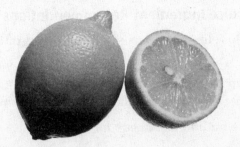

BEAUTIFUL BONE SOLUTION

1 organic Golden or Red Delicious apple, washed

1–2 kale leaves, washed

1 handful parsley, rinsed

1 stalk organic celery, washed

$1/4$ small or medium lemon, washed, or peeled if not organic

$1/2$- to 1-inch piece fresh ginger root, washed

Cut the apple into sections that fit your juicer's feed tube. Bunch up the kale and parsley, and push through the feed tube with the apple, celery, lemon, and ginger. Stir the juice, and pour into a glass. Serve at room temperature.

TOMATO FLORENTINE

1 vine-ripened tomato, washed

1 handful organic spinach, washed

2–3 fresh basil leaves (optional)

$1/4$–$1/2$ small or medium lemon, washed, or peeled if not organic

Cut the tomato into sections that will fit your juicer's feed tube. Bunch up the spinach and basil leaves (if using), and push through the feed tube with the tomato and lemon. Stir the juice, and pour into a glass. Serve at room temperature.

SPRING TONIC

1 medium vine-ripened tomato, washed

1 organic cucumber, scrubbed well

8 asparagus stems, washed

$1/4$–$1/2$ small or medium lemon, washed, or peeled if not organic

Cut the tomato into sections that fit your juicer's feed tube. Cut the cucumber in half lengthwise. Juice the tomato, cucumber, asparagus, and lemon. Stir the juice, and pour into a glass. Serve at room temperature.

MAGNESIUM SPECIAL

5 medium carrots, scrubbed well, green tops removed, ends trimmed

2 stalks organic celery with leaves, washed

$1/2$ small beet with leaves and stems, scrubbed well

2 broccoli florets, washed

$1/4$–$1/2$ small or medium lemon, washed, or peeled if not organic

Juice the carrots, celery, beet, broccoli, and lemon. Stir the juice, and pour into a glass. Serve at room temperature.

POPEYE'S POWER

½ medium organic apple, any kind, washed

1 handful organic spinach, washed

1 small handful parsley, rinsed

4 medium carrots, scrubbed well, green tops removed, ends trimmed

1 stalk organic celery with leaves, washed

½ beet with leaves, scrubbed well

Cut the apple into sections that will fit your juicer's feed tube. Bunch up the spinach and parsley, and push them through the feed tube with the apple, carrots, celery, and beet. Stir the juice, and pour into a glass. Serve at room temperature.

Atherosclerosis

See **Cardiovascular Disease.**

Attention Deficit Disorders

Attention deficit disorder (ADD) is defined as a learning disability marked by inappropriately brief attention span and poor concentration for the child's age. This condition affects approximately 3 to 5 percent of school-age children, with boys outnumbering girls, and can also affect adults. ADD is thought to be caused by heavy metal toxicity, nutrient deficiencies, and frequent ear infections. ADD can be also accompanied by hyperactivity, or inattention and impulsiveness. In looking for causes of ADD with hyperactivity (ADHD), scientists have focused on food additives, food allergies, sugar consumption, frequent ear infections, and a genetic thyroid dysfunction. These factors may cause problems in the brain's use of neuotransmitters, the chemical messengers that carry impulses from one brain cell to another.

Over two million school-age boys are on the prescription drug Ritalin, the standard medical treatment for ADD and ADHD. However, according to an article in *Family Practice News*, this drug may not be the best choice. Too many primary care physicians prescribe Ritalin for the symptoms of

ADD and ADHD without first establishing a precise diagnosis, and the drug has little effect on other problems, such as learning or socialization difficulties.

Diet Recommendations

❥ **Eat only fresh, whole foods, and avoid all food additives.** Read labels. The best rule is: If you can't pronounce it, don't buy it! Over 5,000 food additives are used in the United States, including bleaches, colorings, flavor enhancers, preservatives, thickeners, fillers, anticaking agents, and vegetable gums. Dr. Benjamin Feingold was the first doctor to propose that food-additive sensitivity, along with sensitivity to several naturally occurring compounds, causes hyperactivity in about half of those persons with ADHD. Numerous studies have supported Feingold's findings. For more information on healthy eating, see Basic Guidelines for the Juice Lady's Health and Healing Diet (page 313).

❥ **Especially avoid all refined sugar and food colorings.** Studies have found a correlation between consumption of these dietary items and behavior that is aggressive, destructive, and restless. Sugar consumption leads, oddly enough, to low blood-sugar levels, or hypoglycemia, which can promote hyperactivity and aggression (*see* **Hypoglycemia**).

❥ **Drink plenty of fresh juice.** Fresh juice is chock full of vitamins and minerals, and providing the brain with adequate nutrients will help it to function properly. Many cases of ADD may be the result of poor nutritional status. Raw juice offers nutrients in an easily absorbed form that can greatly improve mental performance.

❥ **Identify and avoid all food allergens and sensitivities.** Research has shown an improvement among a large percentage of children with severe hyperactivity when underlying food allergies were addressed. These children usually have many characteristics associated with a condition called allergic tension fatigue syndrome (ATFS), such as headache, irritability, and behavior disorder. Pay particular attention to dairy products if recurrent ear infections are a problem. Milk and other dairy items are common food allergens that can cause ear infections, which in turn can lead to attention deficit problems. (*See* **Allergies;** also see the Elimination Diet, page 321.) I recommend two books, *Is This Your Child?* and *Is This Your Child's World?*, by Dr. Doris Rapp (see Appendix A).

❥ **Use cleansing programs to help remove heavy metals.** A number of studies have shown a relationship between heavy metal toxicity, especially lead, and learning disabilities, behavior disorder, and criminal behavior.

Children should not be put on a strict juice fast unless supervised by a health care specialist. However, consuming fresh juices and a high-fiber diet, along with plenty of antioxidants (see the Nutrient Recommendations), will help cleanse the body of heavy metals. You can also try the Liver Cleanse (see page 333). In addition, choose organically grown foods, since pesticides and chemical fertilizers could be contributing to a possible toxic overload.

Nutrient Recommendations

❥ **Antioxidants** fight the toxic effects of free radicals. The following antioxidants are important for detoxification, memory enhancement, and overall health:

- *Beta-carotene* is a powerful antioxidant. Best juice sources of carotenes (in order of effectiveness): carrots, kale, parsley, spinach, chard, beet greens, watercress, mangoes, cantaloupes, apricots, broccoli, and romaine lettuce.

- *Selenium* helps activate glutathione peroxidase, an enzyme that serves as the body's own antioxidant. Best juice sources of selenium (in order of effectiveness): chard, turnips, garlic, oranges, radishes, grapes, carrots, and cabbage.

- *Vitamin C* helps protect brain cells from free-radical attack. Best juice sources of vitamin C (in order of effectiveness): kale, parsley, broccoli, Brussels sprouts, watercress, cauliflower, cabbage, strawberries, papaya, spinach, citrus fruit, turnips, mangoes, asparagus, and cantaloupes.

- *Vitamin E* helps protect cell membranes. Best juice sources of vitamin E (in order of effectiveness): spinach, watercress, asparagus, carrots, and tomatoes.

❥ **Essential fatty acids (EFAs),** taken in supplement form, may be able to correct fatty-acid imbalances that contribute to attention deficit problems, according to a Purdue University study. The standard American diet is quite deficient in EFAs. Unrefined flaxseed and hemp oil are rich sources of these nutrients; for more information, see the fats and oils section in Basic Guidelines for the Juice Lady's Health and Healing Diet (page 313).

❥ **Iron** deficiency, which is the most common nutrient deficiency in children, may contribute to ADD and ADHD. However, researchers have found that iron supplementation may also help children with these disorders who are not iron deficient. Best juice sources of nonheme iron, the type found in plant foods (in order of effectiveness): parsley, dandelion greens, broccoli, cauliflower, strawberries, asparagus, chard, blackberries, cabbage, beets with greens, carrots, and pineapple.

Juice Ingredient Recommendations

❥ **Celery** juice has a calming effect.

❥ **Fennel** juice has been used as a traditional tonic that has been found to help release endorphins into the bloodstream. These "feel good" chemicals create a mood of euphoria, and dampen anxiety and fear.

❥ **Parsley** juice is a rich source of beta-carotene, iron, and vitamin C. Intake should be limited to a safe, therapeutic dose of $1/2$ to 1 cup per day. Parsley can be toxic in overdose, and should be especially avoided by pregnant women.

❥ **Pear** can by substituted for apple in any of the juice recipes if apple sensitivity is a problem.

Juice Recipes

WALDORF TWIST

1 organic Red or Golden Delicious apple, washed

3 stalks organic celery with leaves, washed

1/4 small or medium lemon, washed, or peeled if not organic

Cut the apple into sections that will fit your juicer's feed tube, and juice along with the celery and lemon. Stir the juice, and pour into a glass. Serve at room temperature or chilled, as desired.

THE FEEL GOOD COCKTAIL

1/2 pear, washed

4 medium carrots, scrubbed well, green tops removed, ends trimmed

3 fennel stalks with leaves and flowers, washed

1 stalk organic celery with leaves, washed

Cut the pear into sections that fit your juicer's feed tube, and juice along with the carrots, fennel, and celery. Stir the juice, and pour into a glass. Serve at room temperature or chilled, as desired.

POPEYE'S POWER

½ medium organic apple, any kind, washed

1 handful organic spinach, washed

1 small handful parsley, rinsed

4 medium carrots, scrubbed well, green tops removed, ends trimmed

1 stalk organic celery with leaves, washed

½ beet with leaves, scrubbed well

Cut the apple into sections that will fit your juicer's feed tube. Bunch up the spinach and parsley, and push them through the feed tube with the apple, carrots, celery, and beet. Stir the juice, and pour into a glass. Serve at room temperature or chilled, as desired.

THE GINGER HOPPER

½ organic Red or Golden Delicious apple, washed

5 medium carrots, scrubbed well, green tops removed, ends trimmed

½- to 1-inch piece fresh ginger root, washed

Cut the apple into sections, and juice along with the carrots and ginger. Stir the juice, and pour into a glass. Serve at room temperature or chilled, as desired.

MORNING EXPRESS

1 orange, peeled

4–5 carrots, well scrubbed, green tops removed, ends trimmed

Divide the orange into segments that fit your juicer's feed tube, and juice with the carrots. Stir the juice, and pour into a glass. Serve at room temperature or chilled, as desired.

SWEET CALCIUM COCKTAIL

1 three-inch chunk fresh pineapple, scrubbed well or peeled if not organic

1–2 kale leaves, washed

Cut the pineapple into strips that fit your juicer's feed tube. Bunch up the kale, and push through the feed tube with the pineapple. Stir the juice, and pour into a glass. Serve at room temperature or chilled, as desired.

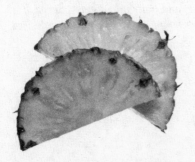

Bladder Infections

Bladder infection, a condition also known as cystitis, occurs when bacteria attack the lining of the bladder, causing inflammation and irritation. Symptoms include urinary urgency, feeling the need to urinate frequently, increased urination at night, burning or other pain with urination, and tenderness in the lower abdomen, just above the pubic bone. The urine may have an unusual odor, and may be cloudy or contain blood. Fever and chills may also occur. Many of these symptoms are similar to those of vaginal infections, urethritis, and some sexually transmitted diseases. Therefore, always see a doctor if you notice these symptoms. Sometimes a bladder infection produces no symptoms, and is only discovered when a urine test is done for other reasons.

Bladder infections are more common in women than in men. That's because the urethra, the tube that carries the urine out of the body, is shorter in women, which gives bacteria a shorter route to the bladder. Menopause and pregnancy are both associated with a greater chance of bladder infection, as is prostate infection in men. Infections can recur, especially if there is a blockage in the urinary tract or if nerve dysfunction prevents the bladder from emptying properly. Recurrent bladder infections can lead to an increased risk of kidney infection, which is a serious health condition.

Diet Recommendations

❥ **Avoid sugar and refined carbohydrates (white flour).** Sugar can depress the immune response for up to five hours after it is consumed. It doesn't matter if the sugar is in refined or natural form; sucrose (table sugar), fructose (fruit sugar), honey, and maple syrup should all be avoided. Even full-strength fruit juice contains too much sugar when you are fighting an infection, and should be diluted by half with water, mineral water, or vegetable juice. Avoid artificial sweeteners, which also depress the immune response. Eating white-flour products leads to a surge in blood-sugar levels.

❥ **Identify food allergies and intolerances.** Any foods you are allergic or sensitive to should be avoided, as these will further tax your immune system. (*See* **Allergies;** also see the Elimination Diet, page 321.)

❥ **Go on juice fasts.** According to Traditional Chinese Medicine, bladder infections can be exacerbated by eating too much food. Therefore, vegetable juices, vegetable broths, and herbal teas are recommended items for a short fast. (See the Juice Fast, page 324.) Vegetable broths that can be especially helpful include those made from adzuki beans, lima beans, celery, carrots, winter squash, potatoes with skins, and asparagus. Add garlic and onions for their antimicrobial and immune-stimulation properties.

❥ **Drink plenty of water.** This means at least eight to twelve 8-ounce glasses of pure water every day when you have a bladder infection. Drinking extra water not only helps to flush bacteria out of the urinary tract, but also will dilute the urine so that it is less uncomfortable to urinate.

❥ **Avoid caffeine and alcohol.** Caffeine, found in coffee, black and green tea, sodas, cola, and chocolate, is a bladder irritant and should be avoided. Alcohol also irritates the bladder.

Nutrient Recommendations

❥ **Vitamin A** and **carotenes** are important for good bladder health. Vitamin A deficiency has been shown to increase susceptibility to infection. This vitamin is important for the regeneration and repair of mucous membranes, such as that which lines the bladder. Certain carotenes, such as beta-carotene, can be converted to vitamin A as needed by the body, and both vitamin A and beta-carotene help fight infections. Best juice sources of carotenes (in order of effectiveness): carrots, kale, parsley, spinach, chard, beet greens, watercress, broccoli, and romaine lettuce.

❥ **Vitamin C** and **bioflavonoids** have been shown to be helpful in battling many types of infections. Vitamin C helps to increase the activity of white blood cells, the primary cells of the immune system. It is also important for keeping tissues strong and healthy. Bioflavonoids are the chemical compounds found in brightly colored fruits and vegetables. They work with vitamin C, making the vitamin's infection-fighting activity more effective. Best juice sources of vitamin C (in order of effectiveness): kale, parsley, broccoli, Brussels sprouts, watercress, cauliflower, cabbage, spinach, citrus fruit, turnips, and asparagus. Best juice sources of bioflavonoids: bell peppers, broccoli, cabbage, parsley, and tomatoes.

❥ **Zinc** is a potent infection fighter. Best juice sources of zinc (in order of effectiveness): ginger root, turnips, parsley, garlic, carrots, spinach, cabbage, lettuce, and cucumbers.

Herb Recommendations

❥ **Bearberry** has an affinity for the urinary tract, and has been used traditionally as a healing herb for the bladder. It is useful for keeping the urinary tract flushed and for diminishing bacterial growth.

❥ **Corn silk** has diuretic properties, and therefore helps flush the urinary tract. It also soothes irritated mucous membranes. Corn silk is most effective when used fresh.

Juice Ingredient Recommendations

❥ **Asparagus** juice is a good diuretic, and a traditional remedy for kidney and bladder problems.

❥ **Berry** juices, particularly those of cranberries, blueberries, lingonberries, and huckleberries, are helpful in healing and preventing bladder infections. The most research has been done on cranberry juice, which has been shown to prevent *E. coli*—the microbe that is the most common bacterial cause of bladder infection—from adhering to the bladder wall. If you wish, you can use unsweetened cranberry concentrate (available at most health food stores) and use $1/2$ teaspoon in place of the cranberries in Cranberry-Apple Cocktail.

❥ **Parsley** juice is a diuretic that also helps decrease inflammation and irritation in the bladder and urethra. A safe, therapeutic dose is $1/2$ to 1 cup of parsley juice per day. Parsley can be toxic in overdose, and should be especially avoided by pregnant women.

❥ **Watermelon** juice helps cleanse the urinary tract.

Juice Recipes

BLADDER TONIC

1 medium vine-ripened tomato, washed

1 organic cucumber, scrubbed well

8 asparagus stems, washed

$1/2$ small or medium lemon, washed, or peeled if not organic

Dash hot sauce

Cut the tomato into sections that fit your juicer's feed tube. Cut the cucumber in half lengthwise. Juice the tomato, cucumber, asparagus, and lemon. Add the hot sauce and stir the juice; pour into a glass. Serve at room temperature or chilled, as desired.

CRANBERRY-APPLE COCKTAIL

2 organic Granny Smith or Pippin apples, washed

1/4 cup fresh or frozen (thawed) cranberries, rinsed

1/4 small or medium lemon, washed, or peeled if not organic

1/2 cup water

Cut the apples into sections that will fit your juicer's feed tube. Juice the apples with the cranberries and lemon. (To keep the cranberries from flying out of the machine, place the cranberries in the juicer first, place an apple section on top of them, and cover with the plunger. Turn on the machine, and push the plunger to begin the juicing process.) Stir the juice, and pour into a glass with the water. Serve at room temperature or chilled, as desired.

ALLERGY RELIEF

1 small bunch parsley, rinsed

2 stalks organic celery with leaves, washed

2–3 large carrots, scrubbed well, green tops removed, ends trimmed

1/4–1/2 small or medium lemon, washed, or peeled if not organic

Bunch up the parsley and push it through the feed tube with the celery, carrots, and lemon. Stir the juice, and pour it into a glass. Serve at room temperature or chilled, as desired.

WATERMELON REFRESHER

1-inch slice watermelon, with seeds and well-scrubbed rind

1/2 cup water

Cut the watermelon into strips that fit your juicer's feed tube. Juice the watermelon, and pour into a glass with the water. Serve at room temperature or chilled, as desired.

BEAUTIFUL BONE SOLUTION

1 organic small Granny Smith or Pippin apple, washed

1–2 kale leaves, washed

1 handful parsley, rinsed

1 stalk organic celery, washed

1/2 small or medium lemon, washed, or peeled if not organic

1/2- to 1-inch piece fresh ginger root, washed

Cut the apple into sections that fit your juicer's feed tube. Bunch up the kale and parsley, and push through the feed tube with the apple, celery, lemon, and ginger. Stir the juice, and pour into a glass. Serve at room temperature or chilled, as desired.

POPEYE'S POWER

1 handful organic spinach, washed
1 small handful parsley, rinsed
5 medium carrots, scrubbed well, green tops removed, ends trimmed
1 stalk organic celery with leaves, washed
½ beet with leaves, scrubbed well

Bunch up the spinach and parsley, and push them through the feed tube with the carrots, celery, and beet. Stir the juice, and pour into a glass. Serve at room temperature or chilled, as desired.

THE MORNING ENERGIZER

5 medium carrots, scrubbed well, green tops removed, ends trimmed
½ small beet with leaves and stems, scrubbed well
½ small or medium lemon, washed, or peeled if not organic
½- to 1-inch piece fresh ginger root, washed

Juice the carrots, beet, lemon, and ginger. Stir the juice, and pour into a glass. Serve at room temperature or chilled, as desired.

THE GINGER HOPPER

5 medium carrots, scrubbed well, green tops removed, ends trimmed
1-inch piece fresh ginger root, washed
½ small or medium lemon, washed, or peeled if not organic

Cut the apple into sections, and juice along with the carrots and ginger. Stir the juice, and pour into a glass. Serve at room temperature or chilled, as desired.

Bronchitis

See **Respiratory Disorders.**

Bruises

A bruise is an injury that does not break the skin, but does rupture under-lying capillaries. This hemorrhaging causes the superficial skin discoloration seen in bruises. If the injury is severe enough, fluid gathers in the affected area, causing swelling, pain, and tenderness.

Easy bruising that occurs with no apparent injury is due to fragile capillaries. These tiny blood vessels can break if their walls are not strong and healthy. While the tendency to bruise easily runs in some families, many people become more prone to this problem as they age or become nutrient deficient.

Diet Recommendations

❥ Make dietary changes to help stop easy bruising and to recover from injury. If your skin bruises easily, or if you are recovering from injuries, eat foods rich in vitamin C and bioflavonoids (see the Nutrient Recommendations and follow the Basic Guidelines for the Juice Lady's Health and Healing Diet, page 313).

Nutrient Recommendations

❥ Bioflavonoids are plant pigments responsible for the bright colors of many fruits and vegetables. Two types of bioflavonoids—proanthocyanidins and procyanidolic oligomers (PCOs, which are large, linked proanthocyanidin molecules)—have been studied for their ability to decrease capillary permeability and fragility. PCOs are considered the most effective bioflavonoid in this regard. Citrus bioflavonoids, including rutin, hesperidin, quercetin, and naringin, have also been found effective in treating easy bruising, capillary fragility, and bruising after sports injuries. In addition, bioflavonoids enhance the actions of vitamin C (see the vitamin C entry on this list). Best juice sources of bioflavonoids: apricots, bell peppers, berries (blueberry, blackberry, and cranberry), broccoli, cabbage, cantaloupes, cherries, citrus fruit, grapes, parsley, plums, prunes, and tomatoes.

❥ Essential fatty acids (EFAs) are recommended for people who bruise easily or are recovering from bruises caused by injury. The body is unable to make EFAs, and so they must be obtained from the diet. Flaxseed and hemp oils are excellent sources of EFAs; one tablespoon per day can be very helpful. For more information, see the fats and oils section in Basic Guidelines for the Juice Lady's Health and Healing Diet (page 313).

❥ Vitamin C strengthens capillary walls by playing a role in the formation and maintenance of collagen, the basis of connective tissue. Healthy collagen is important in maintaining integrity of blood vessels. Best juice sources of vitamin C (in order of effectiveness): kale, parsley, broccoli,

Brussels sprouts, watercress, cauliflower, cabbage, strawberries, papaya, spinach, citrus fruit, turnips, mangoes, asparagus, and cantaloupes.

🌱 **Vitamin E** helps repair tissues. Best juice sources of vitamin E (in order of effectiveness): spinach, watercress, asparagus, carrots, and tomatoes.

Herb Recommendations

🌱 **Arnica,** in tincture, salve, or oil form, can be applied externally to a bruised area. Arnica helps stimulate and dilate blood vessels, thereby helping tissues recover from injury. In stimulating good blood flow, arnica helps remove waste products from a bruised area.

🌱 **Bleeding heart** helps deaden the pain associated with bruises, sprains, and contusions. Apply externally and cover the injured area with a hot, moist towel.

🌱 **Marigold** helps heal wounds, bruises, and strains. Use externally as an ointment, salve, poultice, or compress.

🌱 **Pearly everlasting,** applied externally, helps ease the pain, redness, and swelling associated with bruises.

Traditional Remedy Recommendations

🌱 **Cabbage leaves** have long been used in folk medicine to speed healing of bruises. Wash the outer leaves of an organically grown green cabbage. Then remove and discard the main stems, flatten the leaves with a rolling pin to soften, and apply to the bruise.

Juice Ingredient Recommendations

🌱 **Grape seeds** are a rich source of proanthocyanidins.

🌱 **Parsley** juice is an excellent source of bioflavonoids and vitamin C. Intake should be limited to a safe, therapeutic dose of $1/2$ to 1 cup per day. Parsley can be toxic in overdose, and should be especially avoided by pregnant women.

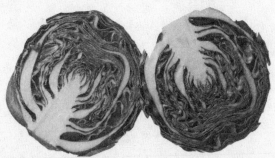

Juice Recipes

POPEYE'S POWER

½ medium organic apple, any kind, washed

1 handful organic spinach, washed

1 small handful parsley, rinsed

4 medium carrots, scrubbed well, green tops removed, ends trimmed

1 stalk organic celery with leaves, washed

½ beet with leaves, scrubbed well

Cut the apple into sections that will fit your juicer's feed tube. Bunch up the spinach and parsley, and push them through the feed tube with the apple, carrots, celery, and beet. Stir the juice, and pour into a glass. Serve at room temperature or chilled, as desired.

SPICY TOMATO ON ICE

2 vine-ripened tomatoes, washed

2 dark green lettuce leaves, such as romaine or green leaf, washed

1 small handful parsley, rinsed

2 radishes with green tops, washed

½ small or medium lime or lemon, washed, or peeled if not organic

Dash hot sauce

Cut the tomato in sections that fit your juicer's feed tube. Bunch up the lettuce leaves and parsley, and push them through the feed tube with the tomatoes, radishes, and lime or lemon. Add a dash of hot sauce, and stir to combine. Pour into tall, ice-filled glasses.

THE COLON CLEANSER

2 organic Granny Smith, McIntosh, or Golden Delicious apples, washed

1 bunch organic spinach, washed

1 handful parsley, rinsed

¼ small or medium lemon, washed, or peeled if not organic

Cut the apples into sections that fit your juicer's feed tube. Bunch up the spinach and parsley, and push them through the feed tube with the apples and lemon. Stir the juice, and pour into a glass. Serve at room temperature or chilled, as desired.

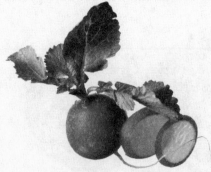

ANTIAGING COCKTAIL

1 small bunch organic purple grapes (about 1 cup) with small stems* and seeds, washed

½ cup blueberries, blackberries, or raspberries, washed

¼ small or medium lemon, washed, or peeled if not organic

½-inch piece fresh ginger root, washed

*Large stems can dull your juicer's blade.

Juice the grapes, berries, lemon, and ginger. Stir the juice, and pour into a glass. Serve at room temperature or chilled, as desired.

SNAPPY GINGER

1 medium orange, peeled

3-inch chunk fresh pineapple, scrubbed well or peeled if not organic

¼ small or medium lemon, washed, or peeled if not organic

1- to 2-inch piece fresh ginger root, washed

Divide the orange into segments, and cut the pineapple into strips that fit your juicer's feed tube. Juice the orange, pineapple, lemon, and ginger. Stir the juice, and pour into two glasses. Serve at room temperature or chilled, as desired.

STRAWBERRY-CANTALOUPE COCKTAIL

½ ripe organic cantaloupe with seeds, washed (peeled if not organic)

1 cup organic strawberries, washed

Cut the cantaloupe into strips that fit your juicer's feed tube. Juice the cantaloupe and strawberries; stir the juice and pour into a glass. Serve at room temperature or chilled, as desired.

Bursitis and Tendinitis

Bursitis is the inflammation of a bursa, a small, fluid-filled cavity found in connecting tissues, usually in places where friction occurs. The most common bursitis locations are the shoulders, elbows, hips, and knees. Symptoms include pain, swelling, and tenderness, along with restricted range of motion. These symptoms can be experienced particularly when stretching or exercising.

Tendinitis is the inflammation of a tendon, the fibrous cord that attaches a muscle to a bone. The condition is painful, and there may be either swelling or a dry, grating sensation. The tendons most often affected are those of the biceps, thumb, knee, inside of the foot, and rotator cuff (shoulder), and the Achilles tendon in the heel.

The most common cause of bursitis or tendinitis is injury or overuse, or sudden excessive tension on a bursa or tendon. This can happen because of poor conditioning, bad posture, or working in an awkward position. Bursitis can also occur as the result of gout (*see* **Gout**), infection, or rheumatoid arthritis (*see* **Rheumatoid Arthritis**). Either condition can become chronic, with the formation of calcium deposits in the affected areas.

Conventional medicine treats bursitis or tendinitis with high doses of nonsteroidal anti-inflammatory drugs (NSAIDs), such as ibuprofen. But these drugs can irritate the gastrointestinal tract. Another common approach is to inject cortisone into the affected area. Dr. Rozbruch of the Mayo Clinic says these injections are not going to eliminate the mechanical problem, though they will temporarily relieve the pain. He suggests taking a more wholistic approach by identifying the underlying cause of the condition, and designing a treatment plan accordingly.

Lifestyle Recommendations

❥ **Rest the affected area.** This is the most important treatment for bursitis or tendinitis. Most often, if you give the affected area a break, the condition will subside. After the inflammation subsides, stretch the affected area before exercising or working to prevent further damage.

❥ **Try alternative treatments.** Acupuncture can bring quick relief of pain as well as a gradual reduction of inflammation. Deep massage can stimulate circulation in the affected area and loosen tight muscles. Chiropractic sessions can help restore the joints' range of motion.

Diet Recommendations

❥ **Eat less meat and more complex carbohydrates.** Animal foods are high in arachidonic acid, a precursor to inflammation-causing substances called prostaglandins. For more information, see Basic Guidelines for the Juice Lady's Health and Healing Diet (page 313).

❥ **Go on juice fasts.** A short juice fast can give your body a chance to remove waste products from inflamed areas. For more information on the healing power of a fast, see the Juice Fast (page 324).

Nutrient Recommendations

❧ **Bioflavonoids** are plant pigments that give fruits and vegetables their bright colors. Two types of flavonoids—quercetin and the anthocyanidins—are of particular interest for people with inflammatory conditions. Quercetin inhibits the secretion of histamine and other inflammatory chemicals, thereby limiting the inflammatory response. Anthocyanidins concentrate in collagen and help repair this protein-based tissue, which is destroyed during bursitis and tendinitis. In addition, bioflavonoids enhance the actions of vitamin C (see vitamin C entry on this list). Best juice sources of bioflavonoids: apricots, bell peppers, berries (blueberry, blackberry, and cranberry), broccoli, cabbage, cantaloupes, cherries, citrus fruit, grapes, parsley, plums, prunes, and tomatoes.

❧ **Essential fatty acids (EFAs),** namely the omega-3 fatty acids, are able to inhibit production of inflammatory substances called PG2 prostaglandins, and thereby lessen inflammation severity. Hemp and flaxseed oils are two of the best sources of EFAs; one to two tablespoons of unrefined hemp or flaxseed oil per day is recommended. For more information on EFAs, see the fats and oils section in Basic Guidelines for the Juice Lady's Health and Healing Diet (page 313).

❧ **Vitamin C** deficiency is associated with inadequate bursa formation. This vitamin is also important in the prevention and repair of tissue damage. In addition, it has anti-inflammatory and antihistamine properties, histamine being one of the primary chemicals involved in inflammation. Best juice sources of vitamin C (in order of effectiveness): kale, parsley, broccoli, Brussels sprouts, watercress, cauliflower, cabbage, strawberries, papaya, spinach, citrus fruit, turnips, mangoes, asparagus, and cantaloupes.

❧ **Zinc** is effective in reducing inflammation and contributing to tissue repair. Best juice sources of zinc (in order of effectiveness): ginger root, turnips, parsley, garlic, carrots, grapes, spinach, cabbage, lettuce, cucumbers, and tangerines.

Herb Recommendations

❧ **Curcumin,** the yellow pigment in turmeric, is able to inhibit inflammatory substances. Curcumin is available in supplement form.

Juice Ingredient Recommendations

❧ **Ginger** juice has anti-inflammatory effects.

❥ **Parsley** juice is an excellent source of bioflavonoids and vitamin C. Intake should be limited to a safe, therapeutic dose of $1/2$ to 1 cup per day. Parsley can be toxic in overdose, and should be especially avoided by pregnant women.

❥ **Pineapple** juice contains bromelain, an enzyme that has demonstrated the ability to inhibit PG2 prostaglandins.

Juice Recipes

SNAPPY GINGER

1 medium orange, peeled

3-inch chunk fresh pineapple, scrubbed well or peeled if not organic

$1/4$ small or medium lemon, washed, or peeled if not organic

1- to 2-inch piece fresh ginger root, washed

Divide the orange into segments, and cut the pineapple into strips that fit your juicer's feed tube. Juice the orange, pineapple, lemon, and ginger. Stir the juice, and pour into two glasses. Serve at room temperature or chilled, as desired.

THE GINGER HOPPER

$1/2$ organic Red or Golden Delicious apple, washed

5 medium carrots, scrubbed well, green tops removed, ends trimmed

$1/2$- to 1-inch piece fresh ginger root, washed

Cut the apple into sections, and juice along with the carrots and ginger. Stir the juice, and pour into a glass. Serve at room temperature or chilled, as desired.

SWEET CALCIUM COCKTAIL

1 three-inch chunk fresh pineapple, scrubbed well or peeled if not organic

1–2 kale leaves, washed

Cut the pineapple into strips that fit your juicer's feed tube. Bunch up the kale, and push through the feed tube with the pineapple. Stir the juice, and pour into a glass. Serve at room temperature or chilled, as desired.

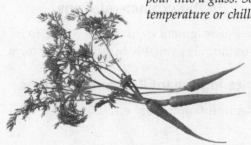

THE MORNING ENERGIZER

½ organic Red or Golden Delicious apple, washed

5 medium carrots, scrubbed well, green tops removed, ends trimmed

½ small beet with leaves and stems, scrubbed well

½ small or medium lemon, washed, or peeled if not organic

½- to 1-inch piece fresh ginger root, washed

Cut the apple into sections that will fit your juicer's feed tube. Juice the apple along with the carrots, beet, lemon, and ginger. Stir the juice, and pour into a glass. Serve at room temperature or chilled, as desired.

MORNING EXPRESS

1 orange, peeled

4–5 carrots, well scrubbed, green tops removed, ends trimmed

Divide the orange into segments that fit your juicer's feed tube, and juice with the carrots. Stir the juice, and pour into a glass. Serve at room temperature or chilled, as desired.

POPEYE'S POWER

½ medium organic apple, any kind, washed

1 handful organic spinach, washed

1 small handful parsley, rinsed

4 medium carrots, scrubbed well, green tops removed, ends trimmed

1 stalk organic celery with leaves, washed

½ beet with leaves, scrubbed well

Cut the apple into sections that will fit your juicer's feed tube. Bunch up the spinach and parsley, and push them through the feed tube with the apple, carrots, celery, and beet. Stir the juice, and pour into a glass. Serve at room temperature or chilled, as desired.

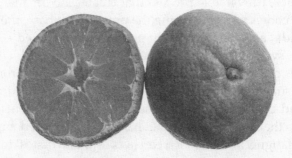

PINK PASSION POTION

1 organic Red Delicious apple, washed

½ cup fresh or frozen (thawed) cranberries, rinsed

1 bunch organic purple grapes, with seeds and small stems,* washed

⅛ small beet (no stems or leaves) for color, scrubbed well (optional)

¼ small or medium lemon, washed, or peeled if not organic

*Large stems can dull your juicer's blade.

Cut the apple into sections that fit your juicer's feed tube. Juice the apple, cranberries, grapes, beet (if using), and lemon. (To prevent the cranberries from flying out of the machine while juicing, place the cranberries in the juicer first, place an apple section on top of them, and cover with the plunger. Turn on the machine, and push the plunger to begin the juicing process.) Stir the juice, and pour into a glass. Serve at room temperature or chilled, as desired.

Cancer

Cancer is a condition in which cells grow unchecked. Cells have an internal governing code, known as homeostatic control, that directs how they reproduce and mature. When cancer develops, this code goes awry—cells divide faster than they mature and reproduce at will, usually producing a tissue mass called a tumor. Cancer cells are malignant, that is, they invade surrounding tissue. There are hundreds of types of cancer. Currently, one in three Americans will develop cancer at some point in his or her life.

A multitude of factors—including genes, diet, lifestyle, environment, hormones, and viruses—can contribute to cancer's development. Most cancers develop in a multistep process that can be broken down into two phases—initiation and promotion. During the initiation phase, there is usually a quick, irreversible process that creates a permanent change in a cell's master code, or DNA. During the promotion phase, the cell is stimulated to divide, and the number of genetically damaged cells increases. The immune system can become overwhelmed and unable to destroy all the cancerous cells, which leads to tumor formation. The promotion phase is gradual, usually requires prolonged exposure to such promoting agents as toxins, and can usually be reversed. Cancer's symptoms are as many and varied as the types of cancer that have been identified, but can include weight loss, fatigue, and pain. Researchers estimate that 80 to 90 percent of all cancers are environmentally related. In that broad category, the National Cancer Institute lists diet as the number-one contributing factor.

Considering that to be the case, doesn't it make sense that diet should be the number-one area to address regarding cancer care? For years nutrition and cancer (a subject on which I did my master's thesis) has been of special interest to me because my mother died of cancer when I was six. I can assure you from all my research that diet—and juicing in particular—will make a tremendous difference in your recovery, in addition to whatever treatments you and your doctor choose. Make dietary changes that give your body, and particularly your immune system, the best chance to destroy cancer cells and heal itself at the cellular level. It is especially important to consume the proper nutrients if you are going through radiation therapy or chemotherapy, as these treatments greatly suppress the immune system. Though the whole subject of nutrition and cancer is far beyond the scope of this book, the information presented here will give you an excellent start. For more information, see the cancer section in Appendix A.

Diet Recommendations

❥ **Eat a low-fat, high-complex carbohydrate diet.** Plant-based diets have been shown in hundreds of studies to be effective against agents that promote cancer. All anticancer diets should include whole grains, such as oats, bran, brown rice, and millet cereal (a good source of vegetable protein); raw nuts (except peanuts) and seeds; and legumes, such as beans, lentils, and split peas. Fruits and vegetables, in particular, help prevent cancer, and are an important part of an overall cancer treatment plan. Eat one serving of cruciferous vegetables—such as broccoli, cauliflower, Brussels sprouts, or cabbage—several times a week. Also choose fruits and vegetables that are deep yellow, orange, or red. They are rich in the cancer-fighting carotenoids (see carotenes under Nutrient Recommendations). For more information on choosing a healthy diet, see Basic Guidelines for the Juice Lady's Health and Healing Diet (page 313).

❥ **Avoid all foods and additives that have been linked with cancer.** These include processed refined foods (white flour products) and packaged foods. Eliminate all saturated fat, hydrogenated vegetable oils, hydrogenated peanut butter, margarine, caffeine, and alcohol. Read labels, and avoid all food additives, preservatives, dyes, fillers, and stabilizers. (A good rule is: If you can't pronounce it, don't buy it.) Avoid peanuts, as they can contain highly carcinogenic aflatoxins. Buy organically grown food as much as possible because pesticides, fungicides, insecticides, and artificial fertilizers can further weaken your immune system. Use kelp and herbal seasonings instead of salt. Completely avoid all barbecued, fried, and smoked foods—the interaction of fat with high heat creates highly carcinogenic byproducts.

❥ **Avoid all sugar.** Sugars have been shown to feed cancer cells, and possibly to contribute to the formation of the protective coating that envelops these cells. Avoid the following: white and brown sugar, dried sugar cane, sugar alcohols such as manitol and sorbitol, honey, maple syrup, and especially all artificial sweeteners, such as aspartame.

❥ **Avoid animal protein.** *Never* eat hot dogs, bacon, luncheon meat, and smoked or cured meats. Avoid red meat and poultry. As your condition improves, you can add a little broiled cold-water fish, such as salmon, tuna, halibut, trout, mackerel, or sardines, to your diet two or three times per week. Too much protein in general is detrimental to health, but is especially so if you have cancer. Restrict your consumption of dairy products; have only a little organic plain yogurt occasionally. Instead, use soy products—soy milk, soy cheese, tofu, and miso. Soy contains phytoestrogens, protease inhibitors, phytosterols, saponins, and isoflavonoids, substances that have all been shown to have an anticancer effect.

❥ **Consider juice, along with raw fruits and vegetables, to be your best friends.** From Dr. Max Gerson, who used carrot-apple juice as the core of his cancer-care program, to famous European health clinics, scores of health practitioners have helped thousands of people successfully make raw fruit and vegetable juices—preferably made from organic produce— an essential part of an anticancer diet. Raw juices do most of the excellent things that solid raw foods do, but with a minimum strain on the digestive system. The alkalinity of raw vegetables and fruits is a particularly powerful ally in your fight against cancer, as this disease develops more easily when the body is too acidic. In addition, raw foods are "alive" with fresh, untouched nutrients that are at the peak of their natural potency. Raw foods are also rich in enzymes, substances that are destroyed by cooking. Enzymes are important for cancer patients; they assist pancreatic enzymes in digesting cooked foods as well as fighting cancer. Pancreatic enzymes have the power to destroy the protective mucous barrier that surrounds cancer cells, as do certain enzymes in fruits and vegetables. Strive for a diet in which 75 percent of your food consists of raw fruits, vegetables, juices, sprouts, seeds, and nuts. Dilute all fruit juices by half with water, and use fruit juices very sparingly to avoid consuming too much fruit sugar. Concentrate on vegetable juices instead.

❥ **Use juice fasts and cleansing programs.** The body eliminates toxins by either directly neutralizing them or excreting them. Toxins the body can't eliminate build up in the tissues, most often in fat cells. It is vitally important that you get rid of stored-up toxins, and that your liver, intestines, and kidneys are all functioning well to assist you in this detoxification process. Studies have shown that people with the poorest detoxification systems are the most susceptible to cancer. Fortunately, detoxification efficiency can be improved through dietary measures and cleansing programs, and a complete detoxification program can help rid the body of toxins. For more information, see the Juice Fast (page 324) and the cleansing programs (pages 323 through 339).

Nutrient Recommendations

❥ **Antioxidants** are found in a number of fruits and vegetables, and have been extensively studied for both their protective and therapeutic actions against cancer. Antioxidants are important because they destroy free radicals, unstable molecules that are always looking to steal electrons from other molecules. This process sets up a chain reaction that leads to cell damage. Free radicals can cause extensive damage over a period of time, damage that can lead to cancer. The following antioxidants bind to free radicals, protecting your cells and greatly enhancing your chances of winning the cancer battle:

• *Bioflavonoids* have been shown to have anticancer, as well as antiviral and anti-inflammatory, properties. They are extremely effective at destroying free radicals. Two flavonoids—nobiletin and tangeretin—boost the activity of a group of enzymes that specialize in ridding the body of such toxins as drugs, heavy metals, and hydrocarbons from auto exhausts. They also enhance the effectiveness of vitamin C (see the vitamin C entry in this list). Best juice sources of bioflavonoids: apricots, bell peppers, berries (blueberry, blackberry, and cranberry), broccoli, cabbage, cantaloupes, cherries, citrus fruit, grapes, parsley, plums, prunes, and tomatoes.

• *Carotenes* are plant pigments that have been found to be quite remarkable in their ability to protect the body against free-radical damage. Diets rich in beta-carotene, one of the most widely studied carotenoids, are associated with a reduced risk of cancers of the lung, cervix, and gastrointestinal tract. Carotenes also have important immune-enhancing capabilities, particularly in stimulating such immune-system cells as helper T cells. Best juice sources of carotenes (in order of effectiveness): carrots, kale, parsley, spinach, chard, beet greens, watercress, mangoes, cantaloupes, apricots, broccoli, and romaine lettuce.

- *Selenium* works with the enzyme glutathione peroxidase, an antioxidant enzyme that is important in the development of many immune-system cells. Best juice sources of selenium (in order of effectiveness): chard, turnips, garlic, oranges, radishes, grapes, carrots, and cabbage.

- *Vitamin C* offers particular immune support for cancer patients; in several studies, it has been shown to increase survival time. It is especially helpful for those going through chemotherapy and radiation, as it appears to enhance the effectiveness of conventional treatment. Best juice sources of vitamin C (in order of effectiveness): kale, parsley, broccoli, Brussels sprouts, watercress, cauliflower, cabbage, strawberries, papaya, spinach, citrus fruit, turnips, mangoes, asparagus, and cantaloupes.

- *Vitamin E* is an antioxidant that supports the immune system. Best juice sources of vitamin E (in order of effectiveness): spinach, watercress, asparagus, carrots, and tomatoes.

- *Zinc* is necessary for enhanced white blood cell functioning, and has been shown to increase production of white cells called T lymphocytes. Best juice sources of zinc (in order of effectiveness): ginger root, turnips, parsley, garlic, carrots, grapes, spinach, cabbage, lettuce, cucumbers, and tangerines.

❥ **Essential fatty acids (EFAs),** especially omega-3s, have powerful anti-cancer properties, especially when they are taken in an oil high in a fiber-based substance called lignan. Lignans appear to be anticarcinogenic, and are similar in chemical structure to estrogens. This allows lignans to bind with estrogen receptors on cells, which can inhibit the growth of estrogen-stimulated cancers. Dr. Johanna Budwig, leading German biochemist and EFA expert, has built an international reputation for treating cancer and other diseases with flaxseed oil, which is rich in omega-3s. For more information on omega-3 rich oils, see the fats and oils section in Basic Guidelines for the Juice Lady's Health and Healing Diet (page 313).

❥ **Iron** tablets should be *avoided* if you have cancer. Excess iron may suppress both the cancer-killing function of the macrophages, immune cells that help in tissue repair, and T- and B-cell activity.

Herb Recommendations

❥ **Astragalus** has been shown to restore immune function when the immune system is suppressed as a side effect of chemotherapy. It has also been shown to increase production of antibodies and interferon, two important immune-system components, and increase the activity of helper T cells. Avoid this herb if you have a fever.

❥ **Echinacea** enhances the immune system. It also acts against viruses, which means it can help you fight off infections if your immune system is not working properly.

Juice Ingredient Recommendations

❥ **Beet** juice has been found in recent clinical experience to reverse and prevent radiation-induced cancers.

❥ **Cabbage** juice contains a high concentration of two substances, indole-3-carbinol and oltipaz, that help increase the activity of enzymes which protect against a wide range of cancers.

❥ **Carrot** juice is one of the richest sources of beta-carotene, which is believed to be one of the substances that can break down the protective mucous membrane around cancer cells. Cancer expert Dr. Virginia Livingston urges her patients to drink two pints of fresh carrot juice each day. Dr. Max Gerson had his patients drink ten 8-ounce glasses of carrot-apple juice daily, alternating with glasses of green juices.

❥ **Garlic** juice has been shown in studies to inhibit tumor growth. Onions have similar properties.

❥ **Green juices,** such as those made from beet greens, spinach, parsley, chard, kale, or sprouts, are rich in chlorophyll. Research at the University of Texas Systems Cancer Center has found that chlorophyll may block the genetic changes that cancer-causing substances produce in cells.

❥ **Parsley** juice is rich in bioflavonoids and vitamin C. Intake should be limited to a safe, therapeutic dose of $^1/_2$ to 1 cup per day. Parsley can be toxic in overdose, and should be especially avoided by pregnant women.

❥ **Tomato** juice is rich in lycopene, a very powerful antioxidant that has been shown to be particularly helpful in protecting against prostate cancer. Tomatoes are also rich in p-coumaric and chlorogenic acid, two phytochemicals that block formation of highly carcinogenic nitrosamine compounds within the body.

❥ **Wheatgrass** juice helps build immunity. Studies have identified a number of substances in wheatgrass juice that are formidable anticancer agents. This juice works best when taken alone, but many people have trouble with the taste. *On a personal note:* Every year I go to what is affectionately called the "wheatgrass clinic"—the Optimum Health Institute (OHI) of San Diego. Their one- to three-week program is an excellent way to cleanse the body and support the healing process. (For information on health institutes that use the raw food and juice-fast plan, see Appendix A.)

Juice Recipes

THE MORNING ENERGIZER

½ organic Red or Golden Delicious apple, washed

5 medium carrots, scrubbed well, green tops removed, ends trimmed

½ small beet with leaves and stems, scrubbed well

½ small or medium lemon, washed, or peeled if not organic

½- to 1-inch piece fresh ginger root, washed

Cut the apple into sections that will fit your juicer's feed tube. Juice the apple along with the carrots, beet, lemon, and ginger. Stir the juice, and pour into a glass. Serve at room temperature or chilled, as desired.

TRIPLE C

¼ small head green cabbage, washed

4 carrots, scrubbed well, green tops removed, and ends trimmed

4 stalks organic celery with leaves, washed

Cut the cabbage into sections that fit your juicer's feed tube. Juice the cabbage along with the carrots and celery. Stir the juice, and pour into a glass. Serve at room temperature or chilled, as desired.

THE GINGER HOPPER

½ organic Red or Golden Delicious apple, washed

5 medium carrots, scrubbed well, green tops removed, ends trimmed

½- to 1-inch piece fresh ginger root, washed

Cut the apple into sections, and juice along with the carrots and ginger. Stir the juice, and pour into a glass. Serve at room temperature or chilled, as desired.

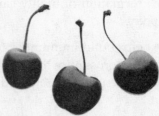

SWEET DREAMS NIGHTCAP

2 romaine lettuce leaves, washed

1 handful parsley, rinsed

4 carrots, scrubbed well, green tops removed, ends trimmed

3 organic celery stalks with leaves, washed

Bunch up the lettuce leaves and parsley, and push through the feed tube with the carrots and celery. Stir the juice, and pour into a glass. Serve at room temperature or chilled, as desired.

TURNIP TIME

1 turnip, scrubbed well

2-inch piece jicama, scrubbed well or peeled if not organic (optional)

1 handful watercress, rinsed

4 carrots, scrubbed well, green tops removed, ends trimmed

1 garlic clove with peel, washed

1/2 small or medium lemon, washed, or peeled if not organic

Cut the turnip and jicama (if using) into strips that fit your juicer's feed tube. Bunch up the watercress, and push through the feed tube with the turnip, jicama, carrots, garlic, and lemon. Stir the juice, and pour into a glass. Serve at room temperature or chilled, as desired.

SPICY TOMATO ON ICE

2 vine-ripened tomatoes, washed

2 dark green lettuce leaves, such as romaine or green leaf, washed

1 small handful parsley, rinsed

2 radishes with green tops, washed

1/2 small or medium lime or lemon, washed, or peeled if not organic

Dash hot sauce

Cut the tomato in sections that fit your juicer's feed tube. Bunch up the lettuce leaves and parsley, and push them through the feed tube with the tomatoes, radishes, and lime or lemon. Add a dash of hot sauce, and stir to combine. Pour into tall, ice-filled glasses.

WHEATGRASS LIGHT

1 organic green apple, washed

1 large handful wheatgrass, rinsed

2–3 sprigs mint, rinsed (optional)

1/4 small or medium lemon, washed, or peeled if not organic

Cut the apple into sections that fit your juicer's feed tube. Bunch up the wheatgrass and mint (if using) and push them through the feed tube with the apple and lemon. Stir the juice, and pour into a glass. Serve at room temperature or chilled, as desired.

PURE GREEN SPROUT DRINK

1 organic cucumber, scrubbed well

1 large handful sunflower sprouts, rinsed

1 small handful buckwheat sprouts, rinsed

1 small handful clover sprouts, rinsed

Cut the cucumber in half lengthwise. Bunch up the sprouts, and push through the feed tube with the cucumber. Stir the juice, and pour into a glass. Serve at room temperature or chilled, as desired.

SANTA FE SALSA COCKTAIL

1 medium vine-ripened tomato, washed

1/2 medium organic cucumber, scrubbed well

1/4 cup cilantro, rinsed

1/4 small or medium lime or lemon, washed, or peeled if not organic

Dash hot sauce (optional)

Cut the tomato into sections that fit your juicer's feed tube. Cut the cucumber in half again lengthwise. Bunch up the cilantro, and push through the feed tube with the tomato, cucumber, and lime or lemon. Pour the juice into a glass, add the hot sauce (if using), and stir. Serve at room temperature or chilled, as desired.

LIVER LIFE TONIC

1/2 organic green apple such as Granny Smith or Pippin, washed

1 handful dandelion greens, washed

5 carrots, scrubbed well, green tops removed, ends trimmed

1/2 small lemon, washed, or peeled if not organic

Cut the apple into wedges that will fit your juicer's feed tube. Bunch up the dandelion greens, and push through the feed tube with the apple, carrots, and lemon. Stir the juice, and pour into a glass. Serve at room temperature or chilled, as desired.

BEAUTIFUL BONE SOLUTION

1 organic green apple, washed

1–2 kale leaves, washed

1 handful parsley, rinsed

1 stalk organic celery, washed

1/4 small or medium lemon, washed, or peeled if not organic

1/2- to 1-inch piece fresh ginger root, washed

Cut the apple into sections that fit your juicer's feed tube. Bunch up the kale and parsley, and push through the feed tube with the apple, celery, lemon, and ginger. Stir the juice, and pour into a glass. Serve at room temperature or chilled, as desired.

POPEYE'S POWER

½ medium organic green apple, washed

1 handful organic spinach, washed

1 small handful parsley, rinsed

4 medium carrots, scrubbed well, green tops removed, ends trimmed

1 stalk organic celery with leaves, washed

½ beet with leaves, scrubbed well

Cut the apple into sections that will fit your juicer's feed tube. Bunch up the spinach and parsley, and push them through the feed tube with the apple, carrots, celery, and beet. Stir the juice, and pour into a glass. Serve at room temperature or chilled, as desired.

JACK & THE BEAN

1 large vine-ripened tomato, washed

2 romaine lettuce leaves, washed

8 organic string beans, washed

3 Brussels sprouts, washed

½ small or medium lemon, washed, or peeled if not organic

Cut the tomato into sections that fit your juicer's feed tube. Bunch up the lettuce leaves, and push through the feed tube with the tomato, string beans, Brussels sprouts, and lemon. Stir the juice, and pour into a glass. Serve at room temperature or chilled, as desired.

Candidiasis

Candidiasis is an infection with any species of the yeast Candida. The most common agent is *Candida albicans*, which is naturally present in the intestines and vaginal area, and on the skin. Candida normally coexists with bacteria that keep it in check, namely bifidobacteria and acidophilus. But if it overgrows, Candida can invade other tissues and create a host of problems. *C. albicans* produces acetaldehyde, a type of alcohol that interferes with normal functioning in various bodily systems. Gastrointestinal symptoms include bloating, gas, cramps, rectal itching, changes in bowel function, and thrush ("white carpet" tongue). Nervous-system reactions include depression, poor memory, irritability, and inability to concentrate. Genitourinary complaints include vaginal yeast infections and recurring bladder infections. Endocrine problems include premenstrual syndrome (PMS) and other menstrual disorders. Immune-system complaints include lowered immunity, allergies, and chemical sensitivities. Overall, candidiasis is characterized by chronic fatigue, loss of sex drive, and malaise.

No single cause is responsible for candidiasis. However, several factors are generally recognized. A suppressed immune system increases the risk for candidiasis. Antibiotic use disturbs the balance of bacteria in the intestines, killing both harmful and beneficial bacteria. Candida overgrowth can also result from the use of other drugs, such as oral contraceptives, antiulcer drugs, and corticosteroids; digestive disorders; or excessive sugar consumption.

Although a complete candidiasis treatment program is beyond the scope of this book, the following guidelines will give you an excellent start in getting the yeast under control. I suffered with candidiasis for a number of years, and I know firsthand that dietary change is a key to recovery.

Diet Recommendations

❥ **Follow the Anti-Candida Diet.** Avoid all sugars—natural, refined, and artificial. This also includes *all* fruit or fruit juice—yeasts love sugars! Avoid all foods that contain yeast or mold, such as raised breads and other raised flour products, cheese, vinegar, olives, peanuts, alcohol, dried fruit, and melons. Don't eat leftovers; they are much more susceptible to mold growth. Choose only organically grown meats and poultry because of the heavy use of antibiotics in the agriculture industry. High-carbohydrate vegetables and grains should be consumed in moderation, no more than one cup per day. This category includes potatoes, yams, corn, winter squash, lentils, peas, millet, rice, and barley. Avoid milk and its products, with the exception of a small amount of butter and a small portion of plain organic yogurt (no more than one-half cup per day). Milk sugars, like other sugars, promote yeast growth. You can generously eat and juice all vegetables, except those specified above, and sprouts; wash the vegetables in biodegradable soap and water. You can also include fish, organically grown lean meat and poultry, seeds, nuts, and nut butters (except peanut butter) in your diet.

❥ **Drink plenty of water.** Increasing your intake of pure water can help your body flush out the toxins released from the yeast. And as the yeasts die off, they need to be removed or you'll feel worse. Adding a teaspoon of fresh lemon juice to each glass of water will help facilitate the cleansing process.

❥ **Increase the use of certain culinary herbs and spices.** Use the following herbs and spices more often in your cooking: anise, cinnamon, fennel, garlic, ginger, lemon balm, licorice, rosemary, and thyme. They have powerful antifungal and antibacterial properties because of their essential oil content. Garlic has been shown to be more active against *C. albicans* than the popular drug nystatin, a common antifungal agent. Cooking can destroy garlic's antifungal compound, allicin, so use garlic fresh in salad dressings, on salads, and in juices.

❥ **Cleanse the liver.** Acetaldehyde, the alcohol produced by *C. albicans*, can cause a person to feel constantly "hung over." The acetaldehyde puts a strain directly on the liver, which must continually detoxify the alcohol. When the liver becomes overloaded, it cannot filter blood properly. The problem is then magnified as the Candida is killed, since this process can release toxins into the bloodstream. Cleansing and supporting the liver is a vital part of Candida treatment; see the Liver Cleanse (page 333). Also, short *vegetable*-juice fasts (no fruit juice!) of one to three days can be quite helpful; see the Juice Fast (page 324).

Nutrient Recommendations

❥ **Caprylic acid,** derived from coconuts, appears to play an important role in combating *C. albicans*. This fatty acid apparently coats the gastrointestinal tract and starves the yeast cells. Caprylic acid is easily absorbed in the intestines. Therefore, it is necessary to take a time-released or enterically coated supplement to get a gradual release along the entire gastrointestinal tract.

❥ **Copper** helps macrophages, white blood cells that get rid of foreign particles, to digest and destroy *C. albicans*. Studies have shown that when there is a copper deficiency, fewer Candida cells are destroyed, and immune-system functions are impaired. Best juice sources of copper (in order of effectiveness): carrots, garlic, ginger root, and turnips.

❥ **Magnesium** plays a role in reestablishing a strong immune system in people who have candidiasis. Best juice sources of magnesium (in order of effectiveness): beet greens, spinach, parsley, dandelion greens, garlic, beets, broccoli, cauliflower, carrots, and celery.

❥ **Selenium** is essential for a healthy immune system. Tests have shown that a selenium deficiency significantly impairs the ability of white blood cells to kill *C. albicans*. Best juice sources of selenium (in order of effectiveness): chard, turnips, garlic, radishes, carrots, and cabbage.

❥ **Vitamin B$_1$ (thiamine)** has been shown to increase the ability of leukocytes, white blood cells that fight infection and tissue damage, to destroy *C. albicans*. Also, vitamin B$_1$ is believed to help combat acetaldehyde production. Best food sources of vitamin B_1 (in order of effectiveness): seeds, nuts, beans, split peas, millet, buckwheat, whole wheat, oatmeal, wild rice, lobster, and cornmeal. It can also be found, in lesser quantities, in sunflower and buckwheat sprouts, and garlic. It is not found in fruits and vegetables.

❥ **Zinc** deficiency is thought to play a role in recurring vaginal candidiasis. Zinc is important to a healthy immune system, and helps detoxify metabolic wastes. Best juice sources of zinc (in order of effectiveness): ginger root, turnips, parsley, garlic, carrots, spinach, cabbage, lettuce, and cucumbers.

Herb Recommendations

❥ **Barberry, goldenseal,** and **Oregon grape** all contain a powerful microbial factor called berberine that is especially effective against *C. albicans*. Do not use any of these herbs if you are pregnant, and do not use them for more than ten days at a time.

❥ **Black walnut** can help eliminate both Candida and parasites, such as worms, commonly found in people who have candidiasis.

❥ **Chamomile** contains compounds that kill Candida. Traditionally, it is used for diarrhea, indigestion, and colic, all common candidiasis symptoms. Be sure to use German chamomile, *Matricaria recutita*, and not Roman chamomile, *Chamaemelum nobile*.

❥ **Pau d' arco,** a Brazilian tree bark, helps eliminate Candida.

Juice Ingredient Recommendations

❥ **Cranberry** juice is commonly used in alleviating bacterial bladder and other urinary tract infections (*see* **Bladder Infections**). Symptoms associated with bladder infection, such as urinary urgency and pain on urination, can be found in people who have candidiasis. If you wish, you can use unsweetened cranberry concentrate (available at most health food stores) and use $1/2$ teaspoon in place of the cranberries in Cranberry-Apple Cocktail.

❥ **Garlic** juice is a potent antifungal agent.

❥ **Parsley** juice is a good source of zinc. Intake should be limited to a safe, therapeutic dose of $1/2$ to 1 cup per day. Parsley can be toxic in overdose, and should be especially avoided by pregnant women.

Juice Recipes

CRANBERRY-APPLE COCKTAIL

2 organic Granny Smith or Pippin apples, washed

¼ cup fresh or frozen (thawed) cranberries, rinsed

¼ small or medium lemon, washed, or peeled if not organic

½ cup water

Cut the apples into sections that will fit your juicer's feed tube. Juice the apples with the cranberries and lemon. (To keep the cranberries from flying out of the machine, place the cranberries in the juicer first, place an apple section on top of them, and cover with the plunger. Turn on the machine, and push the plunger to begin the juicing process.) Stir the juice, and pour into a glass with the water. Serve at room temperature or chilled, as desired.

ANTIVIRAL COCKTAIL

1 organic Granny Smith or Pippin apple, washed

1 turnip, scrubbed well

1 handful watercress, rinsed

5 carrots, scrubbed well, green tops removed, ends trimmed

1 large garlic clove with peel, washed

Cut the apple and turnip into sections that fit your juicer's feed tube. Bunch up the watercress, and juice it with the apple, turnip, carrots, and garlic. Stir the juice, and pour into a glass. Serve at room temperature or chilled, as desired.

PURE GREEN SPROUT DRINK

1 organic cucumber, scrubbed well

1 large handful sunflower sprouts, rinsed

1 small handful buckwheat sprouts, rinsed

1 small handful clover sprouts, rinsed

Cut the cucumber in half lengthwise. Bunch up the sprouts, and push through the feed tube with the cucumber. Stir the juice, and pour into a glass. Serve at room temperature or chilled, as desired.

GINGER TWIST

1 handful parsley, rinsed

5 carrots, scrubbed well, green tops removed, ends trimmed

1-inch piece fresh ginger root, washed

½ small or medium lemon, washed, or peeled if not organic

Bunch up the parsley and push it through the feed tube with the carrots, ginger, and lemon. Stir the juice, and pour into a glass. Serve at room temperature or chilled, as desired.

MAGNESIUM SPECIAL

5 medium carrots, scrubbed well, green tops removed, ends trimmed

2 stalks organic celery with leaves, washed

½ small beet with leaves and stems, scrubbed well

2 broccoli florets, washed

½ small or medium lemon, washed, or peeled if not organic

Juice the carrots, celery, beet, broccoli, and lemon. Stir the juice, and pour into a glass. Serve at room temperature or chilled, as desired.

POPEYE'S POWER

1 handful organic spinach, washed

1 small handful parsley, rinsed

5 medium carrots, scrubbed well, green tops removed, ends trimmed

1 stalk organic celery with leaves, washed

½ beet with leaves, scrubbed well

Bunch up the spinach and parsley, and push them through the feed tube with the carrots, celery, and beet. Stir the juice, and pour into a glass. Serve at room temperature or chilled, as desired.

THYROID TONIC

5 carrots, scrubbed well, green tops removed, ends trimmed

5–6 radishes with green tops, washed

½ small or medium lemon, washed, or peeled if not organic

Juice the carrots, radishes, and lemon. Stir the juice, and pour into a glass. Serve at room temperature or chilled, as desired.

TRIPLE C

¼ small head green cabbage, washed

4 carrots, scrubbed well, green tops removed, and ends trimmed

4 stalks organic celery with leaves, washed

Cut the cabbage into sections that fit your juicer's feed tube. Juice the cabbage along with the carrots and celery. Stir the juice, and pour into a glass. Serve at room temperature or chilled, as desired.

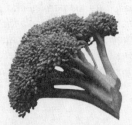
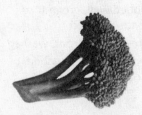

AFTERNOON REFRESHER

1 medium to large organic cucumber, scrubbed well

½ small or medium lemon, washed, or peeled if not organic

Cut the cucumber in half lengthwise, and juice with the lemon. (For an especially cooling version, let the juice splash over a few ice cubes in the juice pitcher.) Stir the juice, and pour into a glass. Serve at room temperature or chilled, as desired.

JACK & THE BEAN

1 large vine-ripened tomato, washed

2 romaine lettuce leaves, washed

8 organic string beans, washed

3 Brussels sprouts, washed

½ small or medium lemon, washed, or peeled if not organic

Cut the tomato into sections that fit your juicer's feed tube. Bunch up the lettuce leaves, and push through the feed tube with the tomato, string beans, Brussels sprouts, and lemon. Stir the juice, and pour into a glass. Serve at room temperature or chilled, as desired.

Canker Sores

Mouth sores, known as canker sores, are small ulcers that can appear on the lips, gums, tongue, or insides of the cheeks. They are surrounded by a reddened border and covered with a white or yellowish membrane, and range in size from a pinhead to a quarter. A burning sensation may precede their development. Canker sores are very painful, and can be single or clustered. They are quite common.

Canker sores can persist for from a few days to nearly two weeks, and larger sores may cause scarring. Possible causes include stress (*see* **Stress**), candidiasis (*see* **Candidiasis**), food sensitivities or allergies, poor dental hygiene, trauma caused by vigorous toothbrushing or by biting the inside of the cheek, or nutrient deficiencies.

Diet Recommendations

❥ **Identify food allergies and sensitivities.** Reactions to offending foods can cause canker sores. Some of the most common offenders are wheat products, dairy products, citrus fruits and juices, and sugars found in such sweets as cakes, pies, cookies, candy, soft drinks, muffins, and gum. (*See* **Allergies;** also see the Elimination Diet, page 321.)

❥ **Eat fewer animal products, and drink less coffee.** Animal proteins and coffee produce excess acid in the body, which contributes to the development of canker sores.

Nutrient Recommendations

❥ **Beta-carotene** helps promote faster healing of the mucous membranes. Best juice sources of carotenes in general (in order of effectiveness): carrots, kale, parsley, spinach, chard, beet greens, watercress, mangoes, cantaloupes, apricots, broccoli, and romaine lettuce.

❥ **Folic acid** deficiencies can cause canker sores to develop. Best juice sources of folic acid (in order of effectiveness): asparagus, spinach, kale, broccoli, cabbage, and blackberries.

❥ **Iron** deficiencies can cause canker sores. Best juice sources of nonheme iron, the type found in plants (in order of effectiveness): parsley, dandelion greens, broccoli, cauliflower, strawberries, asparagus, chard, blackberries, cabbage, beets with greens, carrots, and pineapple.

❥ **Vitamin B$_{12}$ (cobalamin)** deficiencies can cause canker sores. This vitamin is not available in fruit or vegetable juices. The best food sources of vitamin B$_{12}$ are meat, poultry, and fish; it is also available in some fermented soy-based foods, such as tofu and tempeh.

❥ **Zinc** can be beneficial if there is a zinc deficiency. Best juice sources of zinc (in order of effectiveness): ginger root, turnips, parsley, garlic, carrots, grapes, spinach, cabbage, lettuce, cucumbers, and tangerines.

Herb Recommendations

❥ **Common stonecrop** and **water dock** are used to treat mouth ulcers.

Juice Ingredient Recommendations

❥ **Cabbage** juice has been shown to heal peptic ulcers. It may also be helpful for mouth ulcers.

❥ **Parsley** juice is rich in beta-carotene, iron, and zinc. Intake should be limited to a safe, therapeutic dose of $1/2$ to 1 cup per day. Parsley can be toxic in overdose, and should be especially avoided by pregnant women.

Juice Recipes

TRIPLE C

¼ small head green cabbage, washed

4 carrots, scrubbed well, green tops removed, and ends trimmed

4 stalks organic celery with leaves, washed

Cut the cabbage into sections that fit your juicer's feed tube. Juice the cabbage along with the carrots and celery. Stir the juice, and pour into a glass. Serve at room temperature or chilled, as desired.

THE GINGER HOPPER

½ organic Red or Golden Delicious apple, washed

5 medium carrots, scrubbed well, green tops removed, ends trimmed

½- to 1-inch piece fresh ginger root, washed

Cut the apple into sections, and juice along with the carrots and ginger. Stir the juice, and pour into a glass. Serve at room temperature or chilled, as desired.

POPEYE'S POWER

½ medium organic apple, any kind, washed

1 handful organic spinach, washed

1 small handful parsley, rinsed

4 medium carrots, scrubbed well, green tops removed, ends trimmed

1 stalk organic celery with leaves, washed

½ beet with leaves, scrubbed well

Cut the apple into sections that will fit your juicer's feed tube. Bunch up the spinach and parsley, and push them through the feed tube with the apple, carrots, celery, and beet. Stir the juice, and pour into a glass. Serve at room temperature or chilled, as desired.

BEAUTIFUL BONE SOLUTION

1 organic Golden or Red Delicious apple, washed

1–2 kale leaves, washed

1 handful parsley, rinsed

1 stalk organic celery, washed

¼ small or medium lemon, washed, or peeled if not organic

½- to 1-inch piece fresh ginger root, washed

Cut the apple into sections that fit your juicer's feed tube. Bunch up the kale and parsley, and push through the feed tube with the apple, celery, lemon, and ginger. Stir the juice, and pour into a glass. Serve at room temperature or chilled, as desired.

WEIGHT-LOSS BUDDY

1 small Jerusalem artichoke, scrubbed well

4–5 carrots, scrubbed well, green tops removed, ends trimmed

½ small beet with no stems and leaves, scrubbed well

Cut the Jerusalem artichoke into sections that fit your juicer's feed tube. Juice the artichoke along with the carrots and beet. Stir the juice, and pour into a glass. Serve at room temperature or chilled, as desired.

SWEET DREAMS NIGHTCAP

2 romaine lettuce leaves, washed

1 handful parsley, rinsed

4 carrots, scrubbed well, green tops removed, ends trimmed

3 organic celery stalks with leaves, washed

Bunch up the lettuce leaves and parsley, and push through the feed tube with the carrots and celery. Stir the juice, and pour into a glass. Serve at room temperature or chilled, as desired.

Cardiovascular Disease

Cardiovascular disease is a general term for diseases that affect the heart and blood vessels. Vascular disease, commonly called atherosclerosis, is the leading cause of mortality in the United States and in most industrialized countries. In atherosclerosis, fatty plaques build up in the arterial walls and gradually decrease blood flow to the organs such as the heart. Plaque buildup can weaken the vessel wall, causing a rupture, or plaque can break off from the wall to create a blood-vessel obstruction called an embolism. Symptoms can include angina, a squeezing chest pain caused by reduced blood flow to the heart; leg cramps; gradual mental deterioration; weakness; and/or dizziness. Atherosclerosis is also associated with myocardial infarction (heart attack), stroke, and congestive heart failure, which is an inability of the heart to pump blood fast enough to fully meet the body's needs.

The most current theory about how plaque forms is that it follows an injury to the blood-vessel wall. Cholesterol, in the form of low-density lipoproteins (LDLs, the "bad fats"), gathers at the injury site. There, it is oxidized, a process similar to butter going rancid. This process is caused by unstable molecules called free radicals, which can act as toxins within the body.

The major risk factors for atherosclerosis are high blood pressure; elevated LDL levels, especially in relation to levels of high-density lipoproteins (HDLs, the "good fats"); cigarette smoking; diabetes mellitus (*see* **Diabetes Mellitus**); and family history. Men are more often affected than women, and postmenopausal women more than premenopausal women.

In 1990, Dr. Dean Ornish reported from his studies with patients that comprehensive lifestyle changes—such as eating a low-fat vegetarian diet, stopping smoking, practicing stress management, and getting moderate exercise—could regress even severe coronary atherosclerosis. Today, many studies support his claims. Maintaining low LDL levels, for example, can reduce the chances of plaque buildup. Recent findings also indicate that is important to lower levels of homocysteine, a protein byproduct, in the blood. If you follow the recommendations noted in this entry, you should greatly reduce your risk of cardiovascular disease, or strengthen a treatment program for an existing problem.

Lifestyle Recommendations

❥ **If you smoke, stop.** Smoking not only makes the heart work harder, it also promotes the development of artery-clogging plaques (*see* **Cravings**).

❥ **Reduce your stress levels.** Stress causes unhealthy changes in hormone balance that can lead to plaque formation. There are many methods you can use to reduce your stress levels, including meditation, deep breathing, and various kinds of exercises (*see* **Stress**).

❥ **Get more exercise.** Exercise not only tones your heart, it can help you maintain a healthy weight level—another factor in heart disease—and reduce stress.

Diet Recommendations

❥ **Eat a low-fat, high-complex carbohydrate diet.** Fifty percent of your diet should consist of raw fruits, vegetables, sprouts, juices, seeds, and nuts. Studies from all over the world have shown a low incidence of heart disease in places where people eat primarily a high-fiber, low-fat, plant-based diet. This type of diet has been shown to reduce blood cholesterol and LDL levels, and overall reduce the risk of cardiovascular disease. For more information, see Basic Guidelines for the Juice Lady's Health and Healing Diet (page 313).

❥ **Increase your intake of fresh vegetable and fruit juices.** Juices are rich in soluble fiber, such as the pectins found in abundance in apple and pear juice. Soluble fiber has been shown to lower cholesterol and LDL levels. (Oat bran and psyllium seed husk also offer beneficial soluble fiber.) One of the richest sources of pectin is citrus peel, so juice lemons and limes with the peel (organic is best). Do *not* juice orange, grapefruit, and tangerine peels; they contain bitter oils that can cause digestive upset. A one- to three-day juice fast can be very beneficial. See the Juice Fast, page 324.

❥ **Eat more fish.** Fish has been associated with a reduced cardiovascular risk. The best kind are those taken from cold waters—such as salmon, halibut, tuna, cod, trout, and mackerel—as these fish contain relatively large amounts of omega-3 fatty acids. Omega-3s have been shown to decrease platelet clumping, thus preventing the formation of vessel-clogging clots and reducing the formation of atherosclerotic plaques. Studies show that when red meat is replaced by fish in the diet, the composition of fatty acids in the blood changes for the better. Omega-3 fatty acids are also found in flaxseed and hemp oils, which makes these oils an excellent dietary supplement. My recommendation is to supplement your diet with one to two tablespoons of flaxseed or hemp oil per day. For more information, see the fats and oils section in Basic Guidelines for the Juice Lady's Health and Healing Diet (page 313).

❥ **Reduce your consumption of saturated fats.** Saturated fats raise total cholesterol levels and should be avoided. They are found in meats, cheeses, butter, margarine, vegetable shortening, and coconut and palm oil. Cut out all oxidized fats, such as those found in fried and barbecued food. Substitute soy protein, found in tofu, tempeh, soy milk, and miso, for animal protein and fat. Soy protein has been shown to decrease total cholesterol levels and increase the ratio of HDLs to LDLs in the blood.

❥ **Avoid margarine and hydrogenated vegetable oils.** Margarine is made through a process called partial hydrogenation, which produces substances called *trans*-fatty acids. These fatty acids contribute to the development of coronary heart disease and the risk of heart attack. *Trans*-fats in the diet are associated with elevated cholesterol and LDL levels, and with lower HDL levels. When purchasing oils, choose only unrefined, expeller-pressed, or cold-pressed vegetable oils.

❥ **Reduce your salt intake.** Excessive salt intake is a common cause of high blood pressure, particularly in salt-sensitive individuals. Though salt restriction is an effective means of decreasing blood pressure, combining salt restriction with a high-potassium diet of fruits and vegetables will further enhance pressure reduction (*see* **High Blood Pressure**).

❥ **Limit coffee consumption.** Heavy consumption of coffee—more than five cups per day—increases the risk of heart attack in women. Drinking green tea is associated with decreased cholesterol and triglyceride levels, and with increased HDL levels.

❥ **Reduce beer consumption.** One study showed that consumption of high-alcohol (versus low-alcohol) beer results in increased LDL levels.

Nutrient Recommendations

❥ **Antioxidants** reduce the oxidation of fats and decrease the ability of platelets to clump together. Increasing intake of the following antioxidant nutrients has been shown to reduce the risk of premature death from coronary artery disease:

- *Beta-carotene* and *vitamin A* are important for good cardiovascular health. Consumption of foods rich in beta-carotene is associated with a lowered risk of nonfatal heart attacks in women, and this nutrient has reduced cardiovascular disease risk among high-risk men. Beta-carotene, or provitamin A, is the only form of vitamin A found in fruits and vegetables, and is converted by the body to vitamin A as needed. Best juice sources of carotenes in general (in order of effectiveness): carrots, kale, parsley, spinach, chard, beet greens, watercress, mangoes, cantaloupes, apricots, broccoli, and romaine lettuce.

- *Selenium* helps prevent the oxidation of LDL. Best juice sources of selenium (in order of effectiveness): chard, turnips, garlic, oranges, radishes, grapes, carrots, and cabbage.

- *Vitamin C* is involved in breaking down blood triglycerides, a type of fat. It activates enzymes that convert cholesterol into bile acids, which reduces blood cholesterol levels. And it is an important cofactor in the formation of collagen, which strengthens blood-vessel walls. Best juice sources of vitamin C (in order of effectiveness): kale, parsley, broccoli, Brussels sprouts, watercress, cauliflower, cabbage, strawberries, papaya, spinach, citrus fruit, turnips, mangoes, asparagus, and cantaloupes.

- *Vitamin E* has been shown in studies to reduce heart attack risk by decreasing LDL levels. It is also involved in the growth and repair of the inner lining of arterial walls. Best juice sources of vitamin E (in order of effectiveness): spinach, watercress, asparagus, carrots, and tomatoes.

❥ **Coenzyme Q_{10}** is a substance made in the body that inhibits fat oxidation. It also improves the heart's energy production, and has been used supplementally with great success in cases of congestive heart failure. The best food sources are mackerel, salmon, and sardines; it is not available in fruits and vegetables.

❥ **Folic acid** is responsible for converting homocysteine into a nontoxic substance called methionine. A Canadian study showed that low blood levels of folic acid were associated with an increased risk of fatal coronary heart disease. Best juice sources of folic acid (in order of effectiveness): asparagus, spinach, kale, broccoli, cabbage, and blackberries.

❥ **Magnesium** has been shown to be beneficial for congestive heart failure, arrhythmias, and other heart problems. Best juice sources of magnesium (in order of effectiveness): beet greens, spinach, parsley, dandelion greens, garlic, blackberries, beets, broccoli, cauliflower, carrots, and celery.

Herb Recommendations

❥ **Hawthorn** has been used traditionally as a heart tonic. This herb is rich in bioflavonoids, which increase the amount of vitamin C (see Nutrient Recommendations) in the fluid that nourishes the body's cells. These substances also reduce blood pressure and cholesterol levels, and prevent cholesterol from building up in arterial walls. Hawthorn helps improve blood supply to the heart by dilating the coronary blood vessels.

Juice Ingredient Recommendations

❥ **Apple** and **pear** juices contain fiber-rich pectins.

❥ **Berry** juices, along with cherry juice, are rich in bioflavonoids.

❥ **Carrot** juice has factors that can reduce cholesterol levels and increase excretion of fat by way of the stool.

❥ **Garlic** juice contains substances that can help delay stiffening of the aorta, the body's main artery. Garlic can also help other arteries to remain elastic, and has been shown to decrease cholesterol and triglyceride levels.

❥ **Ginger** has been shown to lower cholesterol levels.

❥ **Parsley** juice is rich in bioflavonoids, magnesium, and vitamin C. Intake should be limited to a safe, therapeutic dose of $1/2$ to 1 cup per day. Parsley can be toxic in overdose, and should be especially avoided by pregnant women.

🌶 **Pineapple** juice contains bromelain, an enzyme that inhibits platelet clumping.

Juice Recipes

SWEET & REGULAR

1 pear, washed
1 organic apple, any kind, washed

Cut the pear and apple into sections that fit your juicer's feed tube, and juice them. Stir the juice, and pour into a glass. Serve at room temperature or chilled, as desired.

DIGESTIVE TONIC

1/2 pear, washed
1/2 organic apple, any kind, washed
5 carrots, scrubbed well, green tops removed, ends trimmed

Cut the pear and apple into sections that fit your juicer's feed tube. Juice them with the carrots. Stir the juice, and pour into a glass. Serve at room temperature or chilled, as desired.

ANTIAGING COCKTAIL

1 small bunch organic purple grapes (about 1 cup) with small stems* and seeds, washed
1/2 cup blueberries, blackberries, or raspberries, washed
1/4 small or medium lemon, washed, or peeled if not organic
1/2-inch piece fresh ginger root, washed

Juice the grapes, berries, lemon, and ginger. Stir the juice, and pour into a glass. Serve at room temperature or chilled, as desired.

*Large stems can dull your juicer's blade.

THE GINGER HOPPER

1/2 organic Red or Golden Delicious apple, washed
5 medium carrots, scrubbed well, green tops removed, ends trimmed
1/2- to 1-inch piece fresh ginger root, washed

Cut the apple into sections, and juice along with the carrots and ginger. Stir the juice, and pour into a glass. Serve at room temperature or chilled, as desired.

THE IMMUNE BUILDER

1 organic Golden or Red Delicious
  apple, washed

1 turnip, scrubbed well

1 handful watercress, rinsed
  (optional)

5 carrots, scrubbed well, green tops
  removed, ends trimmed

1 large garlic clove with peel, washed

Cut the apple and turnip into sections that fit your juicer's feed tube. Bunch up the watercress (if using), and push it through the feed tube with the apple, turnip, carrots, and garlic. Stir the juice, and pour into a glass. Serve at room temperature or chilled, as desired.

GINGER TWIST

1 organic Red or Golden Delicious
  apple, washed

1 handful parsley, rinsed

4 carrots, scrubbed well, green tops
  removed, ends trimmed

1-inch piece fresh ginger root, washed

¼ small or medium lemon, washed,
  or peeled if not organic

Cut the apple into sections that fit your juicer's feed tube. Bunch up the parsley and push it through the feed tube with the apple, carrots, ginger, and lemon. Stir the juice, and pour into a glass. Serve at room temperature or chilled, as desired.

SNAPPY GINGER

1 medium orange, peeled

3-inch chunk fresh pineapple,
  scrubbed well or peeled if not
  organic

¼ small or medium lemon, washed,
  or peeled if not organic

1- to 2-inch piece fresh ginger root,
  washed

Divide the orange into segments, and cut the pineapple into strips that fit your juicer's feed tube. Juice the orange, pineapple, lemon, and ginger. Stir the juice, and pour into two glasses. Serve at room temperature or chilled, as desired.

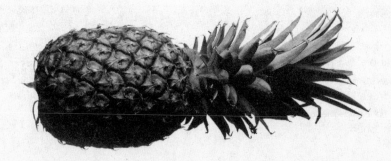

POPEYE'S POWER

½ medium organic apple, any kind, washed

1 handful organic spinach, washed

1 small handful parsley, rinsed

4 medium carrots, scrubbed well, green tops removed, ends trimmed

1 stalk organic celery with leaves, washed

½ beet with leaves, scrubbed well

Cut the apple into sections that will fit your juicer's feed tube. Bunch up the spinach and parsley, and push them through the feed tube with the apple, carrots, celery, and beet. Stir the juice, and pour into a glass. Serve at room temperature or chilled, as desired.

PARSLEY PEP

1 small bunch parsley, rinsed

2 stalks organic celery with leaves, washed

2 large carrots, scrubbed well, green tops removed, ends trimmed

½ small or medium lemon, washed, or peeled if not organic

Bunch up the parsley, and push it through the feed tube with the celery, carrots, and lemon. Stir the juice, and pour it into a glass. Serve at room temperature or chilled, as desired.

MORNING EXPRESS

1 orange, peeled

4–5 carrots, well scrubbed, green tops removed, ends trimmed

Divide the orange into segments that fit your juicer's feed tube, and juice with the carrots. Stir the juice, and pour into a glass. Serve at room temperature or chilled, as desired.

BEAUTIFUL BONE SOLUTION

1 organic Golden or Red Delicious apple, washed

1–2 kale leaves, washed

1 handful parsley, rinsed

1 stalk organic celery, washed

¼ small or medium lemon, washed, or peeled if not organic

½- to 1-inch piece fresh ginger root, washed

Cut the apple into sections that fit your juicer's feed tube. Bunch up the kale and parsley, and push through the feed tube with the apple, celery, lemon, and ginger. Stir the juice, and pour into a glass. Serve at room temperature or chilled, as desired.

TOMATO FLORENTINE

1 vine-ripened tomato, washed

1 handful organic spinach, washed

2–3 fresh basil leaves (optional)

1/2 small or medium lemon, washed, or peeled if not organic

Cut the tomato into sections that will fit your juicer's feed tube. Bunch up the spinach and basil leaves (if using), and push through the feed tube with the tomato and lemon. Stir the juice, and pour into a glass. Serve at room temperature or chilled, as desired.

ORANGE VELVET

1/2 small jicama, scrubbed well or peeled if not organic

1 orange, peeled

1/4 lime, washed or peeled if not organic

Cut the jicama into sections, and divide the orange into segments, that fit your juicer's feed tube. Juice the jicama and orange along with the lime. Stir the juice, and pour into a glass. Serve at room temperature or chilled, as desired.

SWEET CALCIUM COCKTAIL

1 three-inch chunk fresh pineapple, scrubbed well or peeled if not organic

1–2 kale leaves, washed

Cut the pineapple into strips that fit your juicer's feed tube. Bunch up the kale, and push through the feed tube with the pineapple. Stir the juice, and pour into a glass. Serve at room temperature or chilled, as desired.

MAGNESIUM SPECIAL

5 medium carrots, scrubbed well, green tops removed, ends trimmed

2 stalks organic celery with leaves, washed

1/2 small beet with leaves and stems, scrubbed well

2 broccoli florets, washed

1/2 small or medium lemon, washed, or peeled if not organic

Juice the carrots, celery, beet, broccoli, and lemon. Stir the juice, and pour into a glass. Serve at room temperature or chilled, as desired.

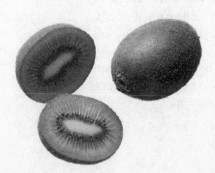

Carpal Tunnel Syndrome

Carpal tunnel syndrome (CTS) is a nerve disorder of the arm and hand. The median nerve in the arm passes through the carpal tunnel, a narrow bony passage in the wrist that also contains tendons and ligaments. CTS occurs when this nerve becomes compressed or damaged. Common CTS symptoms include soreness, tenderness, and weakness of the thumb muscles, and/or aching, numbness, tingling, and burning in the fingers. Pain and tingling may extend up the forearm and into the shoulder. Symptoms often worsen with repetitive motion and at night. Women are three to six times more likely to have CTS than men, and most people who develop this disorder are between the ages of forty and sixty.

CTS can result from a variety of causes, including wrist injury, hormone imbalances, rheumatoid arthritis (*see* **Rheumatoid Arthritis**), systemic diseases, tumors, blood-vessel changes, nutritional deficiencies, and hyperthyroidism (overactive thyroid). Repetitive activities—such as those used in typing, massage, carpentry, warehouse work (and other jobs that require lifting and carrying), or jackhammer use—may result in irritation of the nerve and/or tendons. With the rise in computer use at work, the incidence of occupationally related CTS (OCTS) is also on the rise. Healing becomes difficult if prolonged or continuous irritation occurs. Dietary and lifestyle changes can help ease CTS considerably.

Lifestyle Recommendations

❥ **Avoid taking birth control pills.** It has been found that the use of birth control pills is associated with an increased risk of developing CTS, and that they deplete the body's stores of vitamin B_6, a nutrient that is vitally important in fighting this condition (see the Nutrient Recommendations).

❥ **Wear a wrist splint (or splints) at night, at least during the acute phase.** These splints, available in any pharmacy, contain a metal insert that keeps the wrists bent, palm out, while you sleep. This position takes stress off the affected tendons, which reduces the chance that you will wake up with numb, painful hands.

Diet Recommendations

❥ **Eat more oats.** Oats help nourish nerve tissue. They can be added to juice (after soaking—see the package directions), or can be eaten as a muesli, a breakfast made with uncooked oats soaked in juice, milk, or soy milk along with nuts and dried fruit. Wheat germ can provide extra vitamin B_6. I include a muesli recipe in my cookbook, *The Healthy Gourmet* (see Appendix A).

❦ **Avoid eating excess protein.** The body needs vitamin B_6 to properly break down proteins. If there is a B_6 deficiency, proteins can break down into toxic substances.

❦ **Avoid all foods that contain yellow dyes.** Such dyes are vitamin B_6-depleting substances.

Nutrient Recommendations

❦ **Vitamin B_2 (riboflavin)** converts vitamin B_6 into an active form. Best juice sources of vitamin B_2 (in order of effectiveness): collard greens, kale, parsley, broccoli, beet greens, and prunes.

❦ **Vitamin B_6 (pyridoxine)** deficiency has been found to be a factor that contributes to CTS. (This may explain the increased incidence of CTS during pregnancy, a time of increased nutrient demands.) As you can see from the lifestyle and diet recommendations, the environment is full of substances that can deplete the body's B_6 stores. Studies show that supplementing the diet with extra vitamin B_6 increases pain thresholds and reduces swelling associated with CTS. Improvement is usually noted within a few weeks to three months. Dosages of between 50 and 300 mg a day are needed, which far exceeds the Recommended Daily Allowance (RDA) of 2 to 2.5 mg. Therefore, you should take this vitamin in supplement form, at least until the CTS is under control, and supplement with B_6-rich juices for maintenance. Best juice sources of vitamin B_6 (in order of effectiveness): kale, spinach, turnip greens, bell peppers, and prunes.

❦ **Vitamin C** supports connective-tissue health. Best juice sources of vitamin C (in order of effectiveness): kale, parsley, broccoli, Brussels sprouts, watercress, cauliflower, cabbage, strawberries, papaya, spinach, citrus fruit, turnips, mangoes, asparagus, and cantaloupes.

Herb Recommendations

❦ **Willow bark** oil, applied externally, decreases inflammation and eases pain.

Juice Ingredient Recommendations

❦ **Ginger** juice has anti-inflammatory properties. It is delicious when juiced with fruits or vegetables.

❥ Parsley juice is rich in vitamins B_6 and C. Intake should be limited to a safe, therapeutic dose of $1/2$ to 1 cup per day. Parsley can be toxic in overdose, and should be especially avoided by pregnant women.

❥ Pineapple juice contains bromelain, an enzyme that helps decrease inflammation and relax smooth muscle.

Juice Recipes

SNAPPY GINGER

1 medium orange, peeled
3-inch chunk fresh pineapple, scrubbed well or peeled if not organic
1/4 small or medium lemon, washed, or peeled if not organic
1- to 2-inch piece fresh ginger root, washed

Divide the orange into segments, and cut the pineapple into strips that fit your juicer's feed tube. Juice the orange, pineapple, lemon, and ginger. Stir the juice, and pour into two glasses. Serve at room temperature or chilled, as desired.

SWEET CALCIUM COCKTAIL

1 three-inch chunk fresh pineapple, scrubbed well or peeled if not organic
1–2 kale leaves, washed

Cut the pineapple into strips that fit your juicer's feed tube. Bunch up the kale, and push through the feed tube with the pineapple. Stir the juice, and pour into a glass. Serve at room temperature or chilled, as desired.

BEAUTIFUL BONE SOLUTION

1 organic Golden or Red Delicious apple, washed
1–2 kale leaves, washed
1 handful parsley, rinsed
1 stalk organic celery, washed
1/4 small or medium lemon, washed, or peeled if not organic
1/2- to 1-inch piece fresh ginger root, washed

Cut the apple into sections that fit your juicer's feed tube. Bunch up the kale and parsley, and push through the feed tube with the apple, celery, lemon, and ginger. Stir the juice, and pour into a glass. Serve at room temperature or chilled, as desired.

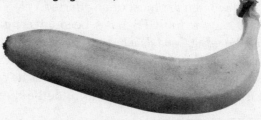

SWEET DREAMS NIGHTCAP

2 romaine lettuce leaves, washed

1 handful parsley, rinsed

4 carrots, scrubbed well, green tops removed, ends trimmed

3 organic celery stalks with leaves, washed

Bunch up the lettuce leaves and parsley, and push through the feed tube with the carrots and celery. Stir the juice, and pour into a glass. Serve at room temperature or chilled, as desired.

STRAWBERRY-CANTALOUPE COCKTAIL

½ ripe organic cantaloupe with seeds, washed (peeled if not organic)

1 cup organic strawberries, washed

Cut the cantaloupe into strips that fit your juicer's feed tube. Juice the cantaloupe and strawberries; stir the juice and pour into a glass. Serve at room temperature or chilled, as desired.

Cataracts

See **Eye Disorders.**

Chronic Fatigue Syndrome

Chronic fatigue syndrome (CFS) is an illness with a multitude of flulike symptoms, including extreme fatigue, recurring sore throat, tender lymph nodes, depression, headaches, muscle aches and soreness, loss of concentration and/or memory, and low-grade fever. Unexplained fatigue that lasts at least six months is the principal means of diagnosis, as currently there is no diagnostic test for CFS. Symptoms are often cyclical, lapsing and recurring. Young women are most often affected.

Many potential causes for CFS have been investigated, such as Epstein-Barr virus, the yeast *Candida albicans*, parasites, allergies, and various immunological disorders. Although many of these conditions are also present with CFS, none has been definitively proved as its cause.

A weakened immune system appears to underlie the symptoms of

CFS. A depleted, exhausted immune system is easy prey for a host of simultaneous infections. CFS can be seen as developing from a combination of nutritional deficiencies, toxicity, poor stress-coping abilities, and systemic infections, all of which lead to a vicious cycle of lowered immune function and more infections.

A multifaceted approach to healing CFS involves dietary changes (especially those that enhance vitamin and mineral intake), exercise, herbal therapies, nutritional supplements, infection treatment, and counseling on stress management in order to revitalize the immune system and restore biochemical balance. To recover, it takes commitment, persistence, faith that you will get well, and a willingness to do whatever it takes to heal. *On a personal note:* I often hear people say in the media that there is no hope for recovery from CFS. There is great hope. I know. In my twenties, and again in 1993, I suffered from such a severe case of CFS that I could not work—I could barely get out of bed. Now, I am well. (I share my recovery from CFS and my journey to health in the Introduction.)

Lifestyle Recommendations

❥ **Control any allergies you may have.** Allergies, whether seasonal-, food-, or drug-related, appear to be a common thread in individuals with CFS. If you have not already done so, have allergy tests performed to pinpoint any problem areas. (*See* **Allergies**; also see the Elimination Diet, page 321.)

❥ **Eliminate yeast, bacterial, and parasitic infections.** Much research is currently focused on the role that *Candida albicans* and other yeasts and parasites play in CFS. Though not the cause of this disorder, intestinal pathogens depress the immune system, making the body more susceptible to infections. *No* fruit or fruit juice is allowed if you have a systemic yeast infection (candidiasis) or parasites. (*See* **Candidiasis** and **Parasitic Infections.**)

Diet Recommendations

❥ **Detoxify your body through cleansing programs.** This is a vital first step toward building a healthy immune system. Toxins, both internal and external, must be reduced in order for the body's natural defenses to facilitate the recovery process. Reduce exposure to environmental chemicals from food, air, and water. Eliminate, as much as possible, drugs, dietary toxins, and allergenic foods. Colon cleansing is one of the keys to detoxification; toxins must be eliminated from the bowel, whether in the form of yeasts, parasites, heavy metals, or mucoid waste matter. In addition, the liver, gallbladder, and kidneys must all be detoxified and supported (see the Cleansing Programs chapter). Massage can be used to encourage draining of the lymphatic system.

❥ **Avoid sugar in all forms.** Sugar will *not* give you more energy—it will throw your blood-sugar levels out of balance and inhibit your immune system. Avoid all forms of processed sugar (white, brown, molasses, corn syrup), either as sweeteners or in processed foods, and avoid both honey and maple syrup. Fruit, which is high in sugar, should only be a small part of your diet—no more than one or two pieces a day. (Avoid fruit completely if you have candidiasis or parasites.) Avoid drinking fruit juices, with the exception of those made with lemon or lime, because of the concentration of fruit sugars.

❥ **Improve your immune function with whole, unprocessed foods.** Diet plays a central role in optimal immune function. Eat only whole, natural, unprocessed foods. "Living foods" provide the freshest, most potent nutrients to improve your energy level. Strive for a diet in which between 50 and 75 percent of your food consists of raw vegetables, vegetable juices, sprouts, nuts, and seeds. (I had to do this in order to get well, and I still do so to maintain my health.) The remainder of your diet should focus on complex carbohydrates, including whole grains such as oats, millet (high in protein), rye, buckwheat, and brown rice, and on legumes, such as beans, lentils, and split peas. You can have moderate amounts of protein—fish, chicken, and soy products such as tofu and tempeh. Minimize your intake of wheat; there's too much of it in the Western diet, and as a result many people are sensitive or allergic to it. As much as possible, your food should be organically grown.

❥ **Avoid stimulants and processed foods.** Avoid all stimulants, including alcohol, caffeine, and tobacco, along with all junk food, fast food, prepared foods, and anything with dyes, preservatives, or additives. These substances can weaken the immune system.

❥ **Drink more water.** Drink eight to ten 8-ounce glasses of clean, purified water each day. (You can benefit from a water purifier.) Adequate water intake is very beneficial to the immune system.

❥ **Use juice fasts to "jump-start" a recovery.** Fasting on vegetable juices for one to three days can give your immune system—indeed your entire body—a powerful boost. Juice fasting for short periods of time is probably the single most effective step you can take toward getting well. No one has been able to explain why drinking only fresh vegetable juices for several days works such a miracle, but "miracle" is the right word. Several studies have shown that the nutrients that occur in optimal proportions and quantities in fresh vegetable juices—along with uncooked vegetables and sprouts—boost production of T and B lymphocytes, key components in the immune response, and so increase resistance to illness. In addition, these juices and foods cleanse the spaces between cells. Waste matter can collect in these spaces when cellular metabolism is not functioning well, and become a breeding ground for bacteria and viruses. Poor cellular metabolism also contributes to fatigue. (See the Juice Fast, page 324.) *On a personal note:* Every year, I take a "health break" at the Optimum Health Institute (OHI) in San Diego for a week of raw foods combined with three days of juice fasting. I've been amazed at the number of CFS sufferers I have met there who have said that this program healed them. (See Appendix A for a list of health institutes that use this program.)

Nutrient Recommendations

❥ **B complex vitamins** are important to well-functioning nervous and immune systems. They provide energy to people who are stressed or fatigued. The best juice sources of B vitamins overall are green leafy vegetables. The best food sources, in addition to green vegetables, are whole grains (especially rye, oats, and brown rice), liver, poultry, fish, eggs, nuts, and beans. Folic acid, one of the B vitamins, has been found to be especially helpful to people with CFS. Best juice sources of folic acid (in order of effectiveness): asparagus, spinach, kale, broccoli, and cabbage.

❥ **Beta-carotene** stimulates the immune system and is converted by the body into vitamin A as needed. Both substances help fight infections. Best juice sources of carotenes in general (in order of effectiveness): carrots, kale, parsley, spinach, chard, beet greens, watercress, broccoli, and romaine lettuce.

❥ **Carnitine,** an amino acid, has been found in low levels in CFS patients. Carnitine plays an essential role in energy production. The best food sources of carnitine are avocado, fish, red meat, tempeh, and wheat. It is not found in most fruits and vegetables.

❥ **Magnesium** affects energy regulation within the body, and it is often found in low amounts in CFS sufferers. Best juice sources of magnesium (in order of effectiveness): beet greens, spinach, parsley, dandelion greens, garlic, beets, broccoli, cauliflower, carrots, and celery.

❥ **Vitamin C** enhances the ability of immune cells to destroy bacteria and viruses. It also increases production of lymphocytes, the cells that play a key role in cellular immunity. Best juice sources of vitamin C (in order of effectiveness): kale, parsley, broccoli, Brussels sprouts, watercress, cauliflower, cabbage, spinach, citrus fruit, turnips, and asparagus.

❥ **Zinc** offers strong support for the immune system and helps the body fight viral infections. Best juice sources of zinc (in order of effectiveness): ginger root, turnips, parsley, garlic, carrots, spinach, cabbage, lettuce, and cucumbers.

Herb Recommendations

❥ **Astragalus** bolsters resistance to disease. Avoid astragalus if you have a fever.

❥ **Echinacea** fights viral infections.

❥ **Goldenseal** supports the liver. Avoid this herb if you are pregnant, and do not use it for more than ten days at a time.

❥ **Licorice root** and **borage** both stimulate the adrenal glands. Avoid licorice if you have high blood pressure, do not use it for prolonged periods of time, and use a medicinal form of the herb, not licorice candy.

❥ **Oat straw** is useful for nervous exhaustion and low fevers.

❥ **Osha root** fights viral infections.

❥ **Siberian ginseng** is used to reduce the effects of physical or mental stress, especially exhaustion and depression. Be sure to use *Eleutherococcus senticosus*, Siberian ginseng, and not *Panax ginseng*, Korean or red ginseng. Avoid this herb if you have an autoimmune disease such as rheumatoid arthritis.

Juice Ingredient Recommendations

❥ **Beet, carrot,** and **cucumber** juices (especially beet juice) help cleanse the liver and gallbladder. Carrot juice is also helpful in treating fatigue.

❥ **Fennel** juice helps relieve CFS-associated depression because it contains compounds that help release endorphins, the "feel-good" chemicals in the brain.

❥ **Garlic** is a strongly antimicrobial herb—effective against bacteria, viruses, and parasites.

❥ **Spinach** and **carrot** juices, taken in combination, help with both blood-sugar regulation and liver cleansing.

❥ **Parsley** juice is a good source of beta-carotene, magnesium, vitamin C, and zinc. Intake should be limited to a safe, therapeutic dose of $1/2$ to 1 cup per day. Parsley can be toxic in overdose, and should be especially avoided by pregnant women.

❥ **Wheatgrass** juice is a powerful immune builder.

Juice Recipes

GALLBLADDER CLEANSING COCKTAIL

$1/2$ organic cucumber, scrubbed well

5 carrots, scrubbed well, green tops removed, ends trimmed

$1/2$ small to medium beet with leaves and stems, scrubbed well

$1/2$ small or medium lemon, washed, or peeled if not organic

Slice the cucumber in half again lengthwise, and juice with the carrots, beet, and lemon. Stir the juice, and pour into a glass. Serve at room temperature or chilled, as desired.

THE MORNING ENERGIZER

5 medium carrots, scrubbed well, green tops removed, ends trimmed

$1/2$ small beet with leaves and stems, scrubbed well

$1/2$ small or medium lemon, washed, or peeled if not organic

$1/2$- to 1-inch piece fresh ginger root, washed

Juice the carrots, beet, lemon, and ginger. Stir the juice, and pour into a glass. Serve at room temperature or chilled, as desired.

THE FEEL GOOD COCKTAIL

4 medium carrots, scrubbed well, green tops removed, ends trimmed

3 fennel stalks with leaves and flowers, washed

1 stalk organic celery with leaves, washed

$1/2$ small or medium lemon, washed, or peeled if not organic

Juice the carrots, fennel, celery, and lemon. Stir the juice, and pour into a glass. Serve at room temperature or chilled, as desired.

ANTIVIRAL COCKTAIL

1 organic **Granny Smith** or **Pippin** apple, washed

1 turnip, scrubbed well

1 handful watercress, rinsed

5 carrots, scrubbed well, green tops removed, ends trimmed

1 large garlic clove with peel, washed

Cut the apple and turnip into sections that fit your juicer's feed tube. Bunch up the watercress, and juice it with the apple, turnip, carrots, and garlic. Stir the juice, and pour into a glass. Serve at room temperature or chilled, as desired.

POPEYE'S POWER

½ medium organic **Granny Smith** or **Pippin** apple, washed

1 handful organic spinach, washed

1 small handful parsley, rinsed

4 medium carrots, scrubbed well, green tops removed, ends trimmed

1 stalk organic celery with leaves, washed

½ beet with leaves, scrubbed well

Cut the apple into sections that will fit your juicer's feed tube. Bunch up the spinach and parsley, and push them through the feed tube with the apple, carrots, celery, and beet. Stir the juice, and pour into a glass. Serve at room temperature or chilled, as desired.

WHEATGRASS LIGHT

1 organic **Granny Smith** or **Pippin** apple, washed

1 large handful wheatgrass, rinsed

2–3 sprigs mint, rinsed (optional)

½ small or medium lemon, washed, or peeled if not organic

Bunch up the wheatgrass and mint (if using) and push them through the feed tube with the lemon. Stir the juice, and pour into a glass. Serve at room temperature or chilled, as desired.

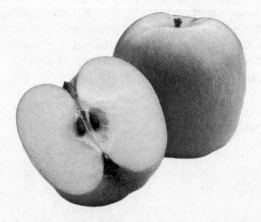

ALLERGY RELIEF

1 small bunch parsley, rinsed

2 stalks organic celery with leaves, washed

2–3 large carrots, scrubbed well, green tops removed, ends trimmed

1/4–1/2 small or medium lemon, washed, or peeled if not organic

Bunch up the parsley and push it through the feed tube with the celery, carrots, and lemon. Stir the juice, and pour it into a glass. Serve at room temperature or chilled, as desired.

SANTA FE SALSA COCKTAIL

1 medium vine-ripened tomato, washed

1/2 medium organic cucumber, scrubbed well

1/4 cup cilantro, rinsed

1/4 small or medium lime or lemon, washed, or peeled if not organic

Dash hot sauce (optional)

Cut the tomato into sections that fit your juicer's feed tube. Cut the cucumber in half again lengthwise. Bunch up the cilantro, and push through the feed tube with the tomato, cucumber, and lime or lemon. Pour the juice into a glass, add the hot sauce (if using), and stir. Serve at room temperature or chilled, as desired.

MEMORY MENDER

2 medium vine-ripened tomatoes, washed

1/4 small head iceberg lettuce, washed

4 cauliflower florets, washed

1/2 small or medium lemon, washed, or peeled if not organic

Cut the tomatoes and lettuce into sections that will fit your juicer's feed tube. Juice the tomatoes and lettuce along with the cauliflower and lemon. Pour into a glass and serve at room temperature or chilled, as desired.

MAGNESIUM SPECIAL

5 medium carrots, scrubbed well, green tops removed, ends trimmed

2 stalks organic celery with leaves, washed

1/2 small beet with leaves and stems, scrubbed well

2 broccoli florets, washed

1/2 small or medium lemon, washed, or peeled if not organic

Juice the carrots, celery, beet, broccoli, and lemon. Stir the juice, and pour into a glass. Serve at room temperature or chilled, as desired.

Sweet Dreams Nightcap

2 romaine lettuce leaves, washed

1 handful parsley, rinsed

4 carrots, scrubbed well, green tops removed, ends trimmed

3 organic celery stalks with leaves, washed

Bunch up the lettuce leaves and parsley, and push through the feed tube with the carrots and celery. Stir the juice, and pour into a glass. Serve at room temperature or chilled, as desired.

Colds

Colds are among the most common illnesses in the world. The common cold can be caused by a variety of viruses (called rhinoviruses) that infect the upper respiratory tract, which consists of the nasal passages, sinuses, and throat. Symptoms include general malaise, fever, sneezing, sore throat, headache, and congestion. Most colds last about a week, although a dry cough may linger afterwards.

The best thing you can do if you have a cold is to support your body's natural defense mechanisms, as opposed to suppressing the symptoms. Actually, the symptoms are a result of the body's attempts to heal itself. For example, the body releases a potent immune-stimulating compound known as interferon during infections, which is responsible for many of the symptoms. As you assist your body nutritionally, you can help it to heal.

While young children can get as many as eight colds a year, that frequency drops off dramatically in adults. By maintaining a healthy immune system, you can protect yourself from getting colds. If you catch more than one or two colds per year, it may be a sign that your immune system needs to be strengthened to prevent future colds.

Diet Recommendations

❥ **Drink plenty of fluids.** Put a special emphasis on drinking juices (primarily vegetable), herbal teas, and vegetable broths. Increasing fluid intake during an infection will prevent dehydration of the respiratory-tract membranes. When these membranes become dehydrated, virus growth accelerates. Increasing fluids also decreases nasal congestion. Doctors believe that if the body is allowed to produce more watery secretions, thicker secretions do not accumulate as easily in the respiratory tract. Inhaling the vapors of spicy soups can help the nasal tissues (as can using a vaporizer).

🌢 **Avoid mucus-forming foods.** This includes dairy products, meat, and wheat products.

🌢 **Go on a short juice fast.** Drinking only juices, especially vegetable juices, for one to three days can accelerate your recovery. This offers your body a chance to rest from digestive activity and instead concentrate on fighting the infection. Also, the "aliveness" of raw juices supports the body at the cellular level to speed up the healing process. (For more information, see the Juice Fast, page 324.)

🌢 **Reduce your fat intake.** Studies have shown that increased levels of cholesterol, nonessential fatty acids, triglycerides, and bile acids—substances all associated with fat intake—inhibit the ability of white blood cells to divide, move to areas of infection, and destroy invading microorganisms.

🌢 **Avoid sugar.** Sugar weakens the immune system. Glucose, the most basic sugar molecule, and vitamin C compete for transport into white blood cells. Excess sugar may outcompete vitamin C, impairing the ability of white cells to engulf viruses and bacteria. Both refined and natural sugars should be avoided. These include sucrose (table sugar), fructose (fruit sugar), honey, maple syrup, sugar alcohols such as manitol or sorbitol, and full-strength fruit juice. Fruit juice, if used at all, should be diluted by half with plain water or unsweetened mineral water. Limit undiluted fruit juice to no more than four to six ounces per day, and stay away from all other forms of sugar during an infection.

🌢 **Avoid alcohol.** Alcohol acts like sugar in the body in that it competes with vitamin C, which weakens the immune cells' ability to fight infections.

Nutrient Recommendations

🌢 **Vitamin A** and **carotenes** heal inflamed mucous membranes and strengthen the immune system. Beta-carotene can help increase the number of helper T cells, cells that play a key role in immunity. The body creates vitamin A from beta-carotene. Best juice sources of carotenes (in order of effectiveness): carrots, kale, parsley, spinach, chard, beet greens, watercress, broccoli, and romaine lettuce.

🌢 **Vitamin C** and **bioflavonoids** have demonstrated the ability to slow cold and flu infections. Vitamin C has been used extensively to prevent colds and to decrease recovery time and alleviate symptoms. Bioflavonoids enhance the uptake of vitamin C into immune cells. Best juice sources of vitamin C (in order of effectiveness): kale, parsley, broccoli, Brussels sprouts, watercress, cauliflower, cabbage, spinach, citrus fruit, turnips, and asparagus. Best juice sources of bioflavonoids: bell peppers, broccoli, cabbage, parsley, and tomatoes.

❥ **Vitamin E** and **selenium** work together to fight infections. Selenium's immune-stimulating effects are enhanced by vitamin E. Studies show these nutrients increase antibody formation. Best juice sources of vitamin E (in order of effectiveness): spinach, watercress, asparagus, carrots, and tomatoes. Best juice sources of selenium (in order of effectiveness): chard, turnips, garlic, radishes, carrots, and cabbage.

❥ **Zinc** shortens the duration and severity of a cold. Zinc blocks the "docking" of the human rhinovirus onto cell membranes, thereby interrupting the infection. Zinc also reduces inflammation. Zinc lozenges are very beneficial when taken at the onset of a cold; the best lozenges are those sweetened with the amino acid glycine. Best juice sources of zinc (in order of effectiveness): ginger root, turnips, parsley, garlic, carrots, spinach, cabbage, lettuce, and cucumbers.

Herb Recommendations

❥ **Astragalus** strengthens the body's resistance to disease, and reduces the incidence and course of infection. Do not use it if you have a fever.

❥ **Echinacea** enhances activity of the natural killer cells, which may be among the principal mechanisms of immunity against viruses early in the course of an infection. Echinacea has been shown to decrease the frequency of infections, and to reduce the duration and severity of symptoms.

❥ **Goldenseal** contains the natural antibiotic berberine. Avoid this herb is you are pregnant, and do not use it for more than ten days.

Juice Ingredient Recommendations

❥ **Apple** juice has antiviral properties. Use tart apples, such as Granny Smiths or Pippins, to avoid consuming too much fruit sugar.

❥ **Garlic** has antiviral effects. In addition to using garlic juice, consume two to three raw cloves three times a day at the onset of an infection.

❥ **Ginger** juice contains anti-inflammatory compounds. Using fresh ginger, in either juice or tea form, at the first sign of a cold may help prevent the cold from occurring, or help to reduce the duration and severity of the symptoms.

❥ **Jerusalem artichoke** juice is rich in inulin, a substance that increases immune-defense mechanisms.

❥ **Parsley** juice is rich in beta-carotene, bioflavonoids, vitamin C, and zinc, nutrients that support the immune system. Intake should be limited to a safe, therapeutic dose of $1/2$ to 1 cup per day. Parsley can be toxic in overdose, and should be especially avoided by pregnant women.

❥ **Wheatgrass** juice is rich in chlorophyll, a powerful blood purifier.

Juice Recipes

ANTIVIRAL COCKTAIL

1 organic Granny Smith or Pippin apple, washed

1 turnip, scrubbed well

1 handful watercress, rinsed

5 carrots, scrubbed well, green tops removed, ends trimmed

1 large garlic clove with peel, washed

Cut the apple and turnip into sections that fit your juicer's feed tube. Bunch up the watercress, and juice it with the apple, turnip, carrots, and garlic. Stir the juice, and pour into a glass. Serve at room temperature.

THE GINGER HOPPER

$1/2$ organic Granny Smith or Pippin apple, washed

5 medium carrots, scrubbed well, green tops removed, ends trimmed

$1/2$- to 1-inch piece fresh ginger root, washed

Cut the apple into sections, and juice along with the carrots and ginger. Stir the juice, and pour into a glass. Serve at room temperature.

WEIGHT-LOSS BUDDY

1 small Jerusalem artichoke, scrubbed well

4–5 carrots, scrubbed well, green tops removed, ends trimmed

$1/2$ small beet with no stems and leaves, scrubbed well

Cut the Jerusalem artichoke into sections that fit your juicer's feed tube. Juice the artichoke along with the carrots and beet. Stir the juice, and pour into a glass. Serve at room temperature.

WHEATGRASS LIGHT

1 organic Granny Smith or Pippin apple, washed

1 small handful wheatgrass, rinsed

2–3 sprigs mint, rinsed (optional)

$\frac{1}{2}$ small or medium lemon, washed, or peeled if not organic

Cut the apple into sections that fit your juicer's feed tube. Bunch up the wheatgrass and mint (if using) and push them through the feed tube with the apple and lemon. Stir the juice, and pour into a glass. Serve at room temperature.

HOT GINGER-LEMON TEA

2-inch piece fresh ginger root, washed

$\frac{1}{2}$ small or medium lemon, washed, or peeled if not organic

2 cups pure water

1 tablespoon loose licorice tea, or 1 tea bag (optional)

1 stick cinnamon, broken

4–5 whole cloves

Dash nutmeg

Dash cardamom

Juice the ginger and lemon. Pour the juice in a small saucepan with the water; add the licorice (if using), cinnamon stick, and cloves. Bring the mixture to a boil, then reduce the heat and simmer for 5 to 10 minutes. Strain and pour into two mugs, add the nutmeg and cardamom, and serve hot.

MAGNESIUM SPECIAL

5 medium carrots, scrubbed well, green tops removed, ends trimmed

2 stalks organic celery with leaves, washed

$\frac{1}{2}$ small beet with leaves and stems, scrubbed well

2 broccoli florets, washed

$\frac{1}{2}$ small or medium lemon, washed, or peeled if not organic

Juice the carrots, celery, beet, broccoli, and lemon. Stir the juice, and pour into a glass. Serve at room temperature.

SINUS SOLUTION

2 medium vine-ripened tomatoes, washed

4 radishes with green tops, washed

$\frac{1}{2}$ small or medium lime or lemon, washed, or peeled if not organic

Cut the tomato into sections that fit your juicer's feed tube. Juice the tomatoes along with the radishes and lime or lemon. Stir the juice, and pour into a glass. Serve at room temperature.

TOMATO FLORENTINE

1 vine-ripened tomato, washed

1 handful organic spinach, washed

2–3 fresh basil leaves (optional)

1/2 small or medium lemon, washed, or peeled if not organic

Cut the tomato into sections that will fit your juicer's feed tube. Bunch up the spinach and basil leaves (if using), and push through the feed tube with the tomato and lemon. Stir the juice, and pour into a glass. Serve at room temperature.

ALLERGY RELIEF

1 small bunch parsley, rinsed

2 stalks organic celery with leaves, washed

2–3 large carrots, scrubbed well, green tops removed, ends trimmed

1/4–1/2 small or medium lemon, washed, or peeled if not organic

Bunch up the parsley and push it through the feed tube with the celery, carrots, and lemon. Stir the juice, and pour it into a glass. Serve at room temperature.

SWEET DREAMS NIGHTCAP

2 romaine lettuce leaves, washed

1 handful parsley, rinsed

4 carrots, scrubbed well, green tops removed, ends trimmed

3 organic celery stalks with leaves, washed

Bunch up the lettuce leaves and parsley, and push through the feed tube with the carrots and celery. Stir the juice, and pour into a glass. Serve at room temperature.

TURNIP TIME

1 turnip, scrubbed well

2-inch piece jicama, scrubbed well or peeled if not organic (optional)

1 handful watercress, rinsed

4 carrots, scrubbed well, green tops removed, ends trimmed

1 garlic clove with peel, washed

1/2 small or medium lemon, washed, or peeled if not organic

Cut the turnip and jicama (if using) into strips that fit your juicer's feed tube. Bunch up the watercress, and push through the feed tube with the turnip, jicama, carrots, garlic, and lemon. Stir the juice, and pour into a glass. Serve at room temperature.

Colitis

The term *colitis* takes in a broad range of intestinal disorders, the two primary ones being irritable bowel syndrome (IBS) and inflammatory bowel disease (IBD). Both disorders are more common in women than in men.

In IBS, food moves through the intestines in an uncoordinated and erratic manner. It is marked by alternating bouts of constipation and diarrhea, persistent gas, bloating, and abdominal pain. The primary cause is a diet low in fiber and high in refined carbohydrates, coupled often with a sedentary lifestyle, stress, and emotional upsets. It has been noted that symptoms of lactose intolerance, or an inability to digest milk sugar, are similar to those of IBS, and lactose intolerance may be a contributing factor in IBS.

IBD is a more severe condition that includes both Crohn's disease and ulcerative colitis. Crohn's disease, or regional enteritis, is an inflammation that can affect any part of the digestive tract, while ulcerative colitis only affects the large intestine. Symptoms include bloody diarrhea, cramps in the lower abdomen, abdominal tenderness, loss of both appetite and weight, flatulence, malaise, low-grade fever, and anal irritation. Anal fissures, hemorrhoids, fistulas (abnormal channels), and abscesses may form. In Crohn's disease, chronic inflammation causes the intestinal walls to become thick and rigid, and the bowels may become narrow and obstructed. IBD is associated with inflammation of the joints, eyes, and/or skin, and with an increased risk of colon cancer.

IBD is believed to be caused by immune-system disturbances and consumption of a typical high-fat, low-fiber Western diet, along with a genetic predisposition. Large-scale population studies show that people suffering with IBD typically eat more refined sugar, butter, margarine, cheese, and meat, and less fruits and vegetables, than healthy individuals. For example, populations in which people eat a traditional, nonprocessed diet have very low rates of Crohn's disease, while the incidence of this disease in the United States has increased by hundreds of percentage points in the last several decades, and rates in Japan have increased markedly with the introduction of Western food.

Lifestyle Recommendations

❥ **Eliminate yeast, bacterial, and parasitic infections.** Parasitic or bacterial infections may be a contributing factor in both IBS and IBD. There is circumstantial evidence that occasional relapses and first attacks of ulcerative colitis are related to infection with bacteria such as *Salmonella*, and bacterial infection has been reported in about 13 percent of Crohn's disease patients. You should be tested to find out if you are harboring disease-causing organisms. If you have a systemic yeast infection (candidiasis) or parasites, *no* fruit or fruit juice is allowed. (*See* **Candidiasis** and **Parasitic Infections**.)

Diet Recommendations

❥ **Eat a high-fiber, low-fat, low-sugar diet to treat IBS and to prevent IBD.** Fiber can help regulate intestinal function. Include high-fiber foods, such as vegetables, fruit, whole grains (except wheat), oat bran, guar gum, and psyllium, in your diet. These high-fiber foods have a positive effect on intestinal flora, the beneficial microbes that are essential to proper digestion. Avoid wheat bran, which may be too irritating, and avoid all insoluble fiber if you have IBD that is in an active state—these foods are too harsh and must be eliminated until the intestines heal. Also, eliminate fat. Avoid animal proteins as much as possible except for fish, which contains the healing omega-3 fatty acids (see the Nutrient Recommendations). Avoid sugar in all forms (cakes, pies, pastries, ice cream), butter, margarine, dairy products, fried foods, spicy foods, wheat products, and all junk food such as chips, soft drinks, and coffee. These foods encourage the secretion of intestinal mucus and prevent the uptake of nutrients. For more information on a healthy diet plan, see Basic Guidelines for the Juice Lady's Health and Healing Diet (page 313).

❥ **Drink plenty of fresh juice and water.** Anyone with IBS and, especially, IBD is at an increased risk for malnourishment. Fresh juices are nutrient-rich and very helpful in keeping people with either form of colitis well-nourished. Juices are easily digested and contain high concentrations of vitamins, minerals, and enzymes. Juices also contain phytonutrients that may help protect against colon cancer. Carotene-rich juices, such as carrot, kale, parsley, and spinach, help heal the intestinal mucosa (see the Nutrient Recommendations). In addition, include at least one quart of purified water in your daily diet; herbal teas can make up part of your water intake. Avoid caffeine and alcohol. If you have a weak digestive system, be sure to drink all fluids at room temperature.

❥ **If you have Crohn's disease, be especially sure to avoid all soft drinks.** One study found an increase in Crohn's disease among people who consumed large amounts of soft drinks. Also iced and carbonated beverages stimulate peristalsis, or the movement that propels food through the intestines.

❥ **Identify food allergies and intolerances.** Allergies and intolerances to dairy products, corn, wheat, and foods that contain carageenan, a stabilizer used in processed foods, can contribute to IBD and IBS. If you are allergic to wheat and have IBS, switch to oat or rice bran cereals, flours, and breads. For more information, *see* **Allergies** and the Elimination Diet, page 321.

❥ **Try colon cleansing and juice fasting.** There have been a number of case reports of people who have experienced considerable relief from colitis after a short juice fast. See the Juice Fast (page 324) and the Intestinal Cleanse (page 332).

Nutrient Recommendations

❥ **Beta-carotene** and **chlorophyll** help heal the intestinal tract. Best juice sources of carotenes (in order of effectiveness): carrots, kale, parsley, spinach, chard, beet greens, watercress, mangoes, cantaloupes, apricots, broccoli, and romaine lettuce. Best juice sources of chlorophyll: all dark green vegetables.

❥ **Glutamine,** an amino acid, is needed for the production of rapidly dividing cells such as those lining the intestines. It has been shown to prevent atrophy of the intestines' mucosal lining. Glutamine is available in most fruit and vegetable juices.

❥ **Omega-3 fatty acids,** especially eicosapentaenoic acid (EPA), have been shown to reduce inflammation. In IBD there is an increased level of chemicals derived from inflammatory fatty acids in the colon, serum, and stools. Omega-3s fight this effect. One double-blind study showed a reduced rate in relapse in Crohn's disease when nine enterically coated fish-oil capsules were taken every day. Flaxseed and hemp oils are richer in omega-3 and omega-6 fatty acids. For more information on omega-3 oils, see the fats and oils section in Basic Guidelines for the Juice Lady's Health and Healing Diet (page 313).

❥ **Vitamin C** is particularly important in preventing fistula formation, such as fistulas between the colon and bladder. Also, vitamin C is an important antistress nutrient, and so is helpful for IBS patients. Best juice sources of vitamin C (in order of effectiveness): kale, parsley, broccoli, Brussels sprouts, watercress, cauliflower, cabbage, strawberries, papaya, spinach, citrus fruit, turnips, mangoes, asparagus, and cantaloupes.

Herb Recommendations for Crohn's Disease

❥ **Boswellia serrata** is an herb used in Ayurvedic, or traditional Indian, medicine for its anti-inflammatory effects.

Herb Recommendations for IBS

❥ **Chamomile, lemon balm, rosemary,** and **valerian** aid the gastrointestinal tract.

❥ **Peppermint** oil, in enterically coated capsules, relieves IBS symptoms by inhibiting gastrointestinal contractions and relieving gas. The enteric capsule coating is important, as it allows the oil to pass undigested through the stomach and reach the colon.

Herb Recommendations for Ulcerative Colitis

❥ **Irish moss, marshmallow root,** and **slippery elm** are traditional remedies that soothe irritated intestinal mucous membranes. Avoid Irish moss if you are allergic to carageenan.

Juice Ingredient Recommendations for Crohn's Disease

❥ **Cabbage** juice has been scientifically documented to heal ulcers. It also contains phytonutrients that inhibit tumor growths and strengthen the immune system.

❥ **Daikon radish** juice is used in traditional Oriental medicine to help dissolve hardened accumulations in the intestines.

❥ **Tomato** juice is packed with lycopene, a powerful antioxidant that helps protect against digestive tract cancers.

❥ **Parsley** juice is rich in beta-carotene and vitamin C. Intake should be limited to a safe, therapeutic dose of $1/2$ to 1 cup per day. Parsley can be toxic in overdose, and should be especially avoided by pregnant women.

❥ **Pear** and **carrot** juices combine to form a traditional remedy for a weak digestive system.

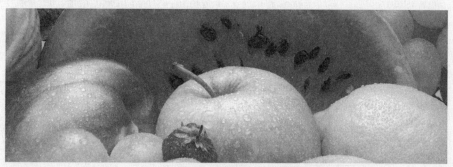

Juice Recipes for Crohn's Disease

TRIPLE C

¼ small head green cabbage, washed

4 carrots, scrubbed well, green tops removed, and ends trimmed

4 stalks organic celery with leaves, washed

Cut the cabbage into sections that fit your juicer's feed tube. Juice the cabbage along with the carrots and celery. Stir the juice, and pour into a glass. Serve at room temperature.

ANTIULCER CABBAGE EXPRESS

3–4 pounds green cabbage, washed (spring or summer cabbage is best)

1 tomato, washed, or 1 orange or lemon, peeled

1 pound organic celery with leaves, washed

Cut the cabbage and tomato or fruit into sections that fit your juicer's feed tube, and juice with the celery. Stir the juice, and pour into a container. Refrigerate in the covered container, and drink throughout the day. Allow juice to reach room temperature before drinking.

ORIENT EXPRESS

2-inch chunk jicama, scrubbed or peeled if not organic (optional)

5 carrots, scrubbed well, green tops removed, ends trimmed

2-inch piece daikon radish, scrubbed well, without green top or end

½-inch piece fresh ginger root, washed

Cut the jicama into strips (if using) that fit your juicer's feed tube. Juice the jicama with the carrots, radish, and ginger. Stir the juice, and pour into a glass. Serve at room temperature. This is a very hot-tasting drink because of the radish and ginger, so you may want to dilute it by half with water.

SANTA FE SALSA COCKTAIL

1 medium vine-ripened tomato, washed

½ medium organic cucumber, scrubbed well

¼ cup cilantro, rinsed

¼ small or medium lime or lemon, washed, or peeled if not organic

Dash hot sauce (optional)

Cut the tomato into sections that fit your juicer's feed tube. Cut the cucumber in half again lengthwise. Bunch up the cilantro, and push through the feed tube with the tomato, cucumber, and lime or lemon. Pour the juice into a glass, add the hot sauce (if using), and stir. Serve at room temperature.

DIGESTIVE TONIC

½ pear, washed

½ organic apple, any kind, washed

5 carrots, scrubbed well, green tops removed, ends trimmed

Cut the pear and apple into sections that fit your juicer's feed tube. Juice them with the carrots. Stir the juice, and pour into a glass. Serve at room temperature.

THE MORNING ENERGIZER

½ organic Red or Golden Delicious apple, washed

5 medium carrots, scrubbed well, green tops removed, ends trimmed

½ small beet with leaves and stems, scrubbed well

½ small or medium lemon, washed, or peeled if not organic

½- to 1-inch piece fresh ginger root, washed

Cut the apple into sections that will fit your juicer's feed tube. Juice the apple along with the carrots, beet, lemon, and ginger. Stir the juice, and pour into a glass. Serve at room temperature.

GINGER TWIST

1 organic Red or Golden Delicious apple, washed

1 handful parsley, rinsed

4 carrots, scrubbed well, green tops removed, ends trimmed

1-inch piece fresh ginger root, washed

¼ small or medium lemon, washed, or peeled if not organic

Cut the apple into sections that fit your juicer's feed tube. Bunch up the parsley and push it through the feed tube with the apple, carrots, ginger, and lemon. Stir the juice, and pour into a glass. Serve at room temperature.

Juice Ingredient Recommendations for IBS

❥ **Carrot** juice is rich in beta-carotene.

❥ **Fennel** and **mint** juices promote digestion and relieve gas, and can help to ease the intestinal spasms common in IBS.

❥ **Ginger** juice aids in the absorption of nutrients, and is excellent for easing indigestion, colic, and flatulence. It is an anti-inflammatory agent.

❥ **Pineapple** contains the enzyme bromelain, which aids digestion.

Juice Recipes for IBS

TROPICAL TREAT

2 firm kiwi fruit, washed

1 small organic green apple, washed

1-inch chunk fresh pineapple, scrubbed well or peeled if not organic

1-inch piece fresh ginger root, washed

Cut the kiwis and apple into sections, and the pineapple into strips, that fit your juicer's feed tube. Juice the kiwi, apple, pineapple, and ginger. Stir the juice, and pour into a glass. Serve at room temperature.

THE FEEL GOOD COCKTAIL

½ pear, washed

4 medium carrots, scrubbed well, green tops removed, ends trimmed

3 fennel stalks with leaves and flowers, washed

1 stalk organic celery with leaves, washed

Cut the pear into sections that fit your juicer's feed tube, and juice along with the carrots, fennel, and celery. Stir the juice, and pour into a glass. Serve at room temperature.

MINT MEDLEY

2 organic apples, any kind, washed

1 small handful mint, rinsed

2 fennel stalks with leaves and flowers, washed

1-inch piece fresh ginger root, washed

Cut the apples into sections that fit your juicer's feed tube. Bunch up the mint, and push through the feed tube with the apple, fennel, and ginger. Stir the juice, and pour into a glass. Serve at room temperature.

THE GINGER HOPPER

½ organic Red or Golden Delicious apple, washed

5 medium carrots, scrubbed well, green tops removed, ends trimmed

½- to 1-inch piece fresh ginger root, washed

Cut the apple into sections, and juice along with the carrots and ginger. Stir the juice, and pour into a glass. Serve at room temperature.

Juice Ingredient Recommendations for Ulcerative Colitis

❧ **Beet green** juice is rich in chlorophyll, a blood purifier.

❧ **Cabbage** juice has been shown to be effective in healing ulcers.

❥ **Carrot** juice is rich in beta-carotene, which helps heal the digestive tract.

❥ **Mango, papaya,** and **pineapple** juices are all rich in enzymes that help digestion. Studies have shown that bromelain, an enzyme in pineapple, and papain, an enzyme in papaya, aid digestion, reduce inflammation, and enhance wound healing.

❥ **Parsley** juice is rich in beta-carotene and vitamin C. Intake should be limited to a safe, therapeutic dose of $^1/_2$ to 1 cup per day. Parsley can be toxic in overdose, and should be especially avoided by pregnant women.

❥ **Wheatgrass** juice is loaded with chlorophyll and beta-carotene. Both compounds have healing properties that are especially beneficial for the intestinal mucosa.

Juice Recipes for Ulcerative Colitis

POPEYE'S POWER

$^1/_2$ medium organic apple, any kind, washed

1 handful organic spinach, washed

1 small handful parsley, rinsed

4 medium carrots, scrubbed well, green tops removed, ends trimmed

1 stalk organic celery with leaves, washed

$^1/_2$ beet with leaves, scrubbed well

Cut the apple into sections that will fit your juicer's feed tube. Bunch up the spinach and parsley, and push them through the feed tube with the apple, carrots, celery, and beet. Stir the juice, and pour into a glass. Serve at room temperature.

TRIPLE C

$^1/_4$ small head green cabbage, washed

4 carrots, scrubbed well, green tops removed, and ends trimmed

4 stalks organic celery with leaves, washed

Cut the cabbage into sections that fit your juicer's feed tube. Juice the cabbage along with the carrots and celery. Stir the juice, and pour into a glass. Serve at room temperature.

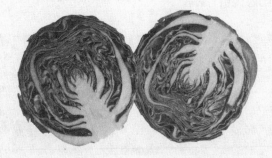

TROPICAL TREAT

2 firm kiwi fruit, washed

1 small organic green apple, washed

1-inch chunk fresh pineapple, scrubbed well, or peeled if not organic

1-inch piece fresh ginger root, washed

Cut the kiwis and apple into sections, and the pineapple into strips, that fit your juicer's feed tube. Juice the kiwi, apple, pineapple, and ginger. Stir the juice, and pour into a glass. Serve at room temperature.

WHEATGRASS LIGHT

1 organic Golden or Red Delicious apple, washed

1 small handful wheatgrass, rinsed

2–3 sprigs mint, rinsed (optional)

1/4 small or medium lemon, washed, or peeled if not organic

Cut the apple into sections that fit your juicer's feed tube. Bunch up the wheatgrass and mint (if using) and push them through the feed tube with the apple and lemon. Stir the juice, and pour into a glass. Serve at room temperature.

THE FEEL GOOD COCKTAIL

1/2 pear, washed

4 medium carrots, scrubbed well, green tops removed, ends trimmed

3 fennel stalks with leaves and flowers, washed

1 stalk organic celery with leaves, washed

Cut the pear into sections that fit your juicer's feed tube, and juice along with the carrots, fennel, and celery. Stir the juice, and pour into a glass. Serve at room temperature.

SWEET DREAMS NIGHTCAP

2 romaine lettuce leaves, washed

1 handful parsley, rinsed

4 carrots, scrubbed well, green tops removed, ends trimmed

3 organic celery stalks with leaves, washed

Bunch up the lettuce leaves and parsley, and push through the feed tube with the carrots and celery. Stir the juice, and pour into a glass. Serve at room temperature.

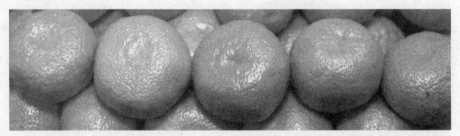

Constipation

Constipation is the infrequent passage of small, hard, and dry bowel movements that are usually difficult and painful. When constipated, a person may feel sluggish, bloated, and uncomfortable. Surveys indicate that constipation affects over four million Americans, who spend $725 million on laxatives yearly.

The most common causes of constipation are eating a low-fiber diet, drinking too little water, and not getting enough exercise. Highly refined, low-fiber foods, such as those which most Americans eat, in conjunction with inadequate fluid intake and exercise, is the main reason so many Americans suffer from this condition. Other causes include food sensitivities, bacterial overgrowth or parasitic infection (*see* **Parasitic Infections**), pregnancy, use of iron tablets or other medications, pesticide exposure, and changes in routine that disrupt bodily rhythms, such as travel. In most cases, constipation is temporary and not serious. However, chronic constipation can persist for months and even years. If this happens, the person is at risk for digestive disorders, including diverticulitis, hemorrhoids, and indigestion, due to wastes and toxins being absorbed back into the bloodstream. Chronic constipation can also cause other problems, such as bad breath, fatigue, and headaches.

Lifestyle Recommendations

❥ **Get regular exercise.** To reverse or prevent constipation, you need to exercise at least thirty minutes a day, three days a week. Aerobic exercise, such as walking, swimming, or aerobic dancing, helps keep the bowels regular.

Diet Recommendations

❥ **Eat a high-fiber, complex-carbohydrate diet.** A diet rich in whole grains, fruits, vegetables, and legumes (beans, lentils, split peas) helps prevent and treat constipation. Rice or oat bran is a good addition to whole-grain cereals, and one study found that barley bran flour was quite effective in reversing constipation. For more information, see Basic Guidelines for the Juice Lady's Health and Healing Diet (page 313).

❥ **Cut down on foods high in fat and refined foods.** Fatty foods include red meat and dark-meat poultry, eggs, and dairy products. Especially reduce intake of cheese, margarine, fried foods, and most fast foods.

Refined sugar products include table sugar, powdered sugar, brown sugar, and such corn-based sweeteners as corn syrup, as well as prepared foods that contain these sugars. Refined flour products include all items made with white flour, such as bread, crackers, pasta, and pizza dough. These foods do not contain enough fiber to keep food moving through the intestines.

❧ **Drink plenty of water.** That means at least one quart per day.

❧ **Use juicing, juice fasting, and colon cleansing.** Many people have told me that once they started drinking any combination of fresh juices, they became very regular. (See the Juice Fast, page 324, and the Intestinal Cleanse, page 332.) A couple of juices are especially helpful in treating constipation. Prune juice is a well-known laxative; you can juice the plums that are used to make prunes, if you can find them. Boysenberry juice is another gentle laxative. (If you have a weak digestive system, drink juices only at room temperature.) Juice fasting and colon cleansing can be very helpful in correcting constipation.

Herb Recommendations

❧ **Psyllium seed,** a bulking agent, is a common herbal remedy for constipation. Make sure you take it with water; see the package directions.

Juice Ingredient Recommendations

❧ **Apple, parsley, pear,** and **radish** juices stimulate intestinal motion. Parsley juice intake should be limited to a safe, therapeutic dose of $1/2$ to 1 cup per day. Parsley can be toxic in overdose, and should be especially avoided by pregnant women.

❧ **Spinach** and **apple** juices cleanse and rejuvenate the intestinal tract.

Juice Recipes

Sweet & Regular

1 pear, washed
1 organic apple, any kind, washed

Cut the pear and apple into sections that fit your juicer's feed tube, and juice them. Stir the juice, and pour into a glass. Serve at room temperature or chilled, as desired.

SINUS SOLUTION

2 medium vine-ripened tomatoes, washed

4 radishes with green tops, washed

1/2 small or medium lime or lemon, washed, or peeled if not organic

Cut the tomato into sections that fit your juicer's feed tube. Juice the tomatoes along with the radishes and lime or lemon. Stir the juice, and pour into a glass. Serve at room temperature or chilled, as desired.

THE COLON CLEANSER

2 organic Granny Smith, McIntosh, or Golden Delicious apples, washed

1 bunch organic spinach, washed

1 handful parsley, rinsed

1/4 small or medium lemon, washed, or peeled if not organic

Cut the apples into sections that fit your juicer's feed tube. Bunch up the spinach and parsley, and push them through the feed tube with the apples and lemon. Stir the juice, and pour into a glass. Serve at room temperature or chilled, as desired.

DIGESTIVE TONIC

1/2 pear, washed

1/2 organic apple, any kind, washed

5 carrots, scrubbed well, green tops removed, ends trimmed

Cut the pear and apple into sections that fit your juicer's feed tube. Juice them with the carrots. Stir the juice, and pour into a glass. Serve at room temperature or chilled, as desired. (If your digestive system is weak, serve at room temperature only.)

POPEYE'S POWER

1/2 medium organic apple, any kind, washed

1 handful organic spinach, washed

1 small handful parsley, rinsed

4 medium carrots, scrubbed well, green tops removed, ends trimmed

1 stalk organic celery with leaves, washed

1/2 beet with leaves, scrubbed well

Cut the apple into sections that will fit your juicer's feed tube. Bunch up the spinach and parsley, and push them through the feed tube with the apple, carrots, celery, and beet. Stir the juice, and pour into a glass. Serve at room temperature or chilled, as desired.

Cravings

Over time, human beings have learned that certain tastes, especially sweet and salt, signal the presence of important nutrients; salt is essential for the body's water balance, while sweet foods are rich in the calories needed for energy. This attraction to sweet and salt was vital for our ancient ancestors, who lived in a hunter-gatherer environment. Because these tastes were so important to early humankind's survival, they involve more than just the taste buds, and are associated with changes in brain chemistry and hormone balance as well.

Cravings for such strange items as dirt, starch, or paint are referred to as *pica*. Recorded for centuries, this phenomenon has been explained as a need for minerals. And that's the current explanation for most familiar cravings—a deficiency of specific nutrients. Cravings can also be due to food allergies (*see* **Allergies**), blood-sugar imbalances (*see* **Hypoglycemia**), candidiasis (*see* **Candidiasis**), or hormonal changes during the premenstrual phase of the menstrual cycle (*see* **Menstrual Disorders**). Or, of course, pregnancy!

Most people have experienced frustrating urges for things like potato chips, chocolate ice cream, or peanut butter, and know firsthand Webster's definition of *crave*, which is to "want greatly." Getting rid of food urges means getting to the root of the cause. Even though you think you are hungry for a quart of strawberry cheesecake ice cream or a bag of honey mustard pretzels, that isn't what your body needs. In this section, find what you crave most often, and put into practice the recommendations for modifying your diet. And the next time an uncontrollable urge to munch strikes, make a big glass of one of the recommended juice recipes to get to the root of your hunger.

Alcohol and Cigarette Cravings/Addictions. These cravings appear to lessen, even disappear, when a diet high in raw foods is introduced. Dr. John Douglas, who worked with addiction patients at the Kaiser-Permanente Medical Center in Los Angeles, discovered that such a diet, eaten over a span of several weeks, caused his patients not to want as many cigarettes or alcoholic drinks as before. He concluded that a diet rich in such raw foods as vegetables, fruits, juices, sprouts, seeds, and nuts must sensitize the body to what is good for it and what is not. He noted that raw sunflower seeds were particularly effective in depressing the cravings associated with addiction. Sunflower sprouts, which should have the same effect, can be juiced. Supplemental L-glutamine, an amino acid, has also been used to help reduce cravings for alcohol and sugar.

Juice Recipes

PURE GREEN SPROUT DRINK

1 organic cucumber, scrubbed well

1 large handful sunflower sprouts, rinsed

1 small handful buckwheat sprouts, rinsed

1 small handful clover sprouts, rinsed

Cut the cucumber in half lengthwise. Bunch up the sprouts, and push through the feed tube with the cucumber. Stir the juice, and pour into a glass. Serve at room temperature or chilled, as desired.

THE GINGER HOPPER

½ organic Red or Golden Delicious apple, washed

5 medium carrots, scrubbed well, green tops removed, ends trimmed

½- to 1-inch piece fresh ginger root, washed

Cut the apple into sections, and juice along with the carrots and ginger. Stir the juice, and pour into a glass. Serve at room temperature or chilled, as desired.

POPEYE'S POWER

½ medium organic apple, any kind, washed

1 handful organic spinach, washed

1 small handful parsley, rinsed

4 medium carrots, scrubbed well, green tops removed, ends trimmed

1 stalk organic celery with leaves, washed

½ beet with leaves, scrubbed well

Cut the apple into sections that will fit your juicer's feed tube. Bunch up the spinach and parsley, and push them through the feed tube with the apple, carrots, celery, and beet. Stir the juice, and pour into a glass. Serve at room temperature or chilled, as desired.

Carbohydrate Cravings. If you desire sweets, refined grains (breads, crackers, pasta), and such starchy vegetables as potatoes and corn, you have a carbohydrate craving. This can contribute to a state known as hyperinsulinemia, in which there is too much insulin in the bloodstream. Hyperinsulinemia is characterized by a cycle of carbohydrate craving and insulin resistance, a condition in which the body cannot use insulin effectively. This cycle creates a metabolic imbalance and further exacerbates chronic hyperinsulinemia. It can also lead to obesity and sabotage attempts at dieting and hunger control. Carbohydrate craving is fairly common during the premenstrual phase due to hormone imbalances.

Often a craving for sweets is caused by a deficiency of the mineral chromium. Chromium helps regulate blood sugar and improves glucose tolerance by increasing insulin's efficiency. Eat more foods rich in chromium, such as oysters, chicken, eggs, broccoli, and whole grains (barley in particular). Best juice sources of chromium (in order of effectiveness): apples, parsnips, spinach, carrots, lettuce, string beans, and cabbage. If after increasing your intake of these foods and juices you still crave sweets, try a chromium supplement of from 50 to 200 mcg. (Liquid, trivalent organic chromium is best.) Vitamin E, vanadium (a trace mineral), and evening primrose oil may also be helpful. Best juice sources of vitamin E: spinach, watercress, asparagus, carrots, and tomatoes. Best juice sources of vanadium: parsley, green beans, carrot, cabbage, garlic, tomatoes, and radishes. Evening primrose oil is best taken in supplement form.

Strict vegans can be protein deficient, which also causes a craving for sweets. If this applies to you, make sure you eat at least two cups of legumes (beans, lentils, or split peas) with an equal complement of whole grains each day.

Juice Recipes

THE GINGER HOPPER

½ organic Red or Golden Delicious apple, washed

5 medium carrots, scrubbed well, green tops removed, ends trimmed

½- to 1-inch piece fresh ginger root, washed

Cut the apple into sections, and juice along with the carrots and ginger. Stir the juice, and pour into a glass. Serve at room temperature or chilled, as desired.

BEAUTIFUL SKIN, HAIR, AND NAIL SOLUTION

1 medium organic cucumber, scrubbed well

1 medium parsnip, scrubbed well

3 carrots, scrubbed well, green tops removed, ends trimmed

½ small or medium lemon, washed, or peeled if not organic

¼ small green bell pepper, washed

Cut the cucumber in half lengthwise, and juice with the parsnip, carrots, lemon, and bell pepper. Stir the juice, and pour into a glass. Serve at room temperature or chilled, as desired.

TRIPLE C

¼ small head green cabbage, washed

4 carrots, scrubbed well, green tops removed, and ends trimmed

4 stalks organic celery with leaves, washed

Cut the cabbage into sections that fit your juicer's feed tube. Juice the cabbage along with the carrots and celery. Stir the juice, and pour into a glass. Serve at room temperature or chilled, as desired.

SINUS SOLUTION

2 medium vine-ripened tomatoes, washed

4 radishes with green tops, washed

¼ small or medium lime or lemon, washed, or peeled if not organic

Cut the tomato into sections that fit your juicer's feed tube. Juice the tomatoes along with the radishes and lime or lemon. Stir the juice, and pour into a glass. Serve at room temperature or chilled, as desired.

TOMATO FLORENTINE

1 vine-ripened tomato, washed

1 handful organic spinach, washed

2–3 fresh basil leaves (optional)

½ small or medium lemon, washed, or peeled if not organic

Cut the tomato into sections that will fit your juicer's feed tube. Bunch up the spinach and basil leaves (if using), and push through the feed tube with the tomato and lemon. Stir the juice, and pour into a glass. Serve at room temperature or chilled, as desired.

SPRING TONIC

1 medium vine-ripened tomato, washed

1 organic cucumber, scrubbed well

8 asparagus stems, washed

½ small or medium lemon, washed, or peeled if not organic

Cut the tomato into sections that fit your juicer's feed tube. Cut the cucumber in half lengthwise. Juice the tomato, cucumber, asparagus, and lemon. Stir the juice, and pour into a glass. Serve at room temperature.

Ice Cravings (Pogophagia). If you continually reach for ice cubes to crunch, you may have what is known as pogophagia. A craving for ice is often a sign of anemia. Anemia can be the result of iron, vitamin B_{12} (cobalamin), and/or folic acid deficiency (*see* **Anemia**). Best juice sources of nonheme iron, the type found in plants (in order of effectiveness): parsley, dandelion greens, broccoli, cauliflower, strawberries, asparagus, chard, blackberries, cabbage, beets with greens, carrots, and pineapple. Best juice sources of folic acid: asparagus, spinach, kale, broccoli, cabbage, and blackberries. Vitamin B_{12} is not available in fruits and vegetables. The best food sources of B_{12} are meat, poultry, and fish; it is also available in some fermented soy-based foods, such as tofu and tempeh. Note that parsley juice intake should be limited to a safe, therapeutic dose of $1/2$ to 1 cup per day. Parsley can be toxic in overdose, and should be especially avoided by pregnant women.

Juice Recipes

POPEYE'S POWER

$1/2$ medium organic apple, any kind, washed

1 handful organic spinach, washed

1 small handful parsley, rinsed

4 medium carrots, scrubbed well, green tops removed, ends trimmed

1 stalk organic celery with leaves, washed

$1/2$ beet with leaves, scrubbed well

Cut the apple into sections that will fit your juicer's feed tube. Bunch up the spinach and parsley, and push them through the feed tube with the apple, carrots, celery, and beet. Stir the juice, and pour into a glass. Serve at room temperature or chilled, as desired.

THE MORNING ENERGIZER

$1/2$ organic Red or Golden Delicious apple, washed

5 medium carrots, scrubbed well, green tops removed, ends trimmed

$1/2$ small beet with leaves and stems, scrubbed well

$1/2$ small or medium lemon, washed, or peeled if not organic

$1/2$- to 1-inch piece fresh ginger root, washed

Cut the apple into sections that will fit your juicer's feed tube. Juice the apple along with the carrots, beet, lemon, and ginger. Stir the juice, and pour into a glass. Serve at room temperature or chilled, as desired.

TRIPLE C

$1/4$ small head green cabbage, washed

4 carrots, scrubbed well, green tops removed, and ends trimmed

4 stalks organic celery with leaves, washed

Cut the cabbage into sections that fit your juicer's feed tube. Juice the cabbage along with the carrots and celery. Stir the juice, and pour into a glass. Serve at room temperature or chilled, as desired.

BEAUTIFUL BONE SOLUTION

1 organic Golden or Red Delicious apple, washed

1–2 kale leaves, washed

1 handful parsley, rinsed

1 stalk organic celery, washed

$1/4$ small or medium lemon, washed, or peeled if not organic

$1/2$- to 1-inch piece fresh ginger root, washed

Cut the apple into sections that fit your juicer's feed tube. Bunch up the kale and parsley, and push through the feed tube with the apple, celery, lemon, and ginger. Stir the juice, and pour into a glass. Serve at room temperature or chilled, as desired.

Peanut Butter Cravings. Do you ever find yourself scooping out spoonsful of peanut butter, never even bothering to spread it on crackers or bread before you eat it? Unless you buy the natural brands that contain only peanuts and salt, it may be the corn syrup or other sugars you're actually craving. Or it may be that you are copper deficient, as peanuts are rich in copper. There are better sources of copper, however, that are lower in fat and without the carcinogenic aflatoxins found on peanuts. Best juice sources of copper (in order of effectiveness): carrots, garlic, ginger root, and turnips.

Juice Recipes

THE GINGER HOPPER

$1/2$ organic Red or Golden Delicious apple, washed

5 medium carrots, scrubbed well, green tops removed, ends trimmed

$1/2$- to 1-inch piece fresh ginger root, washed

Cut the apple into sections, and juice along with the carrots and ginger. Stir the juice, and pour into a glass. Serve at room temperature or chilled, as desired.

ANTIVIRAL COCKTAIL

1 organic Golden or Red Delicious apple, washed

1 turnip, scrubbed well

1 handful watercress, rinsed

5 carrots, scrubbed well, green tops removed, ends trimmed

1 large garlic clove with peel, washed

Cut the apple and turnip into sections that fit your juicer's feed tube. Bunch up the watercress, and juice it with the apple, turnip, carrots, and garlic. Stir the juice, and pour into a glass. Serve at room temperature or chilled, as desired.

APPLE SPICE

1 large organic apple, any kind, washed

1 bunch red organic grapes (about 1½ cups) with small stems* and seeds, washed

½- to 1-inch piece fresh ginger root

*Large stems can dull your juicer's blade.

Cut the apple into sections that fit your juicer's feed tube. Juice the apple with the grapes and ginger. Stir the juice, and pour into a glass. Serve at room temperature or chilled, as desired.

Salty-Food Cravings. If potato chips, pretzels, bacon, or salted popcorn is your desire, it may be the salt you're after. Salt cravings can be a symptom of sickle cell anemia, Addison's disease, various muscular disorders, high blood pressure (*see* **High Blood Pressure**), or diabetes (*see* **Diabetes Mellitus**). A common cause of occasional salt cravings is adrenal stress. Caffeine consumption and other lifestyle stressors can weaken the adrenal glands, allowing blood-pressure levels to drop and bringing on fatigue. Increasing salt intake can temporarily help the symptoms, but can have negative long-term results. Also, magnesium deficiency has been shown to cause salt cravings in animals. If you crave salt, reduce your consumption of table salt (sodium chloride), and increase your consumption of magnesium, pantothenic acid, potassium, vitamin B_6 (pyridoxine), vitamin C, and zinc, all of which help to support your adrenal glands. Best juice sources of magnesium (in order of effectiveness): beet greens, spinach, parsley, dandelion greens, garlic, blackberries, beets, broccoli, cauliflower, carrots, and celery. Of pantothenic acid: broccoli, cauliflower, and kale. Of potassium: parsley, chard, garlic, spinach, broccoli, carrots, celery, radishes, cauliflower, watercress, asparagus, and cabbage. Of vitamin B_6: kale, spinach, turnip greens, bell peppers, and prunes. Of vitamin C: kale, parsley, broccoli, Brussels sprouts, watercress, cauliflower, cabbage, strawberries, papaya, spinach, citrus fruit, turnips, mangoes, asparagus, and cantaloupes. Of zinc: ginger root, turnips, parsley, garlic, carrots, grapes, spinach, cabbage, lettuce, cucumbers, and tangerines. Note that parsley juice intake should be limited to a safe, therapeutic dose of $1/2$ to 1 cup per day. Parsley can be toxic in overdose, and should be especially avoided by pregnant women.

Juice Recipes

MAGNESIUM SPECIAL

5 medium carrots, scrubbed well, green tops removed, ends trimmed

2 stalks organic celery with leaves, washed

½ small beet with leaves and stems, scrubbed well

2 broccoli florets, washed

½ small or medium lemon, washed, or peeled if not organic

Juice the carrots, celery, beet, broccoli, and lemon. Stir the juice, and pour into a glass. Serve at room temperature or chilled, as desired.

LIVER LIFE TONIC

½ organic green apple such as Granny Smith or Pippin, washed

1 handful dandelion greens, washed

5 carrots, scrubbed well, green tops removed, ends trimmed

½ small lemon, washed, or peeled if not organic

Cut the apple into wedges that will fit your juicer's feed tube. Bunch up the dandelion greens, and push through the feed tube with the apple, carrots, and lemon. Stir the juice, and pour into a glass. Serve at room temperature or chilled, as desired.

POPEYE'S POWER

½ medium organic apple, any kind, washed

1 handful organic spinach, washed

1 small handful parsley, rinsed

4 medium carrots, scrubbed well, green tops removed, ends trimmed

1 stalk organic celery with leaves, washed

½ beet with leaves, scrubbed well

Cut the apple into sections that will fit your juicer's feed tube. Bunch up the spinach and parsley, and push them through the feed tube with the apple, carrots, celery, and beet. Stir the juice, and pour into a glass. Serve at room temperature or chilled, as desired.

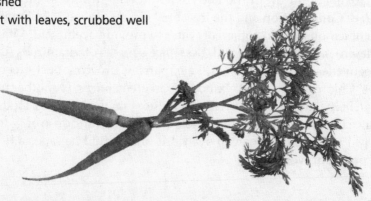

ANTIVIRAL COCKTAIL

1 organic Golden or Red Delicious apple, washed

1 turnip, scrubbed well

1 handful watercress, rinsed

5 carrots, scrubbed well, green tops removed, ends trimmed

1 large garlic clove with peel, washed

Cut the apple and turnip into sections that fit your juicer's feed tube. Bunch up the watercress, and juice it with the apple, turnip, carrots, and garlic. Stir the juice, and pour into a glass. Serve at room temperature or chilled, as desired.

SWEET CALCIUM COCKTAIL

1 three-inch chunk fresh pineapple, scrubbed well or peeled if not organic

1–2 kale leaves, washed

Cut the pineapple into strips that fit your juicer's feed tube. Bunch up the kale, and push through the feed tube with the pineapple. Stir the juice, and pour into a glass. Serve at room temperature or chilled, as desired.

BEAUTIFUL SKIN, HAIR, AND NAIL SOLUTION

1 medium organic cucumber, scrubbed well

1 medium parsnip, scrubbed well

3 carrots, scrubbed well, green tops removed, ends trimmed

$1/2$ small or medium lemon, washed, or peeled if not organic

$1/4$ small green bell pepper, washed

Cut the cucumber in half lengthwise, and juice with the parsnip, carrots, lemon, and bell pepper. Stir the juice, and pour into a glass. Serve at room temperature or chilled, as desired.

Sour-Food Cravings. If you crave lemons, limes, or other sour foods, you may need acetic acid to help detoxify toxins released from undigested proteins. Toxins build up in the body when foods putrefy in the intestinal tract. (*See* **Constipation** and the Intestinal Cleanse, page 332.) Drink a teaspoon of lemon juice in a glass of water to provide acetic acid. Vitamin B_2 (riboflavin) may also be helpful. Best juice sources of vitamin B_2 (in order of effectiveness): collard greens, kale, parsley, broccoli, beet greens, and prunes. Chlorophyll, found abundantly in green juices, is another nutrient that can help detoxify the system and reduce cravings for sour foods. Note that juice intake should be limited to a safe, therapeutic dose of $1/2$ to 1 cup per day. Parsley can be toxic in overdose, and should be especially avoided by pregnant women.

Juice Recipes

SWEET CALCIUM COCKTAIL

1 three-inch chunk fresh pineapple, scrubbed well or peeled if not organic

1–2 kale leaves, washed

Cut the pineapple into strips that fit your juicer's feed tube. Bunch up the kale, and push through the feed tube with the pineapple. Stir the juice, and pour into a glass. Serve at room temperature or chilled, as desired.

MAGNESIUM SPECIAL

5 medium carrots, scrubbed well, green tops removed, ends trimmed

2 stalks organic celery with leaves, washed

$1/2$ small beet with leaves and stems, scrubbed well

2 broccoli florets, washed

$1/2$ small or medium lemon, washed, or peeled if not organic

Juice the carrots, celery, beet, broccoli, and lemon. Stir the juice, and pour into a glass. Serve at room temperature or chilled, as desired.

PURE GREEN SPROUT DRINK

1 organic cucumber, scrubbed well

1 large handful sunflower sprouts, rinsed

1 small handful buckwheat sprouts, rinsed

1 small handful clover sprouts, rinsed

Cut the cucumber in half lengthwise. Bunch up the sprouts, and push through the feed tube with the cucumber. Stir the juice, and pour into a glass. Serve at room temperature or chilled, as desired.

ALLERGY RELIEF

1 small bunch parsley, rinsed

2 stalks organic celery with leaves, washed

2–3 large carrots, scrubbed well, green tops removed, ends trimmed

$1/4$–$1/2$ small or medium lemon, washed, or peeled if not organic

Bunch up the parsley and push it through the feed tube with the celery, carrots, and lemon. Stir the juice, and pour it into a glass. Serve at room temperature or chilled, as desired.

Crohn's Disease

See **Colitis.**

Depression

Depression is a feeling of sadness, gloom, and self-reproach that lasts longer than the passing blue mood. Often, depressed people hide from society and lose interest or pleasure in usual activities. Sex drive may decrease, and they may be irritable. They may tend to sleep a lot or not be able to sleep much at all. They may be unable to get going, or they may become jittery without the ability to concentrate on any one task. They may have no appetite or be constantly hungry. They may have headaches, backaches, or digestive problems, and they may get sick more often, since depression saps the immune system. They may feel worthless, and, if severely depressed, suicidal. For most people, though, depression is not severe; they can still function, but do so more slowly.

The most common cause of depression is thought to be low amounts of the chemical messengers norepinephrine and especially serotonin in the brain. These neurotransmitters are created from the amino acids phenylalanine and tryptophan, amino acids that are not created in the body and so must be present in the diet. Factors that can lead to low serotonin levels include alcohol use, high sugar and/or protein intake, blood-sugar disturbances (*see* **Diabetes Mellitus** and **Hypoglycemia**), candidiasis (*see* **Candidiasis**), poor thyroid or adrenal function, nutrient deficiencies, smoking, food allergies, stress (*see* **Stress**), hormone imbalances, prescription drugs, and environmental toxins.

Doctors fight depression with a wide variety of drugs. However, all of these medications have side effects, some quite severe. Herbs, such as St. John's wort (see Herb Recommendations), are good alternatives. Their advantage is that they have fewer side effects. However, they usually take longer to bring relief. If you are already taking a prescription antidepressant, be sure to see a doctor *before* switching to an herbal agent. And remember, herbal therapy will work best if you follow an overall treatment plan that includes a wholesome, natural diet.

Lifestyle Recommendations

❥ **Get enough sleep.** This helps prevent depression. If you suffer from insomnia, *see* **Insomnia and Jet Lag.**

❥ **Make time for regular exercise.** Exercise not only tones your body, making you feel better physically, it also tones your mind by causing the release of "feel good" brain chemicals called endorphins.

❥ **If you smoke, quit.** Smoking leads to depression by decreasing tryptophan levels. It also decreases vitamin C levels, which can lead to depression. Depression may, in turn, make it more difficult to quit smoking. Thus, by addressing your depression, you may find it easier to kick the habit (*see* **Cravings**).

Diet Recommendations

❥ **Eat a low-fat, high-fiber diet, and eat smaller, more frequent meals.** Depression can be caused by low blood-sugar levels, or hypoglycemia. This disorder develops when there is not enough of the right fuel to keep blood-sugar levels steady. Eliminate all refined carbohydrates and sugars—cakes, cookies, ice cream, such white flour products as breads and rolls, and junk food. This may be difficult if emotional stress leads to a craving for sweets, which provide quick bursts of emotional and physical energy before leaving you feeling burned out. But I recommend you make every effort to avoid them—it will pay off. During times of stress, it is important to eat complex carbohydrates, such as vegetables, whole grains, and legumes, which increase brain serotonin and tryptophan. Also, eat high-energy snacks, such as fruits, fresh juices, raw nuts, and seeds, to keep blood-sugar levels even and ward off depression. For more information, *see* **Hypoglycemia** and Basic Guidelines for the Juice Lady's Health and Healing Diet (page 313).

❥ **Be especially sure to avoid food additives.** These substances are linked with depression. Read food labels, and don't buy what you can't pronounce.

❥ **Combat depression with raw fruits, vegetables, and juices.** Many people who consume a diet high in raw foods and juice have found that these foods lift their spirits. Juice fasting for one to three days can be very helpful; many people have reported a great sense of well-being following a juice fast (see the Juice Fast, page 324).

❥ **Eliminate foods that can cause allergies.** Food allergies can cause you to feel more defensive and depressed. For more information, *see* **Allergies** and the Elimination Diet, page 321.

Nutrient Recommendations

❥ **Essential fatty acids** play an important role in fighting depression. Low levels of omega-3 fatty acids in the diet have been associated with increased rates of depression, and depressed people have been found to have lower blood levels of high-density lipoproteins (HDLs, the "good fats") and higher levels of triglycerides, conditions that respond to the use of omega-3 supplements. Flaxseed and hemp oil both contain omega-3s, as does fish oil and such cold-water fish as salmon and halibut. For more information, see the fats and oils section in Basic Guidelines for the Juice Lady's Health and Healing Diet (page 313).

❥ **Folic acid** and **vitamin B_{12}** (cobalamin) are important depression fighters; deficiencies of either or both are associated with depression. Best juice sources of folic acid (in order of effectiveness): asparagus, spinach, kale, broccoli, cabbage, and blackberries. Vitamin B_{12} is not available in fruits and vegetables. The best food sources of B_{12} are meat, poultry, and fish; it is also available in some fermented soy-based foods, such as tofu and tempeh.

❥ **Phenylalanine** and **tyrosine** are amino acids used by the body to make norepinephrine, and are good alternatives to antidepressant drugs. When used in supplement form, they work most effectively when taken with carbohydrates, such as a glass of fresh juice. Tyramine is an amino-acid precursor to tyrosine. Best juice sources of tyramine: potato, spinach, and tomatoes.

❥ **Tryptophan, vitamin B_3 (niacin),** and **vitamin B_6 (pyridoxine)** work together to fight depression. In order to gain real benefits from tryptophan, the amino acid precursor to serotonin, it must be taken in combination with vitamins B_3 and B_6. Tryptophan is found most abundantly in tuna, turkey, and yogurt. Best food sources of vitamin B_3 (in order of effectiveness): brewer's yeast, rice and wheat bran, peanuts, turkey, chicken, and fish. Best juice sources of vitamin B_6: kale, spinach, turnip greens, bell peppers, and prunes.

❥ **Vitamin C** and **bioflavonoids,** especially rutin, have been known to help people with depression. Best juice sources of vitamin C (in order of effectiveness): kale, parsley, broccoli, Brussels sprouts, watercress, cauliflower, cabbage, strawberries, papaya, spinach, citrus fruit, turnips, mangoes, asparagus, and cantaloupes. Best juice sources of bioflavonoids:

apricots, bell peppers, berries (blueberry, blackberry, and cranberry), broccoli, cabbage, cantaloupes, cherries, citrus fruit, grapes, parsley, plums, prunes, and tomatoes.

Herb Recommendations

❧ **Ginkgo biloba** fights both depression and stress, and helps sharpen mental functioning.

❧ **Gotu kola, hops, lavender, lemon balm, passionflower,** and **valerian** have all been used in traditional medicine for their antidepressant effects.

❧ **Kava-kava** is a good choice for depression that is accompanied by anxiety. Unlike most herbal remedies, it is fairly fast-acting.

❧ **Schisandra** is another stress-fighting herb that also helps support the liver. This allows the liver to more readily rid the body of toxins, including substances that contribute to depression.

❧ **Siberian ginseng** helps the body balance and regulate itself. It also supports the adrenal glands, which often don't function well in people with depression. Be sure to use *Eleutherococcus senticosus*, Siberian ginseng, and not *Panax ginseng*, Korean or red ginseng. Avoid this herb if you have an autoimmune disease such as rheumatoid arthritis.

❧ **St. John's wort,** one of the most well-documented herbal antidepressants, has been shown in a number of studies to fight depression with far fewer side effects than conventional medicines.

Juice Ingredient Recommendations

❧ **Dark green** juices are rich in chlorophyll, a good source of many nutrients, and have shown themselves to be very helpful for depression.

❧ **Fennel** juice has been used as a traditional tonic to help release endorphins into the bloodstream. Endorphins create a mood of euphoria, and help dampen anxiety and fear.

❧ **Mango** juice is known as a folk remedy that helps relieve depression. Mangoes do not juice very well, but they blend well in smoothies.

❧ **Parsley** juice is rich in bioflavonoids, chlorophyll, and vitamin C. Intake should be limited to a safe, therapeutic dose of $1/2$ to 1 cup per day. Parsley can be toxic in overdose, and should be especially avoided by pregnant women.

Juice Recipes

PURE GREEN SPROUT DRINK

1 organic cucumber, scrubbed well

1 large handful sunflower sprouts, rinsed

1 small handful buckwheat sprouts, rinsed

1 small handful clover sprouts, rinsed

Cut the cucumber in half lengthwise. Bunch up the sprouts, and push through the feed tube with the cucumber. Stir the juice, and pour into a glass. Serve at room temperature or chilled, as desired.

THE FEEL GOOD COCKTAIL

½ pear, washed

4 medium carrots, scrubbed well, green tops removed, ends trimmed

3 fennel stalks with leaves and flowers, washed

1 stalk organic celery with leaves, washed

Cut the pear into sections that fit your juicer's feed tube, and juice along with the carrots, fennel, and celery. Stir the juice, and pour into a glass. Serve at room temperature or chilled, as desired.

MANGO MON

1 ripe mango, peeled

1 orange, peeled, divided into segments

1 ripe banana, peeled

6 ice cubes

Cut the mango flesh away from the pit, and add it to a blender with the orange, banana, and ice cubes. Blend until smooth, pour into two glasses, and serve.

MINT MEDLEY

2 organic apples, any kind, washed

1 small handful mint, rinsed

2 fennel stalks with leaves and flowers, washed

1-inch piece fresh ginger root, washed

Cut the apples into sections that fit your juicer's feed tube. Bunch up the mint, and push through the feed tube with the apple, fennel, and ginger. Stir the juice, and pour into a glass. Serve at room temperature.

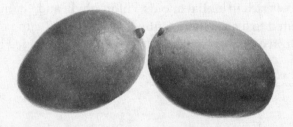

SWEET CALCIUM COCKTAIL

1 three-inch chunk fresh pineapple, scrubbed well or peeled if not organic

1–2 kale leaves, washed

Cut the pineapple into strips that fit your juicer's feed tube. Bunch up the kale, and push through the feed tube with the pineapple. Stir the juice, and pour into a glass. Serve at room temperature or chilled, as desired.

GRAPE EXPECTATIONS

3 plums, washed, stones removed

½ pound organic purple grapes with small stems* and seeds, washed

8 organic strawberries with caps, washed

¼ small or medium lemon, washed, or peeled if not organic

*Large stems can dull your juicer's blade.

Cut the plums in half, and juice with the grapes, strawberries, and lemon. Stir the juice, and pour into a glass. Serve at room temperature or chilled, as desired.

ANTIAGING COCKTAIL

1 small bunch organic purple grapes (about 1 cup) with small stems* and seeds, washed

½ cup blueberries, blackberries, or raspberries, washed

¼ small or medium lemon, washed, or peeled if not organic

½-inch piece fresh ginger root, washed

*Large stems can dull your juicer's blade.

Juice the grapes, berries, lemon, and ginger. Stir the juice, and pour into a glass. Serve at room temperature or chilled, as desired.

POPEYE'S POWER

½ medium organic apple, any kind, washed

1 handful organic spinach, washed

1 small handful parsley, rinsed

4 medium carrots, scrubbed well, green tops removed, ends trimmed

1 stalk organic celery with leaves, washed

½ beet with leaves, scrubbed well

Cut the apple into sections that will fit your juicer's feed tube. Bunch up the spinach and parsley, and push them through the feed tube with the apple, carrots, celery, and beet. Stir the juice, and pour into a glass. Serve at room temperature or chilled, as desired.

BEAUTIFUL SKIN, HAIR, AND NAIL SOLUTION

1 medium organic cucumber, scrubbed well

1 medium parsnip, scrubbed well

3 carrots, scrubbed well, green tops removed, ends trimmed

1/2 small or medium lemon, washed, or peeled if not organic

1/4 small green bell pepper, washed

Cut the cucumber in half lengthwise, and juice with the parsnip, carrots, lemon, and bell pepper. Stir the juice, and pour into a glass. Serve at room temperature or chilled, as desired.

SANTA FE SALSA COCKTAIL

1 medium vine-ripened tomato, washed

1/2 medium organic cucumber, scrubbed well

1/4 cup cilantro, rinsed

1/4 small or medium lime or lemon, washed, or peeled if not organic

Dash hot sauce (optional)

Cut the tomato into sections that fit your juicer's feed tube. Cut the cucumber in half again lengthwise. Bunch up the cilantro, and push through the feed tube with the tomato, cucumber, and lime or lemon. Pour the juice into a glass, add the hot sauce (if using), and stir. Serve at room temperature or chilled, as desired.

Diabetes Mellitus

Diabetes mellitus is a condition in which the body cannot properly regulate blood-sugar levels. This gives rise to symptoms that include fatigue and an increase in thirst. Diabetes mellitus includes several conditions. In type 1 diabetes, also known as insulin-dependent or juvenile-onset diabetes, the body's own immune system destroys cells in the pancreas called beta cells. Beta cells secrete insulin, the hormone that helps most of the body's cells take in glucose—the cells' main fuel source—from the blood. Because there is little or no insulin in the blood, the person must take insulin in order to survive. Type 1 diabetes generally develops sometime in childhood, but can occur in adults.

In type 2 diabetes, also known as adult-onset or non-insulin-dependent diabetes, the pancreas secretes insulin, but there is a problem with the insulin receptors on the body's cells—there may not be a enough receptors, or the receptors may be insensitive to insulin. This condition usually develops after a person reaches age forty. It can be controlled by diet and, in some cases, by medication. But if type 2 diabetes is not controlled, it can progress to the point that additional insulin is required.

A third type of diabetes is known as gestational diabetes mellitus (GDM). It occurs for the first time during pregnancy and usually disappears after a woman gives birth. GDM is usually controlled well with dietary changes. These changes must continue after delivery, though, because women who develop GDM have a much higher chance of developing type 2 diabetes later in life.

Diabetes can have a number of long-term complications, including atherosclerosis, susceptibility to infection, and damage to the eyes, nerves, and kidneys. Therefore, it is important to control your blood-sugar levels even if you are not experiencing any symptoms.

Diet Recommendations

❥ **Avoid sweets and other simple carbohydrates.** This includes cookies, candies, cakes, pies, ice cream, and items made with processed white flour. Fruit also contains simple carbohydrates, so do not eat more than one or two pieces per day. Limit your intake of fruit juice, and dilute juice by half with water. Avoid alcohol, as it is a simple carbohydrate and acts like sugar in the body.

❥ **Eat complex carbohydrates and whole, unprocessed foods.** Vegetables, whole grains, and legumes (beans, lentils, split peas) are made up of complex carbohydrates. These carbohydrates require more time for your digestive system to break them down into fuel. Since digestion takes more time, glucose is released into the bloodstream more slowly and evenly than is the case with simple carbohydrates, which tend to dump glucose into your bloodstream all at once. Whole foods are good sources of fiber, which also helps regulate blood sugar. Limit consumption to no more than 1 cup per day of such starchy vegetables as potatoes, yams, peas, and corn; they are processed into fuel more quickly than other vegetables.

❥ **Eat more of your vegetables raw, and drink fresh vegetable juices.** Dr. John Douglas of the Kaiser-Permanente Medical Center in Los Angeles found that raw vegetables are better tolerated by diabetics than cooked vegetables, and that raw foods help stabilize blood-sugar levels. Dr. Max Bircher-Benner, of the European Bircher-Benner clinic, successfully used raw vegetable juices in treating diabetics. For more information, see the section on raw foods and Basic Guidelines for the Juice Lady's Health and Healing Diet, page 313.

❥ **Eat smaller, more frequent meals, and include protein at each meal or snack.** Diabetics do best eating several small meals throughout the day, rather than two or three large meals. Eating more frequently, and eating a little protein at each meal or snack, helps keep blood sugar at a relatively constant level, which is far better than inducing big surges in blood sugar by eating a substantial meal. One way to accomplish this goal is to save a portion of each meal and eat it later as a snack.

❥ **Reduce your consumption of animal products.** Research shows that a healthy vegetarian diet lowers the risk of developing severe diabetes complications when compared with a diet that includes high amounts of animal products. If you do not wish to eat a strictly vegetarian diet, eat fish more often, and eat only small quantities of meat and poultry. Cold-water fish, such as salmon, tuna, halibut, cod, trout, and sardines, contain oils called essential fatty acids that can help make cells more receptive to insulin.

Nutrient Recommendations

❥ **Chromium** makes insulin more effective at the cellular level. It is a component of glucose tolerance factor (GTF), which helps the cells take up glucose and helps regulate blood-sugar levels. Best juice sources of chromium (in order of effectiveness): green pepper, parsnips, spinach, carrots, lettuce, string beans, and cabbage.

❥ **Copper** deficiency may impair glucose tolerance. Best juice sources of copper (in order of effectiveness): carrots, garlic, ginger root, and turnips.

❥ **Magnesium** deficiency is the most common mineral deficiency seen in type 1 diabetes. Magnesium can improve glucose tolerance and may also help prevent some diabetes complications. Best juice sources of magnesium (in order of effectiveness): beet greens, spinach, parsley, dandelion greens, garlic, beets, broccoli, cauliflower, carrots, and celery.

❥ **Vitamin B_3 (niacin),** like chromium, is a component of GTF. Best food sources of vitamin B_3 (in order of effectiveness): brewer's yeast, rice and wheat bran, peanuts, turkey, chicken, and fish. It is not available in vegetables and fruits.

❥ **Vitamin C** metabolism can be disrupted by diabetes, and a deficiency can lead to problems with glucose regulation. Vitamin C levels are typically lower in people with diabetes, even when they take supplemental C. Best juice sources of vitamin C (in order of effectiveness): kale, parsley, broccoli, Brussels sprouts, watercress, cauliflower, cabbage, spinach, citrus fruit, turnips, and asparagus.

❥ **Vitamin E** needs increase with diabetes, and this vitamin can help to decrease the amount of insulin required. Best juice sources of vitamin E (in order of effectiveness): spinach, watercress, asparagus, carrots, and tomatoes.

Herb Recommendations

❥ **Gymnema sylvestre** is an herb used in Ayurevedic, or traditional Indian, medicine. In animal studies, it has been shown to reduce blood-sugar levels in individuals with high sugar levels while not affecting those individuals with normal levels.

Traditional Remedy Recommendations

❥ **Bitter melon** is a green melon that can be found in Asian produce markets. It has been used for centuries by the Chinese and East Indians to treat diabetes, since it enhances glucose metabolism and lowers blood-sugar levels. Bitter melon is prepared by juicing the fruit with the seeds and mixing the juice with other desired juices and water.

Juice Ingredient Recommendations

❥ **Asparagus, cucumber, lemon,** and **parsley** juices all act as natural diuretics. Cantaloupe and watermelon juices also have diuretic properties, but have higher amounts of sugars (especially watermelon), and should be avoided by diabetics.

❥ **Cabbage** juice was found in one study to help diabetics; it is suspected of having an insulinlike activity.

❥ **Garlic** juice lowers blood-sugar levels. It also helps the body fight off infections, which tend to occur more frequently when diabetes is present.

❥ **Jerusalem artichoke** juice helps stabilize blood-sugar levels.

❥ **String bean** juice has been used to support the pancreas. It is recommended that five cups of string bean juice be consumed throughout the day—one cup with breakfast, lunch, dinner, and two snacks. Green bean juice is very strong tasting and should be mixed with milder-tasting juices, such as carrot and celery.

Juice Recipes

NATURAL DIURETIC COCKTAIL

1 medium vine-ripened tomato, washed

1 small handful parsley, rinsed

1 organic cucumber, scrubbed well

4 asparagus stems, washed

½ small or medium lemon, washed, or peeled if not organic

Cut the tomato into sections that fit your juicer's feed tube. Bunch up the parsley, and juice with the cucumber, asparagus, and lemon. Stir the juice, and pour into a glass. Serve at room temperature or chilled, as desired.

BEAUTIFUL SKIN, HAIR, AND NAIL SOLUTION

1 medium organic cucumber, scrubbed well

1 medium parsnip, scrubbed well

3 carrots, scrubbed well, green tops removed, ends trimmed

½ small or medium lemon, washed, or peeled if not organic

¼ small green bell pepper, washed

Cut the cucumber in half lengthwise, and juice with the parsnip, carrots, lemon, and bell pepper. Stir the juice, and pour into a glass. Serve at room temperature or chilled, as desired.

TRIPLE C

¼ small head green cabbage, washed

4 carrots, scrubbed well, green tops removed, and ends trimmed

4 stalks organic celery with leaves, washed

Cut the cabbage into sections that fit your juicer's feed tube. Juice the cabbage along with the carrots and celery. Stir the juice, and pour into a glass. Serve at room temperature or chilled, as desired.

WEIGHT-LOSS BUDDY

1 small Jerusalem artichoke, scrubbed well

4–5 carrots, scrubbed well, green tops removed, ends trimmed

½ small beet with no stems and leaves, scrubbed well

Cut the Jerusalem artichoke into sections that fit your juicer's feed tube. Juice the artichoke along with the carrots and beet. Stir the juice, and pour into a glass. Serve at room temperature or chilled, as desired.

JACK & THE BEAN

1 large tomato, washed

2 romaine lettuce leaves, washed

8 organic string beans*

3 Brussels sprouts, washed

1/2 small or medium lemon, washed, or peeled if not organic

*Add extra string (green) beans to make one cup of green bean juice in addition to the other juices. About 4 cups of string beans makes about one cup of juice.

Juice the string beans first to make one cup of bean juice. Cut the tomato into sections that fit your juicer's feed tube. Bunch up the lettuce leaves and juice with the tomato, string beans, Brussels sprouts, and lemon. Stir the juice, and pour into a glass. Serve at room temperature or chilled, as desired.

THE MORNING ENERGIZER

5 medium carrots, scrubbed well, green tops removed, ends trimmed

1/2 small beet with leaves and stems, scrubbed well

1/2 small or medium lemon, washed, or peeled if not organic

1/2- to 1-inch piece fresh ginger root, washed

Juice the carrots, beet, lemon, and ginger. Stir the juice, and pour into a glass. Serve at room temperature, or chilled, as desired.

TOMATO FLORENTINE

1 vine-ripened tomato, washed

1 handful organic spinach, washed

2–3 fresh basil leaves (optional)

1/2 small or medium lemon, washed, or peeled if not organic

Cut the tomato into sections that will fit your juicer's feed tube. Bunch up the spinach and basil leaves (if using), and push through the feed tube with the tomato and lemon. Stir the juice, and pour into a glass. Serve at room temperature or chilled, as desired.

ANTIVIRAL COCKTAIL

1 organic Granny Smith or Pippin apple, washed

1 turnip, scrubbed well

1 handful watercress, rinsed

5 carrots, scrubbed well, green tops removed, ends trimmed

1 large garlic clove with peel, washed

Cut the apple and turnip into sections that fit your juicer's feed tube. Bunch up the watercress, and juice it with the apple, turnip, carrots, and garlic. Stir the juice, and pour into a glass. Serve at room temperature or chilled, as desired.

MAGNESIUM SPECIAL

5 medium carrots, scrubbed well, green tops removed, ends trimmed

2 stalks organic celery with leaves, washed

½ small beet with leaves and stems, scrubbed well

2 broccoli florets, washed

½ small or medium lemon, washed, or peeled if not organic

Juice the carrots, celery, beet, broccoli, and lemon. Stir the juice, and pour into a glass. Serve at room temperature or chilled, as desired.

Diverticulitis and Diverticulosis

Diverticulosis is a condition in which little pouches called diverticula develop along the intestinal walls, generally those of the large intestine. Intestinal outpouchings occur at weak points, such as between fibers in the intestinal muscles or where arteries enter the bowel wall. Diverticulitis is a condition in which the diverticula become inflamed. Symptoms of diverticulitis include cramping, lower abdominal pain, alternating bouts of constipation and diarrhea, and fever. Abscesses can form, as can fistulas, or abnormal connections between the bowel and other organs. Diverticulosis is usually symptomless, although there may be rectal bleeding and vague feelings of intestinal distress. Both conditions tend to develop after middle age.

Diverticula are created when pressure is exerted against the intestinal wall. This pressure is strongest in the sigmoid area, the place where the large intestine is narrowest. Not surprisingly, the sigmoid area is also the place where most diverticula are found. Diverticulosis is often a consequence of chronic constipation (*see* **Constipation**), as dry, hard stools require more force to pass.

Chronic gastrointestinal diseases, such as diverticulitis, may result in malnutrition, which impairs both digestion and absorption of nutrients. Nutrient insufficiency leads to a decrease in digestive enzyme production and decreased cell growth. A high-fiber diet can ease both malnutrition and the underlying diverticulitis.

Diet Recommendations

❥ **Eat a high-fiber diet.** Diverticular disease was rare in the United States prior to the twentieth century, since people used to eat a diet that contained a lot more fiber. Roughage is vital for digestive-tract health. Both soluble and insoluble fibers hold water and increase fecal bulk, and soluble fiber combines with water to form a gel that lubricates the stool. These actions make stools softer and easier to pass. Insoluble fiber generally decreases transit time, the time it takes food to travel from one end of the digestive tract to the other, and soluble fiber normalizes transit time. The importance of eating a high-fiber diet rich in vegetables, fruits, sprouts, whole grains, and legumes (beans, lentils, split peas) cannot be overemphasized. For more information on dietary goals, see Basic Guidelines for the Juice Lady's Health and Healing Diet (page 313).

❥ **Take supplemental fiber.** Use pectin, psyllium husk, guar gum, or oat bran, along with acidophilus, the friendly bacteria that aid digestion. Together, they help prevent constipation. Avoid supplemental fiber, though, during a period of active inflammation, as fiber can aggravate the problem.

❥ **Juice fast during an acute phase.** Juice fasting gives the bowel a rest, and juice is rich in soluble fibers. Carrot, cabbage, and green juices are especially healing for the intestinal tract (see the Juice Fast on page 324). If you have a weak digestive system, drink the juices at room temperature—do *not* chill. The Intestinal Cleanse can also be quite beneficial (see page 332).

❥ **Avoid irritating foods.** Nuts and seeds can become trapped in the diverticula, causing inflammation. Dairy products, especially cheese (small amounts of plain yogurt are acceptable), red meat, fried foods, spices, sugar, refined flour products, and processed foods can cause intestinal irritation and/or constipation.

Nutrient Recommendations

❥ **Beta-carotene** helps heal the mucous membranes that line the intestine. Best juice sources of carotenes in general (in order of effectiveness): carrots, kale, parsley, spinach, chard, beet greens, watercress, mangoes, cantaloupes, apricots, broccoli, and romaine lettuce.

❥ **Vitamin K** deficiency has been linked to intestinal disorders. Best juice sources of vitamin K (in order of effectiveness): turnip greens, broccoli, lettuce, cabbage, spinach, watercress, asparagus, and string beans.

Herb Recommendations

❥ **Fenugreek seed, flaxseed, licorice, marshmallow root,** and **psyllium seed** soothe and protect the mucosa that lines the intestines. Avoid licorice if you have high blood pressure, do not use for prolonged periods of time, and use a medicinal form of the herb, not licorice candy.

Juice Ingredient Recommendations

❥ **Parsley** juice is a rich source of beta-carotene. Intake should be limited to a safe, therapeutic dose of $1/_2$ to 1 cup per day. Parsley can be toxic in overdose, and should be especially avoided by pregnant women.

❥ **Pear** juice has been used traditionally for weak digestive systems; pear and apple juices are rich in pectins (soluble fiber), which help improve elimination.

Juice Recipes

DIGESTIVE TONIC

½ pear, washed
½ organic apple, any kind, washed
5 carrots, scrubbed well, green tops removed, ends trimmed

Cut the pear and apple into sections that fit your juicer's feed tube. Juice them with the carrots. Stir the juice, and pour into a glass. Serve at room temperature.

SWEET & REGULAR

1 pear, washed
1 organic apple, any kind, washed

Cut the pear and apple into sections that fit your juicer's feed tube, and juice them. Stir the juice, and pour into a glass. Serve at room temperature.

TROPICAL TREAT

2 firm kiwi fruit, washed
1 small organic green apple, washed
1-inch chunk fresh pineapple, scrubbed well or peeled if not organic
1-inch piece fresh ginger root, washed

Cut the kiwis and apple into sections, and the pineapple into strips, that fit your juicer's feed tube. Juice the kiwi, apple, pineapple, and ginger. Stir the juice, and pour into a glass. Serve at room temperature.

THE MORNING ENERGIZER

½ organic Red or Golden Delicious apple, washed

5 medium carrots, scrubbed well, green tops removed, ends trimmed

½ small beet with leaves and stems, scrubbed well

½ small or medium lemon, washed, or peeled if not organic

½- to 1-inch piece fresh ginger root, washed

Cut the apple into sections that will fit your juicer's feed tube. Juice the apple along with the carrots, beet, lemon, and ginger. Stir the juice, and pour into a glass. Serve at room temperature.

NATURAL DIURETIC COCKTAIL

1 medium vine-ripened tomato, washed

1 small handful parsley, rinsed

1 organic cucumber, scrubbed well

4 asparagus stems, washed

½ small or medium lemon, washed, or peeled if not organic

Cut the tomato into sections that fit your juicer's feed tube. Bunch up the parsley, and juice with the cucumber, asparagus, and lemon. Stir the juice, and pour into a glass. Serve at room temperature.

THE COLON CLEANSER

2 organic Granny Smith, McIntosh, or Golden Delicious apples, washed

1 bunch organic spinach, washed

1 handful parsley, rinsed

¼ small or medium lemon, washed, or peeled if not organic

Cut the apples into sections that fit your juicer's feed tube. Bunch up the spinach and parsley, and push them through the feed tube with the apples and lemon. Stir the juice, and pour into a glass. Serve at room temperature.

Eczema (Atopic Dermatitis)

Eczema is an intensely itchy, inflammatory skin disorder that is commonly found on the hands, face, wrists, elbows, and knees. It can occur at any age, but is most common in infants and often disappears by eighteen months of age (although it can recur later in life). Eczema is characterized by patches of red, itchy skin that is dry and thickened. There are various types of lesions—scratches, papules, red patches, weeping areas, and scaly areas with small blisters. Eczema leaves the skin vulnerable to bacterial and/or viral infection.

The causes of eczema can be linked to a host of factors, including heredity, diet, stress (*see* **Stress**), candidiasis (*see* **Candidiasis**), and environmental pollutants and irritants. (Another type of eczema, contact dermatitis, is most often caused by exposure to poison ivy or oak.) Many eczema sufferers have a personal or family history of such allergic conditions as hay fever or hives. Although it is known that certain genetic factors may be involved in eczema, some experts say that heredity may be more related to familial environment, that is, similar diet and lifestyle. Since World War II, the numbers of new cases of eczema have continued to rise steadily. This suggests that environmental pollution, along with consumption of refined and fast foods, may be strong factors in its development.

Breast milk is the best food for a infant who has eczema (or any infant, for that matter). If you or an older child is prone to this condition, the following suggestions can help.

Lifestyle Recommendations

❥ **Reduce exposure to irritating metals.** Several studies have found a correlation between eczema and allergy to gold or nickel. Not wearing gold jewelry is an obvious start, but it is also important to avoid gold fillings or gold in cosmetics. Common sources of nickel include chocolate, soybeans, oatmeal, almonds, legumes (bean, lentils, split peas), and stainless steel cookware.

Diet Recommendations

❥ **Eat a high-fiber diet that includes plenty of raw fruits, vegetables, and juices.** A high-fiber diet greatly facilitates elimination, and good elimination is vital in easing eczema. Drinking plenty of fresh juices (and water) is also important for proper elimination (*see* **Constipation**).

❥ **Avoid sugar and refined (white) flour.** Limit or avoid all sugars (such as table sugar, fruit sugar, honey, and maple syrup) and refined flour products (such as white bread, rolls, and pasta). These substances can contribute to a weakening of the immune system, and abnormalities associated with eczema originate in the immune system.

❥ **Eliminate food allergens.** Many studies have demonstrated a strong correlation between the onset of eczema and consumption of such foods as milk and dairy products, wheat, corn, soy, peanuts, and eggs. There are many accounts in which skin rash has been alleviated when allergenic foods were eliminated from the diet. (*See* **Allergies**; also see the Elimination Diet, page 321.)

❥ Increase the good bacteria in your intestines. Lactobacillis and bifidus are the "friendly" bacteria that live in your intestines and aid the digestive process. Supplementing the diet with cultures of these bacteria, as well as eating foods like plain nonfat yogurt and miso, will help restock the gastrointestinal tract with these beneficial microbes. This is important because many Americans have an overgrowth of disease-promoting pathogens, such as the yeast *Candida albicans* or parasites, in their intestinal tracts, and such overgrowths can lead to the development of eczema (*see* **Candidiasis** and **Parasitic Infections**).

❥ Use juice fasting and cleansing diets to rid your body of toxins. One to three days of juice fasting will help cleanse the lymphatic system, which is an important part of treating eczema. The skin—also known as the "third lung"—is partially responsible for clearing toxins from the body, but cannot perform this vital function if the lymphatic system is sluggish. The liver is another important elimination organ. When it is overtaxed, it becomes incapable of doing its job correctly, and waste products build up in the bloodstream and lymph. Excess waste contributes to inflammation and thus to outbreaks of eczema. For more information, see the Juice Fast (page 324) and the Liver and Skin Cleanses (pages 333 and 338).

Nutrient Recommendations

❥ Bioflavonoids help to control factors involved in inflammation and allergic reactions. Best juice sources of bioflavonoids: apricots, bell peppers, berries (blueberry, blackberry, and cranberry), broccoli, cabbage, cantaloupes, cherries, citrus fruit, grapes, parsley, plums, prunes, and tomatoes.

❥ Essential fatty acids (EFAs) are vital to your skin's health. Researchers stress the importance of eating a diet that is rich in essential fatty acids (EFAs)—which exist in two forms, omega-3 and omega-6 fatty acids—in the treatment of eczema, with omega-3s being the most important ones. Studies have shown that the breast milk of mothers whose children have eczema is low in EFAs. EFAs can be found in such cold-water fish as salmon, trout, tuna, mackerel, halibut, and sardines. They are also plentiful in flaxseed and hemp oils. For more information, see the fats and oils section in Basic Guidelines for the Juice Lady's Health and Healing Diet (page 313).

❥ **Vitamin A** deficiency can cause a thickening of the skin, a condition typically found in eczema. Carotenes, found in fruits and vegetables, are converted in the body to vitamin A. Best juice sources of carotenes (in order of effectiveness): carrots, kale, parsley, spinach, chard, beet greens, watercress, mangoes, cantaloupes, apricots, broccoli, and romaine lettuce.

❥ **Zinc** is necessary for the conversion of EFAs into anti-inflammatory substances called prostaglandins. Best juice sources of zinc (in order of effectiveness): ginger root, turnips, parsley, garlic, carrots, grapes, spinach, cabbage, lettuce, cucumbers, and tangerines.

Supplement Recommendations

❥ **Digestive enzymes** improve digestion and may help decrease eczema's severity. Ness Formula enzymes are the best supplemental enzymes I've found; they are available through some doctors' offices. Also, Arise & Shine offers a papaya enzyme supplement (see Appendix A). Bitter leafy green vegetables, such as kale, mustard greens, and dandelion greens, also help promote the flow of digestive juices. They can be juiced, mixed with milder tasting juices (such as carrot and apple, pear, and/or pineapple), and drunk prior to eating.

Herb Recommendations

❥ **Burdock root, dandelion root, garlic, goldenseal,** and **red clover** are all lymph-cleansing herbs. Avoid goldenseal if you are pregnant, and do not use it for more than ten days at a time.

Juice Ingredient Recommendations

❥ **Beet, cabbage, carrot, celery, cucumber, parsley,** and **spinach** juices all help cleanse the lymphatic system. Cucumber juice can also relieve itching when applied directly to the skin.

❥ **Green juices,** such as wheatgrass, parsley, kale, and spinach, are rich in chlorophyll, which is a blood purifier.

❥ **Parsley** juice is rich in beta-carotene and zinc. Intake should be limited to a safe, therapeutic dose of $1/2$ to 1 cup per day. Parsley can be toxic in overdose, and should be especially avoided by pregnant women.

Juice Recipes

MAGNESIUM SPECIAL

5 medium carrots, scrubbed well, green tops removed, ends trimmed

2 stalks organic celery with leaves, washed

½ small beet with leaves and stems, scrubbed well

2 broccoli florets, washed

½ small or medium lemon, washed, or peeled if not organic

Juice the carrots, celery, beet, broccoli, and lemon. Stir the juice, and pour into a glass. Serve at room temperature or chilled, as desired.

POPEYE'S POWER

½ medium organic apple, any kind, washed

1 handful organic spinach, washed

1 small handful parsley, rinsed

4 medium carrots, scrubbed well, green tops removed, ends trimmed

1 stalk organic celery with leaves, washed

½ beet with leaves, scrubbed well

Cut the apple into sections that will fit your juicer's feed tube. Bunch up the spinach and parsley, and push them through the feed tube with the apple, carrots, celery, and beet. Stir the juice, and pour into a glass. Serve at room temperature or chilled, as desired.

PURE GREEN SPROUT DRINK

1 organic cucumber, scrubbed well

1 large handful sunflower sprouts, rinsed

1 small handful buckwheat sprouts, rinsed

1 small handful clover sprouts, rinsed

Cut the cucumber in half lengthwise. Bunch up the sprouts, and push through the feed tube with the cucumber. Stir the juice, and pour into a glass. Serve at room temperature or chilled, as desired.

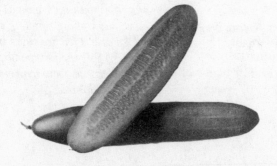

WHEATGRASS LIGHT

1 organic Golden or Red Delicious
  apple, washed

1 small handful wheatgrass, rinsed

2–3 sprigs mint, rinsed (optional)

1/4 small or medium lemon, washed,
  or peeled if not organic

Cut the apple into sections that fit your juicer's feed tube. Bunch up the wheatgrass and mint (if using) and push them through the feed tube with the apple and lemon. Stir the juice, and pour into a glass. Serve at room temperature or chilled, as desired.

SWEET CALCIUM COCKTAIL

1 three-inch chunk fresh pineapple,
  scrubbed well or peeled if not
  organic

1–2 kale leaves, washed

Cut the pineapple into strips that fit your juicer's feed tube. Bunch up the kale, and push through the feed tube with the pineapple. Stir the juice, and pour into a glass. Serve at room temperature or chilled, as desired.

ALLERGY RELIEF

1 small bunch parsley, rinsed

2 stalks organic celery with leaves,
  washed

2–3 large carrots, scrubbed well,
  green tops removed, ends
  trimmed

1/4–1/2 small or medium lemon,
  washed, or peeled if not organic

Bunch up the parsley and push it through the feed tube with the celery, carrots, and lemon. Stir the juice, and pour it into a glass. Serve at room temperature or chilled, as desired.

AFTERNOON REFRESHER

1 medium to large organic cucumber,
  scrubbed well

1/2 small or medium lemon, washed,
  or peeled if not organic

Cut the cucumber in half lengthwise, and juice with the lemon. (For an especially cooling version, let the juice splash over a few ice cubes in the juice pitcher.) Stir the juice, and pour into a glass. Serve at room temperature or chilled, as desired.

PINK PASSION POTION

1 organic Red Delicious apple, washed

½ cup fresh or frozen (thawed) cranberries, rinsed

1 bunch organic purple grapes, with seeds and small stems,* washed

⅛ small beet (no stems or leaves) for color, scrubbed well (optional)

¼ small or medium lemon, washed, or peeled if not organic

*Large stems can dull your juicer's blade.

Cut the apple into sections that fit your juicer's feed tube. Juice the apple, cranberries, grapes, beet (if using), and lemon. (To prevent the cranberries from flying out of the machine while juicing, place the cranberries in the juicer first, place an apple section on top of them, and cover with the plunger. Turn on the machine, and push the plunger to begin the juicing process.) Stir the juice, and pour into a glass. Serve at room temperature or chilled, as desired.

THE MORNING ENERGIZER

½ organic Red or Golden Delicious apple, washed

5 medium carrots, scrubbed well, green tops removed, ends trimmed

½ small beet with leaves and stems, scrubbed well

½ small or medium lemon, washed, or peeled if not organic

½- to 1-inch piece fresh ginger root, washed

Cut the apple into sections that will fit your juicer's feed tube. Juice the apple along with the carrots, beet, lemon, and ginger. Stir the juice, and pour into a glass. Serve at room temperature or chilled, as desired.

THE GINGER HOPPER

½ organic Red or Golden Delicious apple, washed

5 medium carrots, scrubbed well, green tops removed, ends trimmed

½- to 1-inch piece fresh ginger root, washed

Cut the apple into sections, and juice along with the carrots and ginger. Stir the juice, and pour into a glass. Serve at room temperature or chilled, as desired.

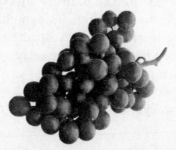

GINGER TWIST

1 organic Red or Golden Delicious apple, washed

1 handful parsley, rinsed

4 carrots, scrubbed well, green tops removed, ends trimmed

1-inch piece fresh ginger root, washed

1/4 small or medium lemon, washed, or peeled if not organic

Cut the apple into sections that fit your juicer's feed tube. Bunch up the parsley and push it through the feed tube with the apple, carrots, ginger, and lemon. Stir the juice, and pour into a glass. Serve at room temperature or chilled, as desired.

TRIPLE C

1/4 small head green cabbage, washed

4 carrots, scrubbed well, green tops removed, and ends trimmed

4 stalks organic celery with leaves, washed

Cut the cabbage into sections that fit your juicer's feed tube. Juice the cabbage along with the carrots and celery. Stir the juice, and pour into a glass. Serve at room temperature or chilled, as desired.

Epilepsy and Seizures

Seizures involve uncontrolled electrical discharges from nerve cells, called neurons, in the brain. Seizures can cause loss of consciousness and uncontrolled muscle movements called convulsions, as well as tingling, temporary loss of speech, staring, and inattentiveness. Epilepsy is a disease characterized by recurring seizures. Some people have daily attacks, while others have long periods of time—up to a year or two—between episodes. Many children diagnosed with epilepsy outgrow their seizures.

If a seizure affects many different areas of the brain at once, a generalized seizure occurs. This can cause a loss of consciousness and convulsions. If only one small part of the brain is affected, a partial seizure occurs. A partial seizure causes less dramatic symptoms, the exact nature of which depends on the location of the misfiring neurons. Within both basic categories are many forms of epileptic seizures, each characterized by a specific pattern of symptoms.

Possible causes of epilepsy include lesions of the central nervous system, food sensitivities, heavy metal toxicity, cell damage by toxins called free radicals, pesticide poisoning, head injuries, hypoglycemia (*see* **Hypo-glycemia**), and malnutrition. A healthy diet can address a number of these factors.

Diet Recommendations

❥ **Eat a high-fat, low-carbohydrate diet (the MCT diet).** A number of studies have shown that a high-fat, low-carbohydrate diet has been used effectively in controlling seizures. Clinical trials are now confirming that this treatment works "better than any other regimen," according to Dr. John Freeman, director of the Pediatric Epilepsy Clinic at the Children's Center in Baltimore, who created the Ketogenic Diet based on that principle (see *The Epilepsy Diet Treatment: An Introduction to the Ketogenic Diet,* in Appendix A). I recommend the MCT (medium-chain fatty acids) diet, used by Children's Hospital in Boston. This is a modified ketogenic diet in which more carbohydrates and proteins are used (to reduce the problems associated with a high fat intake) without sacrificing the benefits of the high-fat diet (see Appendix A for information on MCT oil).

❥ **Choose a gluten-free diet as well.** A significant percentage of epileptic patients are sensitive to a protein called gluten, and avoiding foods that contain gluten has been beneficial for many epileptics. Therefore, eliminate wheat, buckwheat, oats, rye, and barley from your diet. Instead, use rice, potatoes, corn, cornmeal, rice flour, and potato flour, and gluten-free breads and flour products. Also avoid such vegetables as beans, cabbage, turnips, dried peas, and cucumbers.

❥ **Switch, to the extent possible, to an organically produced diet.** More organic foods means less of the heavy metals and pesticide residues that have been implicated in epilepsy (see page 14).

❥ **Avoid the artificial sweetener aspartame.** Findings are inconclusive on aspartame's contribution to seizures. However, according to the National Cancer Institute, there has been a significant increase in aspartame-related seizures and malignant brain tumors since 1985, about two years after aspartame was introduced on the market. Foods containing aspartame include: soft drinks, gum, ice cream, frozen yogurt, cookies, candy, and other dessert items.

❥ **Avoid caffeine.** Studies show that caffeine may affect seizure frequency, making epilepsy more difficult to control. Foods containing caffeine include coffee, green and black tea, soft drinks, and chocolate. Some medications contain caffeine as well.

Nutrient Recommendations

❥ **Glutamine** and **glycine** are amino acids that can help prevent seizures. The best food sources of glycine: almonds, turkey, and wheat germ; best juice sources: carrots and celery. Glutamine is available in most fruit and vegetable juices.

❥ **Manganese** is a mineral that has been found in low levels in the blood and hair of epileptics. Those with the lowest levels of manganese typically have the highest number of seizures. Best juice sources of manganese (in order of effectiveness): spinach, beet greens, Brussels sprouts, carrots, broccoli, cabbage, peaches, tangerines, beets, apples, oranges, and pears.

❥ **Selenium** is important in certain enzyme reactions that may play a role in protecting nerve cells from free-radical damage. Selenium deficiency may be an important triggering factor for seizures, and subsequent nerve damage, in people with epilepsy. Best juice sources of selenium (in order of effectiveness): chard, turnips, garlic, oranges, radishes, grapes, carrots, and cabbage.

❥ **Sodium,** known to many people as a substance to avoid, may actually help people who are prone to seizures. Studies have shown that epileptics with the lowest sodium concentrations in their bloodstreams have the highest number of seizures. I don't recommend that you increase your use of table salt (sodium chloride), but rather that you eat more fresh sodium-rich vegetables and drink their juices. Best juice sources of sodium (in order of effectiveness): chard, beets with greens, celery, spinach, watercress, turnips, carrots, parsley, sunflower sprouts, cabbage, garlic, and broccoli.

❥ **Vitamin B_6 (pyridoxine)** is important for the production of an amino acid called gamma-aminobutyric acid (GABA) in the brain. A reduction in GABA levels increases the chance of seizures. Some doctors have used an intravenous form of this vitamin for a week, followed by supplemental use, to completely control seizures in their patients. Best juice sources of vitamin B_6 (in order of effectiveness): kale, spinach, turnip greens, bell peppers, and prunes.

❥ **Zinc** levels have been shown in studies to be lower in epileptics than in other people. Best juice sources of zinc (in order of effectiveness): ginger root, turnips, parsley, garlic, carrots, grapes, spinach, cabbage, lettuce, cucumbers, and tangerines.

Juice Ingredient Recommendations

❥ **Parsley** juice is a good source of both sodium and zinc. Intake should be limited to a safe, therapeutic dose of $1/2$ to 1 cup per day. Parsley can be toxic in overdose, and should be especially avoided by pregnant women.

Juice Recipes

THE MORNING ENERGIZER

$1/2$ organic Red or Golden Delicious apple, washed

5 medium carrots, scrubbed well, green tops removed, ends trimmed

$1/2$ small beet with leaves and stems, scrubbed well

$1/2$ small or medium lemon, washed, or peeled if not organic

$1/2$- to 1-inch piece fresh ginger root, washed

Cut the apple into sections that will fit your juicer's feed tube. Juice the apple along with the carrots, beet, lemon, and ginger. Stir the juice, and pour into a glass. Serve at room temperature or chilled, as desired.

POPEYE'S POWER

$1/2$ medium organic apple, any kind, washed

1 handful organic spinach, washed

1 small handful parsley, rinsed

4 medium carrots, scrubbed well, green tops removed, ends trimmed

1 stalk organic celery with leaves, washed

$1/2$ beet with leaves, scrubbed well

Cut the apple into sections that will fit your juicer's feed tube. Bunch up the spinach and parsley, and push them through the feed tube with the apple, carrots, celery, and beet. Stir the juice, and pour into a glass. Serve at room temperature or chilled, as desired.

THE GINGER HOPPER

$1/2$ organic Red or Golden Delicious apple, washed

5 medium carrots, scrubbed well, green tops removed, ends trimmed

$1/2$- to 1-inch piece fresh ginger root, washed

Cut the apple into sections, and juice along with the carrots and ginger. Stir the juice, and pour into a glass. Serve at room temperature or chilled, as desired.

MORNING EXPRESS

1 orange, peeled
4–5 carrots, well scrubbed, green tops removed, ends trimmed

Divide the orange into segments that fit your juicer's feed tube, and juice with the carrots. Stir the juice, and pour into a glass. Serve at room temperature or chilled, as desired.

SWEET CALCIUM COCKTAIL

1 three-inch chunk fresh pineapple, scrubbed well or peeled if not organic
1–2 kale leaves, washed

Cut the pineapple into strips that fit your juicer's feed tube. Bunch up the kale, and push through the feed tube with the pineapple. Stir the juice, and pour into a glass. Serve at room temperature or chilled, as desired.

JUST PEACHY

1 ripe organic peach, washed, or peeled if not organic
1 pear, washed
$\frac{1}{2}$- to 1-inch piece fresh ginger root, washed

Cut the peach and pear into sections that fit your juicer's feed tube. Juice them along with the ginger. Stir the juice, and pour into a glass. Serve at room temperature or chilled, as desired.

WALDORF TWIST

1 organic Red or Golden Delicious apple, washed
3 stalks organic celery with leaves, washed
$\frac{1}{4}$ small or medium lemon, washed, or peeled if not organic

Cut the apple into sections that will fit your juicer's feed tube, and juice along with the celery and lemon. Stir the juice, and pour into a glass. Serve at room temperature or chilled, as desired.

Eye Disorders

The eye is subject to a number of disorders. Some, such as near- and far-sightedness, are produced by problems with the structure of the eye itself. Other disorders are caused by damage that accumulates over time, damage often caused by toxins called free radicals. Cataracts and macular degeneration are both damage-related disorders.

A cataract is a loss of transparency or a clouding of the eye's lens. This clouding is often caused by free-radical damage to some of the proteins and fats in the lens, damage that causes white spots to develop. When this happens, the lens cannot transmit light to the retina at the back of the eyeball, a situation that causes progressively blurred vision. Cataracts can result from eye diseases, surgery, or injury; systemic diseases; or exposure to ultraviolet light or radiation, or to toxins. Diabetics run an increased risk of cataract development (*see* **Diabetes Mellitus**). Cataracts affect about 50 percent of all Americans over age seventy-five.

Like cataracts, macular degeneration occurs more often in older people. This disorder is marked by damage to a spot called the macula, which lies at the center of the retina. In dry macular degeneration, the damage is caused by pigment deposits. In wet degeneration, the leakage of blood or other fluid causes scarring in the macula. Symptoms include dim or distorted vision, especially while reading, with a gradual loss of precise central vision and blank spots in the field of central vision. Systemic disease and toxin exposure contribute to macular degeneration.

Research indicates that a diet rich in antioxidants can help prevent and even, in some cases, partially reverse these disorders.

Lifestyle Recommendations

❥ **If you smoke, stop.** Tobacco contains significant amounts of cadmium, and high amounts of cadmium in the eye lens have been linked with both cataracts and macular degeneration. Cigarette smoke also is loaded with free radicals and aldehydes, which attack proteins and fats in the eye.

Diet Recommendations

❥ **Eat more fruits and vegetables, especially spinach and other dark leafy greens, and drink fresh juices.** Studies show that people who ate spinach and other dark greens five or more times per week reduced their risk of developing cataracts by between 47 and 65 percent. Dark greens and corn are rich in what is known as oxycarotenoids, specifically lutein and zeaxanthin, substances that are important antioxidants. In addition, tomatoes are associated with lower risk of cataracts. That's because tomatoes also contain carotenoids, and the carotenoid family in general is associated with a significantly reduced risk of macular degeneration (see the Nutrient Recommendations).

❥ **Reduce fat and salt intake.** Studies show an increased risk of cataracts is associated with elevated fat and salt consumption. A low-fat diet may offer protection from cataracts.

❥ **Avoid sweets.** Sugars promote osmotic pressure (swelling of the lens) and increase the risk of free-radical damage.

Nutrient Recommendations

❥ **Antioxidants** help fight degenerative eye disorders by limiting free-radical damage. In studies, people who have been treated for degeneration of the retina with high doses of beta-carotene and vitamin E have reported an improvement in vision. In other studies, patients with acute macular degeneration were treated with vitamin C, vitamin E, beta-carotene, and selenium; this treatment halted or reversed degenerative changes in 60 percent of the participants. The following antioxidants can help prevent, slow, halt, or even partially reverse degenerative eye problems:

- *Carotenes* destroy free radicals, and help prevent both cataracts and macular degeneration. A number of diverse studies show carotenes to be helpful in preventing and treating retinal disorders. One study shows that supplementation with vitamin A and carotenes can halt or reverse blindness in children with vitamin A deficiency, which shows a definite link between these substances and proper vision. *On a personal note:* I received a letter several years ago from a lady who said she had been declared legally blind, but once she started following the dietary program from my book *Juicing for Life* (see Appendix A), her vision was restored to normal. I can only speculate that she may have been deficient in vitamin A, and juicing the vegetables highest in beta-carotene, which the body uses to create vitamin A, restored her vision. Best juice sources of carotenes (in order of effectiveness): carrots, kale, parsley, spinach, chard, beet greens, watercress, mangoes, cantaloupes, apricots, broccoli, and romaine lettuce.

- *Glutathione* is a protein that plays an important role in protecting cells against free-radical damage. It has been shown to help prevent cataract formation. Best juice sources of glutathione: asparagus, broccoli, citrus fruit, peaches, strawberries, tomatoes, and watermelon.

- *Quercetin,* a bioflavonoid, can help prevent diabetic cataracts by decreasing the accumulation of sorbitol, a toxin formed from glucose, in the lens. Best juice sources of quercetin: berries, citrus fruit, and parsley.

- *Selenium* can, when taken in supplement form, restore the cellular activity of glutathione. Studies have shown that a large number of people with cataracts have low levels of selenium. Best juice sources of selenium (in order of effectiveness): chard, turnips, garlic, oranges, radishes, grapes, carrots, and cabbage.

- *Vitamin C* can slow the development of both cataracts and macular degeneration. The Nurses Health Study, conducted through Tufts University, found that those nurses who supplemented their diet with vitamin C for at least ten years had the lowest prevalence of cataracts. Best juice sources of vitamin C (in order of effectiveness): kale, parsley, broccoli, Brussels sprouts, watercress, cauliflower, cabbage, strawberries, papaya, spinach, citrus fruit, turnips, mangoes, asparagus, and cantaloupes.

- *Vitamin E* helps prevent both cataracts and macular degeneration. It is also helpful in halting and reversing the progress of these conditions. Best juice sources of vitamin E (in order of effectiveness): spinach, watercress, asparagus, carrots, and tomatoes.

Herb Recommendations

❧ Curcumin is a phytonutrient that helps protect the eye lens from degeneration. It is available in supplement form, and is present in both ginger root and turmeric.

Juice Ingredient Recommendations

❧ Apricot juice helps improve eyesight.

❧ Carrot juice is very helpful for strengthening the eyes and improving vision.

Juice Recipes

APRICOT NECTAR

2 organic apples, any kind, washed
2 apricots, washed, pits removed

Cut the apples and apricots into sections that fit your juicer's feed tube, and juice. Stir the juice, and pour into a glass. Serve at room temperature or chilled, as desired.

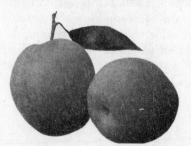

THE MORNING ENERGIZER

½ organic Red or Golden Delicious apple, washed

5 medium carrots, scrubbed well, green tops removed, ends trimmed

½ small beet with leaves and stems, scrubbed well

½ small or medium lemon, washed, or peeled if not organic

½- to 1-inch piece fresh ginger root, washed

Cut the apple into sections that will fit your juicer's feed tube. Juice the apple along with the carrots, beet, lemon, and ginger. Stir the juice, and pour into a glass. Serve at room temperature or chilled, as desired.

THE GINGER HOPPER

½ organic Red or Golden Delicious apple, washed

5 medium carrots, scrubbed well, green tops removed, ends trimmed

½- to 1-inch piece fresh ginger root, washed

Cut the apple into sections, and juice along with the carrots and ginger. Stir the juice, and pour into a glass. Serve at room temperature or chilled, as desired.

MORNING EXPRESS

1 orange, peeled

4–5 carrots, well scrubbed, green tops removed, ends trimmed

Divide the orange into segments that fit your juicer's feed tube, and juice with the carrots. Stir the juice, and pour into a glass. Serve at room temperature or chilled, as desired.

TURNIP TIME

1 turnip, scrubbed well

2-inch piece jicama, scrubbed well or peeled if not organic (optional)

1 handful watercress, rinsed

4 carrots, scrubbed well, green tops removed, ends trimmed

1 garlic clove with peel, washed

½ small or medium lemon, washed, or peeled if not organic

Cut the turnip and jicama (if using) into strips that fit your juicer's feed tube. Bunch up the watercress, and push through the feed tube with the turnip, jicama, carrots, garlic, and lemon. Stir the juice, and pour into a glass. Serve at room temperature or chilled, as desired.

ANTIAGING COCKTAIL

1 small bunch organic purple grapes (about 1 cup) with small stems* and seeds, washed

1/2 cup blueberries, blackberries, or raspberries, washed

1/4 small or medium lemon, washed, or peeled if not organic

1/2-inch piece fresh ginger root, washed

*Large stems can dull your juicer's blade.

Juice the grapes, berries, lemon, and ginger. Stir the juice, and pour into a glass. Serve at room temperature or chilled, as desired.

Fibrocystic Breast Disease

Fibrocystic breast disease (FBD) is a benign cystic condition of the breasts that is fairly common, especially among women from the ages of thirty to fifty. The lumps that characterize FBD can be either firm or soft, and move freely beneath the skin. These lumps form when fibrous tissue surrounds cysts and thickens like scar tissue, which causes pain. There is rapid fluctuation in the size of the masses at different times in a woman's hormonal cycle, with tenderness and lumpiness often increasing during the premenstrual phase. Symptoms vary in severity, ranging from mild discomfort to severe pain.

FBD is usually caused by a hormone imbalance. High estrogen levels can cause excess breast tissue growth, especially if the body doesn't produce enough progesterone, a hormone that limits estrogen's activity. Excess dietary estrogens have been implicated in FBD—women who eat meat have estrogen levels that are 50 percent higher than those found in vegetarian women. While all animal protein contains some estrogen, this problem is intensified when cows, chickens, and turkeys are fed hormone growth stimulants, as this causes estrogens to be passed on to people when the meat is ingested. Iodine deficiency and abnormal breast milk production have also been linked to FBD.

A diet that reduces estrogen levels can help ease the pain and discomfort of FBD. You should note that while most breast lumps are benign, *any* lumps within the breast should be brought to a doctor's attention.

Diet Recommendations

❥ **Eat a low-saturated-fat, high-complex-carbohydrate diet.** This diet should be mostly vegetarian, except for fish. (If you can find organically grown meat, chicken, or turkey, eating small amounts of these foods occasionally may be acceptable once the FBD is controlled.) The idea is to exclude dietary animal estrogens. In addition, a diet that consists of whole grains, vegetables, fruit, and legumes has been shown to decrease symptoms of premenstrual breast tenderness and swelling (*see also* **Menstrual Disorders**). The fiber in such a diet is beneficial because fiber decreases the time it takes food to move through the colon. The longer waste material stays in the intestinal tract, the more estrogen is reabsorbed into the bloodstream. For more information, see Basic Guidelines for the Juice Lady's Health and Healing Diet (page 313).

❥ **Eat more soy products.** Soy foods include tofu, tempeh, miso, and soy milk. Studies show that the phytoestrogens, or plant-based estrogens, in soy products stabilize estrogen levels in the body.

❥ **Avoid caffeine.** Caffeine is known to stimulate overproduction of fibrous tissue and cyst fluid. Caffeine is found in coffee, black and green tea, chocolate, cola, and some medications. One study showed nearly a 98-percent improvement in women with FBD who eliminated caffeine from their diets.

❥ **Use juice fasting and liver cleansing.** Juice fasting will help to cleanse the system and also give it a complete rest from all animal estrogens. In addition, cleansing the liver can help alleviate FBD symptoms. See the Juice Fast (page 324) and the Liver Cleanse (page 333).

Nutrient Recommendations

❥ **Iodine** is required by the body for production of thyroid hormone, and there is an association between low thyroid function and FBD. Iodine is especially abundant in seafood, fish, and sea vegetables. Best juice sources of iodine (in order of effectiveness): pineapple, lettuce, spinach, and green bell pepper.

❥ **Vitamin A** has helped reduce breast pain and decrease breast cysts in some women. The body can convert beta-carotene, found in fruits and vegetables, to vitamin A. Best juice sources of beta-carotene (in order of effectiveness): carrots, kale, parsley, spinach, chard, beet greens, watercress, mangoes, cantaloupes, apricots, broccoli, and romaine lettuce.

❥ **Vitamin E** works to ease fibrocystic disease by normalizing abnormal hormone levels. Best juice sources of vitamin E (in order of effectiveness): spinach, watercress, asparagus, carrots, and tomatoes.

Herb Recommendations

🌶 **Gotu kola** has been used by naturopaths to treat FBD.

🌶 **Vitex agnus castus,** also known as chaste tree fruit, has been shown to normalize hormone levels.

Juice Ingredient Recommendations

🌶 **Asparagus, cantaloupe (with seeds), cucumber, lemon, parsley,** and **watermelon** juices are natural diuretics, or substances that remove excess water from the body.

🌶 **Beet** juice is a good liver cleanser, as is the juice of artichoke leaf.

🌶 **Parsley** juice is a rich source of beta-carotene. Intake should be limited to a safe, therapeutic dose of $1/2$ to 1 cup per day. Parsley can be toxic in overdose, and should be especially avoided by pregnant women.

Juice Recipes

THE MORNING ENERGIZER

$1/2$ organic Red or Golden Delicious apple, washed

5 medium carrots, scrubbed well, green tops removed, ends trimmed

$1/2$ small beet with leaves and stems, scrubbed well

$1/2$ small or medium lemon, washed, or peeled if not organic

$1/2$- to 1-inch piece fresh ginger root, washed

Cut the apple into sections that will fit your juicer's feed tube. Juice the apple along with the carrots, beet, lemon, and ginger. Stir the juice, and pour into a glass. Serve at room temperature or chilled, as desired.

WATERMELON REFRESHER

1-inch slice watermelon, with seeds and well-scrubbed rind

Cut the watermelon into strips that fit your juicer's feed tube. Juice the watermelon, and pour into a glass. Serve at room temperature or chilled, as desired.

STRAWBERRY-CANTALOUPE COCKTAIL

½ ripe organic cantaloupe with seeds, washed, or peeled if not organic

1 cup organic strawberries, washed

Cut the cantaloupe into strips that fit your juicer's feed tube. Juice the cantaloupe and strawberries; stir the juice and pour into a glass. Serve at room temperature or chilled, as desired.

AFTERNOON REFRESHER

1 medium to large organic cucumber, scrubbed well

½ small or medium lemon, washed, or peeled if not organic

Cut the cucumber in half lengthwise, and juice with the lemon. (For an especially cooling version, let the juice splash over a few ice cubes in the juice pitcher.) Stir the juice, and pour into a glass. Serve at room temperature or chilled, as desired.

NATURAL DIURETIC COCKTAIL

1 medium vine-ripened tomato, washed

1 small handful parsley, rinsed

1 organic cucumber, scrubbed well

4 asparagus stems, washed

½ small or medium lemon, washed, or peeled if not organic

Cut the tomato into sections that fit your juicer's feed tube. Bunch up the parsley and juice with the cucumber, asparagus, and lemon. Stir the juice, and pour into a glass. Serve at room temperature or chilled, as desired.

MAGNESIUM SPECIAL

5 medium carrots, scrubbed well, green tops removed, ends trimmed

2 stalks organic celery with leaves, washed

½ small beet with leaves and stems, scrubbed well

2 broccoli florets, washed

½ small or medium lemon, washed, or peeled if not organic

Juice the carrots, celery, beet, broccoli, and lemon. Stir the juice, and pour into a glass. Serve at room temperature or chilled, as desired.

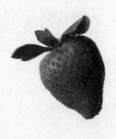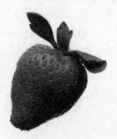

BEAUTIFUL BONE SOLUTION

1 organic Golden or Red Delicious apple, washed

1–2 kale leaves, washed

1 handful parsley, rinsed

1 stalk organic celery, washed

¼ small or medium lemon, washed, or peeled if not organic

½- to 1-inch piece fresh ginger root, washed

Cut the apple into sections that fit your juicer's feed tube. Bunch up the kale and parsley, and push through the feed tube with the apple, celery, lemon, and ginger. Stir the juice, and pour into a glass. Serve at room temperature or chilled, as desired.

POPEYE'S POWER

½ medium organic apple, any kind, washed

1 handful organic spinach, washed

1 small handful parsley, rinsed

4 medium carrots, scrubbed well, green tops removed, ends trimmed

1 stalk organic celery with leaves, washed

½ beet with leaves, scrubbed well

Cut the apple into sections that will fit your juicer's feed tube. Bunch up the spinach and parsley, and push them through the feed tube with the apple, carrots, celery, and beet. Stir the juice, and pour into a glass. Serve at room temperature or chilled, as desired.

SWEET CALCIUM COCKTAIL

1 three-inch chunk fresh pineapple, scrubbed well or peeled if not organic

1–2 kale leaves, washed

Cut the pineapple into strips that fit your juicer's feed tube. Bunch up the kale, and push through the feed tube with the pineapple. Stir the juice, and pour into a glass. Serve at room temperature or chilled, as desired.

Fibromyalgia

The symptoms of fibromyalgia are similar to those of chronic fatigue syndrome (CFS; *see* **Chronic Fatigue Syndrome**), with the major difference between the disorders being the musculoskeletal pain associated with fibromyalgia. Symptoms include aches or stiffness that lasts for at least three months and the existence of six or more tender points. These tender points, or points sensitive to pressure, usually occur in specific areas of the back, buttocks, elbows, knees, neck, rib cage, and thighs. The pain is accompanied by at least four of the following symptoms: fatigue, chronic headache, sleep disturbances, neurological and psychological complaints, joint swelling, tingling sensations or numbness, and irritable bowel syndrome (*see* **Colitis**).

Like CFS, fibromyalgia is more common among women than men, generally women between the ages of twenty and fifty. Also like CFS, there is no definitive test for fibromyalgia, with the diagnosis being made on the basis of the symptoms and after other disorders are ruled out. Symptoms of fibromyalgia can be triggered or aggravated by a number of conditions, including overwork, depression or anxiety, and fluctuations in temperature or humidity levels. The cause of fibromyalgia is unknown, but evidence points to both immune- and nervous-system factors.

Good nutrition is important in fighting any disease, but especially if you are dealing with a condition as difficult to treat as fibromyalgia. Making the dietary changes suggested here can go a long way in helping you recover.

Diet Recommendations

❥ **Avoid simple carbohydrates (sugar and white flour).** It has been found that a significant percentage of fibromyalgia patients have hypoglycemia, or low blood sugar (*see* **Hypoglycemia**), and do not tolerate carbohydrates well. You should eliminate all sweets, such as cakes, pies, frozen yogurt, candy, cookies, and ice cream; all fruit juice (it's too high in fruit sugars); and all refined (white) flour products, such as bread, rolls, and pasta. Completely avoid alcohol and caffeine; alcohol blocks proper glucose (blood sugar) usage, and caffeine alters glucose levels. Limit fruit intake to no more than one or two servings per day. Increase vegetable and protein servings, and choose only whole-grain products. Correction of this condition may lie as much in what you avoid eating as in what you consume. For more information on healthy eating, see Basic Guidelines for the Juice Lady's Health and Healing Diet (page 313). *On a personal note:* Several years ago, while on a lecture tour, I started drinking more of the fruit juices I made on stage. I was thirsty and they were available. I have hypoglycemia and had previously avoided almost all simple carbohydrates, but I was feeling so healthy that I thought myself "invincible" to sugar imbalances. In less than a year, I had developed a full-blown case of fibromyalgia, and my CFS had returned. I felt like nearly every point on my body was a tender spot. I identified the problem and eliminated all fruit juice, as well as all other simple carbohydrates, from my diet. It took about a year to recover. Needless to say, I don't add any fruit (except lemon or lime) to my juices nor do I eat fruit or *anything* sweet.

❥ **Use juices and juice fasting.** Vegetable juices can help tremendously in healing the aching soreness. I suggest three to four glasses per day. Omit the fruit in all recipes, except for lemon or lime (unless they bother you as well). Also, a short vegetable-juice fast of one to three days can be very healing (see the Juice Fast, page 324). I recommend the Optimum Health Institute (OHI) of San Diego or Austin for a very effective juice fast program (see Appendix A). I go there often, and after one week I feel transformed.

Nutrient Recommendations

❥ **Magnesium** levels in fibromyalgia patients have been found to be significantly lower than average. Also, enzymes that depend on vitamin B_1 (see the B_1 entry on this list) require an adequate supply of magnesium. Best juice sources of magnesium (in order of effectiveness): beet greens, spinach, parsley, dandelion greens, garlic, beets, broccoli, cauliflower, carrots, and celery.

❥ **Vitamin B_1 (thiamine)** has helped a number of fibromyalgia sufferers, according to investigative reports. Best food sources of vitamin B_1 (in order of effectiveness): seeds, nuts, beans, split peas, millet, buckwheat, whole wheat, oatmeal, wild rice, lobster, and cornmeal. It can also be found, in lesser quantities, in sunflower and buckwheat sprouts, and garlic. It is not found in fruits and vegetables.

Herb Recommendations

❥ **Burdock** can cleanse the lymphatic system and bloodstream.

❥ **Devil's claw** can reduce inflammation and pain.

❥ **Echinacea** can enhance the immune system.

❥ **Valerian** can improve sleep.

Juice Ingredient Recommendations

❥ **Fennel** juice has been used as a traditional tonic to help release endorphins into the bloodstream. Endorphins create a mood of euphoria, and help dampen anxiety and fear.

❥ **Garlic** juice offers a healthy amount of vitamin B_1, and has antibiotic properties.

❥ **Parsley** juice contains magnesium. Intake should be limited to a safe, therapeutic dose of $1/2$ to 1 cup per day. Parsley can be toxic in overdose, and should be especially avoided by pregnant women.

❥ **Sprout** juice provides the most concentrated natural sources of vitamins, minerals, enzymes, and amino acids. Sprouts are considered by many one of nature's most perfect healing foods.

Juice Recipes

THE FEEL GOOD COCKTAIL

4 medium carrots, scrubbed well, green tops removed, ends trimmed

3 fennel stalks with leaves and flowers, washed

1 stalk organic celery with leaves, washed

$1/2$ small or medium lemon, washed, or peeled if not organic

Juice the carrots, fennel, celery, and lemon. Stir the juice, and pour into a glass. Serve at room temperature or chilled, as desired.

ANTIVIRAL COCKTAIL

1 organic Granny Smith or Pippin apple, washed

1 turnip, scrubbed well

1 handful watercress, rinsed

5 carrots, scrubbed well, green tops removed, ends trimmed

1 large garlic clove with peel, washed

Cut the apple and turnip into sections that fit your juicer's feed tube. Bunch up the watercress, and juice it with the apple, turnip, carrots, and garlic. Stir the juice, and pour into a glass. Serve at room temperature or chilled, as desired.

TURNIP TIME

1 turnip, scrubbed well

2-inch piece jicama, scrubbed well or peeled if not organic (optional)

1 handful watercress, rinsed

4 carrots, scrubbed well, green tops removed, ends trimmed

1 garlic clove with peel, washed

$1/2$ small or medium lemon, washed, or peeled if not organic

Cut the turnip and jicama (if using) into strips that fit your juicer's feed tube. Bunch up the watercress, and push through the feed tube with the turnip, jicama, carrots, garlic, and lemon. Stir the juice, and pour into a glass. Serve at room temperature or chilled, as desired.

PURE GREEN SPROUT DRINK

1 organic cucumber, scrubbed well

1 large handful sunflower sprouts, rinsed

1 small handful buckwheat sprouts, rinsed

1 small handful clover sprouts, rinsed

Cut the cucumber in half lengthwise. Bunch up the sprouts, and push through the feed tube with the cucumber. Stir the juice, and pour into a glass. Serve at room temperature or chilled, as desired.

MAGNESIUM SPECIAL

5 medium carrots, scrubbed well, green tops removed, ends trimmed

2 stalks organic celery with leaves, washed

$1/2$ small beet with leaves and stems, scrubbed well

2 broccoli florets, washed

$1/2$ small or medium lemon, washed, or peeled if not organic

Juice the carrots, celery, beet, broccoli, and lemon. Stir the juice, and pour into a glass. Serve at room temperature or chilled, as desired.

PARSLEY PEP

1 small bunch parsley, rinsed

2 stalks organic celery with leaves, washed

2 large carrots, scrubbed well, green tops removed, ends trimmed

$1/2$ small or medium lemon, washed, or peeled if not organic

Bunch up the parsley, and push it through the feed tube with the celery, carrots, and lemon. Stir the juice, and pour it into a glass. Serve at room temperature or chilled, as desired.

THE MORNING ENERGIZER

5 medium carrots, scrubbed well, green tops removed, ends trimmed

$1/2$ small beet with leaves and stems, scrubbed well

$1/2$ small or medium lemon, washed, or peeled if not organic

$1/2$- to 1-inch piece fresh ginger root, washed

Juice the carrots, beet, lemon, and ginger. Stir the juice, and pour into a glass. Serve at room temperature, or chilled, as desired.

AFTERNOON REFRESHER

1 medium to large organic cucumber, scrubbed well

½ small or medium lemon, washed, or peeled if not organic

Cut the cucumber in half lengthwise, and juice with the lemon. (For an especially cooling version, let the juice splash over a few ice cubes in the juice pitcher.) Stir the juice, and pour into a glass. Serve at room temperature or chilled, as desired.

TOMATO FLORENTINE

1 vine-ripened tomato, washed

1 handful organic spinach, washed

2–3 fresh basil leaves (optional)

½ small or medium lemon, washed, or peeled if not organic

Cut the tomato into sections that will fit your juicer's feed tube. Bunch up the spinach and basil leaves (if using), and push through the feed tube with the tomato and lemon. Stir the juice, and pour into a glass. Serve at room temperature or chilled, as desired.

SPICY TOMATO ON ICE

2 vine-ripened tomatoes, washed

2 dark green lettuce leaves, such as romaine or green leaf, washed

1 small handful parsley, rinsed

2 radishes with green tops, washed

½ small or medium lime or lemon, washed, or peeled if not organic

Dash hot sauce

Cut the tomato in sections that fit your juicer's feed tube. Bunch up the lettuce leaves and parsley, and push them through the feed tube with the tomatoes, radishes, and lime or lemon. Add a dash of hot sauce, and stir to combine. Pour into tall, ice-filled glasses.

THYROID TONIC

5 carrots, scrubbed well, green tops removed, ends trimmed

5–6 radishes with green tops, washed

½ small or medium lemon, washed, or peeled if not organic

Juice the carrots, radishes, and lemon. Stir the juice, and pour into a glass. Serve at room temperature or chilled, as desired.

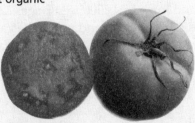

Gallstones

Located directly under the liver, the gallbladder is a small, pear-shaped sac that functions as a reservoir for the bile (created by the liver) that the body uses to digest fats. The gallbladder is connected to the liver and intestines by tiny ducts, called bile ducts. Hard, rocklike accumulations called gallstones can form in the gallbladder and bile ducts. Stones generally form when cholesterol combines with calcium salts and with bile salts and pigments. Gallstones occur more often in women than in men, and a person's chances of developing gallstones increase with age.

Often, gallstones are "silent" and produce no symptoms at all. But a stone can block a bile duct, which usually produces nausea, vomiting, and severe pain that may last for several hours. These symptoms often appear after a high-fat meal. If the gallbladder becomes inflamed, there is severe pain in the upper right abdomen, accompanied by nausea, vomiting, and fever. (This condition must be treated immediately, or it can become life-threatening.) Obesity (*see* **Overweight/Obesity**) is associated with gallstones, as is rapid weight loss caused by a very-low-calorie diet.

Diet Recommendations

❥ **Aim for a diet in which 50 to 75 percent of what you eat consists of high-fiber, low-fat foods, such as raw fruits, vegetables, sprouts, juices, nuts, and seeds.** Include plenty of dark leafy green salads, beets, apples, whole grains, olive oil, and fish, plus a moderate number of organic eggs. A considerable amount of research suggests that a fiber-depleted, refined-foods diet contributes to gallstone development. For more information on healthy eating, see Basic Guidelines for the Juice Lady's Health and Healing Diet (page 313).

❥ **Drink plenty of fresh juices.** Apple, pear, beet, carrot, and lemon juices are all very good. These juices help cleanse the liver and colon, which improves gallbladder function.

❥ **Detoxify your system through cleansing programs.** Follow the Gallbladder, Liver, Kidney, and Intestinal Cleanses (pages 328 to 338). The gallbladder flush can help dissolve stones and purge the gallbladder, a detoxification plan for the liver and colon will support the gallbladder, and the kidney cleanse helps support the liver cleansing program.

❥ **Eat a low-fat diet.** Avoid all animal fat, meat, fried foods, commercial oils, margarine, and spicy foods. Use extra virgin, unrefined olive oil or flaxseed oil.

❥ **Avoid all sweets and refined flours.** Studies show that sugar consumption is higher among people with gallstones. Sugars may influence gallstone composition. Eliminate all sweets, including chocolate, cake, candy, cookies, pie, ice cream, frozen yogurt, and soft drinks. Also avoid refined (white) flour products, including bread, rolls, and pasta. Choose only whole-grain products, including whole-grain pasta (available at health food stores).

❥ **Prevent constipation.** Studies show that transit time, the time it takes food to move through the intestinal tract, is much slower among women with gallstones and could be a contributing factor to gallstone formation. *See* **Constipation.**

Nutrient Recommendations

❥ **Vitamin C** can help prevent gallstone formation. Best juice sources of vitamin C (in order of effectiveness): kale, parsley, broccoli, Brussels sprouts, watercress, cauliflower, cabbage, strawberries, papaya, spinach, citrus fruit, turnips, mangoes, asparagus, and cantaloupes.

Herb Recommendations

❥ **Milk thistle (silymarin)** has been used in traditional medicine to cleanse and support the liver.

Juice Ingredient Recommendations

❥ **Apple** and **spinach** juices are helpful in preventing constipation, and are good for the colon and gallbladder.

❥ **Beet, dandelion,** and **lemon** juices have been used by naturopaths to cleanse the liver.

❥ **Carrot, beet,** and **cucumber** juices have traditionally been used to cleanse the gallbladder.

❥ **Daikon radish** juice is used in Traditional Chinese Medicine to help eliminate excess fat from the body.

❥ **Papaya** and **mango** juices contain enzymes that aid digestion.

❥ **Parsley** juice is a good source of vitamin C. Intake should be limited to a safe, therapeutic dose of $1/2$ to 1 cup per day. Parsley can be toxic in overdose, and should be especially avoided by pregnant women.

❥ **Pear** juice is helpful for preventing constipation, and is good for the gallbladder.

Juice Recipes

THE COLON CLEANSER

2 organic Granny Smith, McIntosh, or Golden Delicious apples, washed

1 bunch organic spinach, washed

1 handful parsley, rinsed

¼ small or medium lemon, washed, or peeled if not organic

Cut the apples into sections that fit your juicer's feed tube. Bunch up the spinach and parsley, and push them through the feed tube with the apples and lemon. Stir the juice, and pour into a glass. Serve at room temperature or chilled, as desired.

THE MORNING ENERGIZER

½ organic Red or Golden Delicious apple, washed

5 medium carrots, scrubbed well, green tops removed, ends trimmed

½ small beet with leaves and stems, scrubbed well

½ small or medium lemon, washed, or peeled if not organic

½- to 1-inch piece fresh ginger root, washed

Cut the apple into sections that will fit your juicer's feed tube. Juice the apple along with the carrots, beet, lemon, and ginger. Stir the juice, and pour into a glass. Serve at room temperature or chilled, as desired.

LIVER LIFE TONIC

½ organic green apple such as Granny Smith or Pippin, washed

1 handful dandelion greens, washed

5 carrots, scrubbed well, green tops removed, ends trimmed

½ small lemon, washed, or peeled if not organic

Cut the apple into wedges that will fit your juicer's feed tube. Bunch up the dandelion greens, and push through the feed tube with the apple, carrots, and lemon. Stir the juice, and pour into a glass. Serve at room temperature or chilled, as desired.

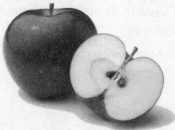

GALLBLADDER CLEANSING COCKTAIL

½ organic cucumber, scrubbed well

5 carrots, scrubbed well, green tops removed, ends trimmed

½ small to medium beet with leaves and stems, scrubbed well

½ small or medium lemon, washed, or peeled if not organic

Slice the cucumber in half again lengthwise, and juice with the carrots, beet, and lemon. Stir the juice, and pour into a glass. Serve at room temperature or chilled, as desired.

ORIENT EXPRESS

2-inch chunk jicama, scrubbed, or peeled if not organic (optional)

5 carrots, scrubbed well, green tops removed, ends trimmed

2-inch piece daikon radish, scrubbed well, without green top or end

½-inch piece fresh ginger root, washed

Cut the jicama into strips (if using) that fit your juicer's feed tube. Juice the jicama with the carrots, radish, and ginger. Stir the juice, and pour into a glass. Serve at room temperature. This is a very hot-tasting drink because of the radish and ginger, so you may want to dilute it by half with water.

TROPICAL SUNRISE

1 three-inch chunk fresh pineapple, scrubbed well or peeled if not organic

1 ripe medium banana, peeled

½ medium papaya, peeled and seeded

½ cup plain or vanilla soy milk, or lowfat dairy milk

¼ teaspoon pure vanilla extract

6 ice cubes

Cut the pineapple into strips that fit your juicer's feed tube, and juice the strips. Pour the juice into a blender, and add the banana, papaya, milk, vanilla, and ice cubes; blend until smooth. Pour the mixture into two glasses and serve immediately.

DIGESTIVE TONIC

½ pear, washed

½ organic apple, any kind, washed

5 carrots, scrubbed well, green tops removed, ends trimmed

Cut the pear and apple into sections that fit your juicer's feed tube. Juice them with the carrots. Stir the juice, and pour into a glass. Serve at room temperature or chilled, as desired.

SWEET & REGULAR

1 pear, washed
1 organic apple, any kind, washed

Cut the pear and apple into sections that fit your juicer's feed tube, and juice them. Stir the juice, and pour into a glass. Serve at room temperature or chilled, as desired.

THE GINGER HOPPER

½ organic Red or Golden Delicious
  apple, washed
5 medium carrots, scrubbed well,
  green tops removed, ends trimmed
½- to 1-inch piece fresh ginger root,
  washed

Cut the apple into sections, and juice along with the carrots and ginger. Stir the juice, and pour into a glass. Serve at room temperature or chilled, as desired.

MAGNESIUM SPECIAL

5 medium carrots, scrubbed well,
  green tops removed, ends trimmed
2 stalks organic celery with leaves,
  washed
½ small beet with leaves and stems,
  scrubbed well
2 broccoli florets, washed
½ small or medium lemon, washed,
  or peeled if not organic

Juice the carrots, celery, beet, broccoli, and lemon. Stir the juice, and pour into a glass. Serve at room temperature or chilled, as desired.

PURE GREEN SPROUT DRINK

1 organic cucumber, scrubbed well
1 large handful sunflower sprouts,
  rinsed
1 small handful buckwheat sprouts,
  rinsed
1 small handful clover sprouts, rinsed

Cut the cucumber in half lengthwise. Bunch up the sprouts, and push through the feed tube with the cucumber. Stir the juice, and pour into a glass. Serve at room temperature or chilled, as desired.

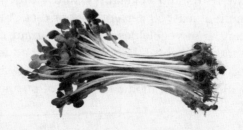

MANGO MON

1 ripe mango, peeled	*Cut the mango flesh away from the pit,*
1 orange, peeled, divided into segments	*and add it to a blender with the*
	orange, banana, and ice cubes. Blend
1 ripe banana, peeled	*until smooth, pour into two glasses,*
6 ice cubes	*and serve.*

Gout

One of the oldest conditions in recorded medical history, gout is a painful arthritic disorder. It is caused by a substance called uric acid, which is produced when the body processes protein-based substances called purines. In gout, the body produces excess uric acid and/or is unable to eliminate uric acid—blood levels of this chemical can reach three to fifteen times the normal level. Excess uric acid crystallizes in the joints and in other tissues. There, it acts as an abrasive, and causes swelling and intense pain. The first joint of the big toe is most often affected, although gout can also attack the ankle, elbow, instep, knee, and wrist. The skin over the affected joint becomes reddish and shiny, and is warm to the touch. Fever, chills, and general malaise often accompany the attack. Gout usually occurs in middle age, and a tendency to develop this disorder runs in some families.

Attacks often occur in the night after a person overeats such purine-rich foods as meat, poultry, fish, alcohol, fried foods, and rich pastries. (Because this diet was beyond the means of most people until the middle of the twentieth century, gout is often called "the rich man's disease.") As the disease progresses, more joints can be affected, attacks can last for longer periods of time, and deformities can develop. There is also a higher risk of kidney dysfunction and kidney stones.

Diet Recommendations

❥ **Eat plenty of raw fruits and vegetables.** Raw fruits, vegetables, and juices should make up at least 50 percent of your diet. A large portion of your diet should consist of vegetables and whole grains, such as brown rice, millet, barley, and buckwheat. Popcorn (without added butter or oil) makes a good snack. Limit your consumption of spinach, asparagus, peas, and mushrooms, which contain moderate levels of purines, and of dried legumes, which contain moderately high levels of purines. For more information, see Basic Guidelines for the Juice Lady's Health and Healing Diet (page 313).

❥ **Avoid all red meat, poultry, fried foods, and fish, especially shellfish, sardines, anchovies, herring, and fish roe.** These foods contain high amount of purines. Also omit gravy, consommé, concentrated sweets, rich pastries, cakes, and pies from your diet. Avoid all white flour products and sugar.

❥ **Restrict fat consumption.** Fats are believed to reduce the normal excretion of uric acid.

❥ **Avoid all alcohol.** Ethanol increases the production of uric acid. Studies of gout sufferers show that many patients consume above-average amounts of alcohol.

❥ **Avoid fruit sugar.** Fruit sugar, or fructose, increases uric acid production. Limit your consumption of fruit juices, except for cherry and strawberry juice.

❥ **Eat half a pound of cherries each day.** Or drink the equivalent in cherry juice every day. Studies show that people with gout who consumed the cherry diet daily had no attacks of gout, and their blood levels of uric acid were reduced to normal. A number of patients reported greater freedom of movement in finger and toe joints. Dark-colored or yellow, sweet or sour—all varieties appear to be equally effective. The effective ingredient in cherries is not known, but keracyanin, the coloring pigment, is suspected to be the beneficial agent. Strawberry and celery juices have also been found to be beneficial.

Nutrient Recommendations

❥ **Vitamin C** may help lower serum uric acid by increasing its excretion. Megadoses of supplemental vitamin C are not recommended, as they can increase uric acid levels in some individuals. Best juice sources of vitamin C (in order of effectiveness): kale, parsley, broccoli, Brussels sprouts, watercress, cauliflower, cabbage, strawberries, citrus fruit, and turnips.

Herb Recommendations

❥ **Couch grass, English ivy (woodbind), horsetail,** and **primrose (cowslip)** have all been used in folk medicine for gout, although the actions of none of these herbs has been scientifically documented.

Juice Ingredient Recommendations

❧ **Cherry** juice contains gout-fighting compounds; strawberry and celery juices have also been found to be beneficial.

❧ **Ginger** juice is an anti-inflammatory agent.

❧ **Parsley** juice is a very good source of vitamin C. Intake should be limited to a safe, therapeutic dose of $1/2$ to 1 cup per day. Parsley can be toxic in overdose, and should be especially avoided by pregnant women.

❧ **Water** can be added to any of the recipes below in order to reduce concentrations of fruit sugar.

Juice Recipes

GOUT-FIGHTING TONIC

$1/2$ small organic green apple, such as Granny Smith or Pippin, washed

$1/2$ pound organic cherries, washed, pits removed

1 cup organic strawberries with caps, washed

Cut the apple in half, and juice with the cherries and strawberries. Stir the juice, and pour into a glass. Serve at room temperature or chilled, as desired.

WALDORF TWIST

1 organic Granny Smith or Pippin apple, washed

3 stalks organic celery with leaves, washed

$1/4$ small or medium lemon, washed, or peeled if not organic

Cut the apple into sections that will fit your juicer's feed tube, and juice along with the celery and lemon. Stir the juice, and pour into a glass. Serve at room temperature or chilled, as desired.

THE GINGER HOPPER

$1/2$ organic Granny Smith or Pippin apple, washed

5 medium carrots, scrubbed well, green tops removed, ends trimmed

$1/2$- to 1-inch piece fresh ginger root, washed

Cut the apple into sections, and juice along with the carrots and ginger. Stir the juice, and pour into a glass. Serve at room temperature or chilled, as desired.

GINGER TWIST

1 handful parsley, rinsed

5 carrots, scrubbed well, green tops removed, ends trimmed

1-inch piece fresh ginger root, washed

1/2 small or medium lemon, washed, or peeled if not organic

Bunch up the parsley and push it through the feed tube with the carrots, ginger, and lemon. Stir the juice, and pour into a glass. Serve at room temperature or chilled, as desired.

BEAUTIFUL BONE SOLUTION

1 organic Granny Smith or Pippin apple, washed

1–2 kale leaves, washed

1 handful parsley, rinsed

1 stalk organic celery, washed

1/4 small or medium lemon, washed, or peeled if not organic

1/2- to 1-inch piece fresh ginger root, washed

Cut the apple into sections that fit your juicer's feed tube. Bunch up the kale and parsley, and push through the feed tube with the apple, celery, lemon, and ginger. Stir the juice, and pour into a glass. Serve at room temperature or chilled, as desired.

WEIGHT-LOSS EXPRESS

1/2 organic cucumber, scrubbed well

1/2 small organic green apple, such as Granny Smith or Pippin, washed

1 small handful parsley, rinsed

5 medium carrots, scrubbed well, green tops removed, ends trimmed

1/4 small or medium lemon, washed, or peeled if not organic

1-inch piece fresh ginger root, washed

Cut the cucumber in half lengthwise and the apple into sections that fit your juicer's feed tube. Bunch up the parsley, and push through the feed tube with the cucumber, apple, carrots, lemon, and ginger. Stir the juice, and pour into a glass. Serve at room temperature or chilled, as desired.

Heart Disease

See **Cardiovascular Disease.**

Hemorrhoids

See **Varicose Veins and Hemorrhoids.**

Herpes

There are several types of herpesviruses, but the most common types are herpes simplex 1 and 2. Type 1 herpes (HSV-1) is most commonly seen as cold sores on the lips, while type 2 (HSV-2) is most commonly found in the genital area, and is also known as genital herpes. Both types cause painful, highly contagious blisters that occur either singly or in multiple clusters. The development of the blisters is often preceded by a burning or itching sensation; the initial infection may be accompanied by mild fever.

After entering the body, the herpesvirus never leaves, although it may be dormant for long periods of time. Recurrences of HSV-1 may be triggered by certain foods, fever, colds, allergies, sunburn, and menstruation. Recurrences of HSV-2 may be triggered by illness, stress, certain foods, sunburn, sexual intercourse, and menstruation. HSV-2 infections can cause serious complications. In women, these infections increase the risk of cervical cancer, so regular Pap smears are recommended. An infected woman can also pass the virus to her baby during childbirth.

Since the herpesvirus cannot be eliminated from the body, it is important to keep the virus in a dormant state. The best way to do this is to control, as much as possible, factors that activate the virus and to build your body's immune defenses.

Diet Recommendations

❥ **Eat a high-fiber, low-fat diet that provides the right amino acids.** Choose foods that are high in lysine, an amino acid that retards growth of the herpesvirus. High-lysine foods include fish, chicken, turkey, eggs, and vegetables. Increase your consumption of lysine-rich foods during outbreaks. Whole grains, legumes, and fruits round out a healthy diet. Also, avoid foods that contain significant amounts of arginine, an amino acid necessary for the herpesvirus to grow. Eat the following high-arginine foods sparingly, and avoid them completely during an outbreak: all nuts, but especially almonds and cashews; peanuts; seeds; and chocolate.

❥ **Eliminate alcohol, caffeine, sugar, soft drinks, white flour products, and processed foods.** These foods inhibit the immune response.

Nutrient Recommendations

❥ **Beta-carotene** increases the action of interferon, an immune-system substance your body uses to stop viruses from reproducing. In addition, beta-carotene stimulates white blood cells to kill more viruses. Best juice sources of carotenes (in order of effectiveness): carrots, kale, parsley, spinach, chard, beet greens, watercress, mangoes, cantaloupes, apricots, broccoli, and romaine lettuce.

❥ **Lysine** is an amino acid that retards the growth of the herpesvirus. The recommended supplement dosage is from 500 to 1,000 mg per day.

❥ **Polyphenols** have inactivated viruses in test tubes, and they have the potential of doing the same thing in the body. Best juice sources of polyphenols: apples, blueberries, and purple grapes.

❥ **Vitamin C** and **bioflavonoids** offer powerful immune system support, and studies show that vitamin C helps reduce blister formation. Best juice sources of vitamin C (in order of effectiveness): kale, parsley, broccoli, Brussels sprouts, watercress, cauliflower, cabbage, strawberries, papaya, spinach, citrus fruit, turnips, mangoes, asparagus, and cantaloupes. Best juice sources of bioflavonoids: apricots, bell peppers, berries (blueberry, blackberry, and cranberry), broccoli, cabbage, cantaloupes, cherries, citrus fruit, grapes, parsley, plums, prunes, and tomatoes.

❥ **Vitamin E** strengthens the immune system. Best juice sources of vitamin E (in order of effectiveness): spinach, watercress, asparagus, carrots, and tomatoes.

❥ **Zinc** stops viruses from reproducing, and supports and strengthens the immune system. Best juice sources of zinc (in order of effectiveness): ginger root, turnips, parsley, garlic, carrots, grapes, spinach, cabbage, lettuce, cucumbers, and tangerines.

Herb Recommendations

❥ **Echinacea** and **goldenseal** support the immune system. Avoid goldenseal if you are pregnant, and do not use it for more than ten days at a time.

Juice Ingredient Recommendations

❥ **Carrot, blueberry, parsley,** and **spinach** juices contain concentrated amounts of the nutrients that are most helpful in controlling herpes infections. Parsley juice intake should be limited to a safe, therapeutic dose of $1/2$ to 1 cup per day. Parsley can be toxic in overdose, and should be especially avoided by pregnant women.

Juice Recipes

THE MORNING ENERGIZER

$1/2$ organic Red or Golden Delicious apple, washed

5 medium carrots, scrubbed well, green tops removed, ends trimmed

$1/2$ small beet with leaves and stems, scrubbed well

$1/2$ small or medium lemon, washed, or peeled if not organic

$1/2$- to 1-inch piece fresh ginger root, washed

Cut the apple into sections that will fit your juicer's feed tube. Juice the apple along with the carrots, beet, lemon, and ginger. Stir the juice, and pour into a glass. Serve at room temperature or chilled, as desired.

POPEYE'S POWER

$1/2$ medium organic apple, any kind, washed

1 handful organic spinach, washed

1 small handful parsley, rinsed

4 medium carrots, scrubbed well, green tops removed, ends trimmed

1 stalk organic celery with leaves, washed

$1/2$ beet with leaves, scrubbed well

Cut the apple into sections that will fit your juicer's feed tube. Bunch up the spinach and parsley, and push them through the feed tube with the apple, carrots, celery, and beet. Stir the juice, and pour into a glass. Serve at room temperature or chilled, as desired.

GINGER TWIST

1 organic Red or Golden Delicious apple, washed

1 handful parsley, rinsed

4 carrots, scrubbed well, green tops removed, ends trimmed

1-inch piece fresh ginger root, washed

$1/4$ small or medium lemon, washed, or peeled if not organic

Cut the apple into sections that fit your juicer's feed tube. Bunch up the parsley and push it through the feed tube with the apple, carrots, ginger, and lemon. Stir the juice, and pour into a glass. Serve at room temperature or chilled, as desired.

TRIPLE C

¼ small head green cabbage, washed

4 carrots, scrubbed well, green tops removed, and ends trimmed

4 stalks organic celery with leaves, washed

Cut the cabbage into sections that fit your juicer's feed tube. Juice the cabbage along with the carrots and celery. Stir the juice, and pour into a glass. Serve at room temperature or chilled, as desired.

TOMATO FLORENTINE

1 vine-ripened tomato, washed

1 handful organic spinach, washed

2–3 fresh basil leaves (optional)

½ small or medium lemon, washed, or peeled if not organic

Cut the tomato into sections that will fit your juicer's feed tube. Bunch up the spinach and basil leaves (if using), and push through the feed tube with the tomato and lemon. Stir the juice, and pour into a glass. Serve at room temperature or chilled, as desired.

THE COLON CLEANSER

2 organic Granny Smith, McIntosh, or Golden Delicious apples, washed

1 bunch organic spinach, washed

1 handful parsley, rinsed

¼ small or medium lemon, washed, or peeled if not organic

Cut the apples into sections that fit your juicer's feed tube. Bunch up the spinach and parsley, and push them through the feed tube with the apples and lemon. Stir the juice, and pour into a glass. Serve at room temperature or chilled, as desired.

THE GINGER HOPPER

½ organic Red or Golden Delicious apple, washed

5 medium carrots, scrubbed well, green tops removed, ends trimmed

½- to 1-inch piece fresh ginger root, washed

Cut the apple into sections, and juice along with the carrots and ginger. Stir the juice, and pour into a glass. Serve at room temperature or chilled, as desired.

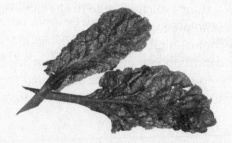

ANTIAGING COCKTAIL

1 small bunch organic purple grapes (about 1 cup) with small stems* and seeds, washed

½ cup blueberries, blackberries, or raspberries, washed

¼ small or medium lemon, washed, or peeled if not organic

½-inch piece fresh ginger root, washed

*Large stems can dull your juicer's blade.

Juice the grapes, berries, lemon, and ginger. Stir the juice, and pour into a glass. Serve at room temperature or chilled, as desired.

High Blood Pressure (Hypertension)

About 60 million Americans have high blood pressure, which occurs when circulating blood exerts too much pressure against the blood-vessel walls. High blood pressure is usually determined as a pressure reading greater than 140/90. The first number is the systolic pressure, or that exerted during heartbeats, and the second is the diastolic pressure, or the pressure exerted between beats.

Although there is no identifiable cause of high blood pressure in most cases, a high cholesterol level and a family history of the disorder are predisposing factors. For most people, the risk of developing this condition is associated with being overweight (*see* **Overweight/Obesity**). Everyday lifestyle choices that can contribute to the development of high blood pressure include caffeine consumption; alcohol intake; a diet that contains too few fruits and vegetables, and too much sugar, fat, and salt; low intake of a number of vitamins, minerals, and essential fatty acids; stress (*see* **Stress**); smoking; and lack of exercise. Some drugs can also contribute to high blood pressure, as can pregnancy.

It is important to control high blood pressure, which often is symptomless, because this condition is a major risk factor for heart attack or stroke. Most borderline to mild cases can be controlled through diet and lifestyle changes. These changes are considered more advantageous than the use of pressure-lowering drugs, which can cause side effects such as fatigue and headaches, and can increase the risk of heart disease.

Lifestyle Recommendations

❥ **If you smoke, stop.** Smoking can contribute to high blood pressure.

❥ **Get regular exercise.** Aerobic exercise—generally, any type that doesn't involve lifting weights—can help lower pressure. Exercise for at least thirty minutes three times a week; walking, swimming, and aerobic dance are all good choices.

❥ **Practice relaxation techniques.** Activities such as deep breathing exercises, biofeedback, and progressive muscle relaxation can all help lower blood pressure. Ask your doctor how to perform these techniques, or look for an adult ed course at your local high school or library.

Diet Recommendations

❥ **Eat a high-fiber, low-fat diet.** Eat at least 50 percent of your diet in the form of raw fruits, vegetables, juices, sprouts, seeds, and nuts. Also, reduce your fat intake. A recent study published in *The New England Journal of Medicine* found that a diet rich in fruits and vegetables, and low in fat, significantly reduced blood pressure. For more information on healthy dietary choices, see Basic Guidelines for the Juice Lady's Health and Healing Diet (page 313).

❥ **Greatly reduce or eliminate sugar and alcohol consumption.** Sugar requires an increase in the body's water stores; for every gram of sugar, three grams of water are needed for transport, storage, and metabolism. This increases fluid volume, which can lead to problems with urine elimination. Also, sugar increases levels of triglycerides and cholesterol, which increases blood viscosity, or stickiness. Alcohol, which acts like sugar in the body, causes the same problems.

❥ **Use salt sparingly.** Studies show that restricted use of sodium chloride, or common table salt, results in a fall in blood pressure and a reduction in the need for medication. If you eat out frequently, you may be ingesting much more salt than you would think, since restaurant food is often heavily salted for flavor. Request salt-free dishes so you can control your salt intake. Vinegar, lemon juice, and herbs make good substitute flavor enhancers. In addition, use potassium to offset the effects of sodium (see the Nutrient Recommendations).

❥ **Use juices to help lower your blood pressure.** Fresh juices are rich in the vitamins and minerals directly related to lowering high blood pressure and maintaining normal pressure. I have received letters from many people who have lowered their blood pressure simply by adding raw juices to their diets.

❥ **Limit or avoid caffeine consumption.** Studies with caffeinated coffee show that eliminating coffee consumption resulted in a significant reduction in blood pressure. Caffeine is also in cola, sodas, chocolate, green and black tea, and some medications. If you have trouble giving up the taste of coffee, switch to water-processed decaf coffee. Or try decaf or herbal tea (see the Herb Recommendations).

Nutrient Recommendations

❥ **Calcium** plays an important role in maintaining normal blood pressure. Best juice sources of calcium (in order of effectiveness): kale, parsley, dandelion greens, watercress, beet greens, broccoli, spinach, romaine lettuce, string beans, oranges, celery, and carrots.

❥ **Essential fatty acids (EFAs)** help control blood pressure. Several studies have shown that fish eaters tend to have lower blood pressures than even vegetarians. This has been attributed to eicosapentaenoic acid (EPA) and docosahexaenoic acid (DHA), two essential fatty acids found in fish. The body can also create EPA and DHA from EFAs found in such plant-based oils as flaxseed and hemp oils. For more information, see the fats and oils section in Basic Guidelines for the Juice Lady's Health and Healing Diet (page 313).

❥ **Magnesium** makes a difference in blood pressure. Studies have shown that people who consume more magnesium-rich foods have lower blood pressures than people who do not. Best juice sources of magnesium (in order of effectiveness): beet greens, spinach, parsley, dandelion greens, garlic, blackberries, beets, broccoli, cauliflower, carrots, and celery.

❥ **Potassium**-rich diets may allow significant reductions in hypertensive medication dosages. Best juice sources of potassium (in order of effectiveness): parsley, chard, garlic, spinach, broccoli, carrots, celery, radishes, cauliflower, watercress, asparagus, and cabbage.

❥ **Vitamin C** can keep blood pressure in the normal range, according to a number of studies. Best juice sources of vitamin C (in order of effectiveness): kale, parsley, broccoli, Brussels sprouts, watercress, cauliflower, cabbage, strawberries, papaya, spinach, citrus fruit, turnips, mangoes, asparagus, and cantaloupes.

Herb Recommendations

❥ **Green tea** has been shown in studies to lower blood pressure. Look for a decaffeinated green tea. If you can find it, look for a tea processed to have extra GABA, a chemical shown to be even more effective in lowering blood pressure.

❥ **Licorice** should be *avoided* if you have high blood pressure.

Juice Ingredient Recommendations

❥ **Beet, blackberry, carrot, celery, cucumber, parsley, raspberry,** and **spinach** juices are all traditional remedies for high blood pressure. Parsley juice intake should be limited to a safe, therapeutic dose of $1/2$ to 1 cup per day. Parsley can be toxic in overdose, and should be especially avoided by pregnant women.

Juice Recipes

POPEYE'S POWER

$1/2$ medium organic apple, any kind, washed

1 handful organic spinach, washed

1 small handful parsley, rinsed

4 medium carrots, scrubbed well, green tops removed, ends trimmed

1 stalk organic celery with leaves, washed

$1/2$ beet with leaves, scrubbed well

Cut the apple into sections that will fit your juicer's feed tube. Bunch up the spinach and parsley, and push them through the feed tube with the apple, carrots, celery, and beet. Stir the juice, and pour into a glass. Serve at room temperature or chilled, as desired.

ANTIAGING COCKTAIL

1 small bunch organic purple grapes (about 1 cup) with small stems* and seeds, washed

$1/2$ cup blueberries, blackberries, or raspberries, washed

$1/4$ small or medium lemon, washed, or peeled if not organic

$1/2$-inch piece fresh ginger root, washed

Juice the grapes, berries, lemon, and ginger. Stir the juice, and pour into a glass. Serve at room temperature or chilled, as desired.

*Large stems can dull your juicer's blade.

MORNING SUNRISE

1 pink, red, or white grapefruit,
   peeled
1 orange, peeled

Divide the grapefruit and orange into segments that fit your juicer's feed tube. Juice the grapefruit and orange, and stir the juice. Pour into a glass and serve at room temperature or chilled, as desired.

STRAWBERRY-CANTALOUPE COCKTAIL

½ ripe organic cantaloupe with seeds,
   washed, or peeled if not organic
1 cup organic strawberries, washed

Cut the cantaloupe into strips that fit your juicer's feed tube. Juice the cantaloupe and strawberries; stir the juice and pour into a glass. Serve at room temperature or chilled, as desired.

AFTERNOON REFRESHER

1 medium to large organic cucumber,
   scrubbed well
½ small or medium lemon, washed,
   or peeled if not organic

Cut the cucumber in half lengthwise, and juice with the lemon. (For an especially cooling version, let the juice splash over a few ice cubes in the juice pitcher.) Stir the juice, and pour into a glass. Serve at room temperature or chilled, as desired.

BEAUTIFUL BONE SOLUTION

1 organic Golden or Red Delicious
   apple, washed
1–2 kale leaves, washed
1 handful parsley, rinsed
1 stalk organic celery, washed
¼ small or medium lemon, washed,
   or peeled if not organic
½- to 1-inch piece fresh ginger root,
   washed

Cut the apple into sections that fit your juicer's feed tube. Bunch up the kale and parsley, and push through the feed tube with the apple, celery, lemon, and ginger. Stir the juice, and pour into a glass. Serve at room temperature or chilled, as desired.

SWEET CALCIUM COCKTAIL

1 three-inch chunk fresh pineapple, scrubbed well or peeled if not organic

1–2 kale leaves, washed

Cut the pineapple into strips that fit your juicer's feed tube. Bunch up the kale, and push through the feed tube with the pineapple. Stir the juice, and pour into a glass. Serve at room temperature or chilled, as desired.

MAGNESIUM SPECIAL

5 medium carrots, scrubbed well, green tops removed, ends trimmed

2 stalks organic celery with leaves, washed

1/2 small beet with leaves and stems, scrubbed well

2 broccoli florets, washed

1/2 small or medium lemon, washed, or peeled if not organic

Juice the carrots, celery, beet, broccoli, and lemon. Stir the juice, and pour into a glass. Serve at room temperature or chilled, as desired.

TOMATO FLORENTINE

1 vine-ripened tomato, washed

1 handful organic spinach, washed

2–3 fresh basil leaves (optional)

1/2 small or medium lemon, washed, or peeled if not organic

Cut the tomato into sections that will fit your juicer's feed tube. Bunch up the spinach and basil leaves (if using), and push through the feed tube with the tomato and lemon. Stir the juice, and pour into a glass. Serve at room temperature or chilled, as desired.

High Cholesterol

See **Cardiovascular Disease.**

Hypoglycemia

Hypoglycemia, or low blood sugar, occurs when too much insulin is secreted by the pancreas, generally in response to sugar consumption. Sugar circulates in the bloodstream as glucose, and excess insulin clears glucose from the blood too quickly. This results in abnormally low blood-glucose levels.

Hypoglycemia is characterized by headaches, dizziness, sweating, tremors, increased heart rate, depression, anxiety, irritability, and hunger, especially cravings for sweets. In more severe cases, there can be blurred vision, mental confusion, incoherent speech, and convulsions. Symptoms generally appear three to five hours after eating sugar. Hypoglycemia is usually diagnosed when an oral glucose tolerance test shows a glucose reading below 50 mg/dl, but some individuals have this condition even though their glucose levels are in the normal range.

Repeatedly eating refined carbohydrate foods, such as sweets and white flour products, creates a great strain on the pancreas, as it is called on repeatedly to secrete insulin in response to high levels of sugar in the bloodstream. If this eating pattern continues, other organs begin to show signs of strain as well. As the presence of insulin causes blood-sugar levels to drop, the liver is signaled to release its glucose stores. The thyroid speeds up to aid the liver. The adrenal glands secrete hormones that cause even more glucose to be released. Eventually, all these glands and organs become overworked. Unless dietary changes are made, this condition can lead to diabetes in some individuals (*see* **Diabetes Mellitus**) and severe hypoglycemia in others.

Diet Recommendations

❥ **Do not eat sugar-rich foods to relieve hypoglycemia symptoms.** Eating something sweet may seem like the logical approach, and indeed this will cause your sugar levels to rise initially. But afterward your sugar levels will plummet again as insulin is oversecreted in response to the sugar. This results in a ping-pong effect that leaves you feeling like you are bouncing off the walls. Hypoglycemia symptoms should be treated by eating complex carbohydrates and a little protein. For example, raw almonds, or other nuts or seeds, make a good, portable protein snack.

❥ **Greatly limit your consumption of simple sugars in general.** Items such as cookies, candies, cakes, pies, doughnuts, and ice cream, and refined white flour products should be completely avoided. Greatly limit natural sugars, such as honey, maple syrup, and dried sugar cane. Brown rice and malt barley syrups (found at health food stores) may be tolerated in small quantities occasionally because they are absorbed more slowly into the bloodstream. Fruit is a source of simple carbohydrates, and you should eat no more than one or two pieces of fresh, whole fruit per day. (If your hypoglycemia is especially severe, do not eat even that much fruit.) Fruit sugar, or fructose, is very sweet—one and a half times as sweet as table sugar. Fruit juice is too high in fruit sugar and should be avoided, or at least consumed in very small quantities and diluted by half with water. *On a personal note:* I finally concluded that I cannot eat fruit regularly because of my hypoglycemia. I rarely eat even fresh fruit and never drink fruit juice, except for lemon or lime juice added to vegetable combinations or in water. I have also found that even brown rice and malt barley syrups affect my immune system adversely in a slow, cumulative way.

❥ **Eat a high-complex-carbohydrate diet.** Complex carbohydrates are vegetables, whole grains, and legumes (beans, lentils, and split peas). Switching to this type of diet is the most important step you can take in controlling hypoglycemia. Complex carbohydrates contain fiber, which causes them to release their sugars much more slowly into the bloodstream than simple carbohydrates (see the next entry for more information). Refined carbohydrates are not only stripped of most of their fiber, but they contain relatively few vitamins, minerals, and other nutrients. For more information on healthy eating, see the Basic Guidelines for the Juice Lady's Health and Healing Diet (page 313).

❥ **Increase the amount of fiber in your diet.** Fiber slows digestion and the release of sugars into the bloodstream. So eating more fiber helps to control blood sugar, but it is important to eat the right type of fiber. Water-soluble fiber is the most beneficial for controlling hypoglycemia. Hemicellulose, mucilages, gums, and pectins are all water-soluble forms of fiber. Good sources of water-soluble fiber are legumes, oat bran, nuts, seeds, and most vegetables and vegetable juices. Pear and apple juices are good sources of soluble fiber, but you should avoid them because of their sugar content.

❥ **Increase your consumption of essential fatty acids and protein.** If you are not overweight, you can benefit from introducing more protein and essential fatty acids (EFAs), the "good fats" vital to good health, into your diet. Raw nuts, seeds, and avocados are good snacks. They provide excellent sources of steady energy, and have a calming effect on hyperactive hypoglycemic states. People who have hypoglycemia often show such signs of EFA deficiency as dry hair and skin, low body weight (although you be both overweight and EFA deficient), depression, nervousness, aches and pains, and cramps. When you increase your intake of complex carbohydrates and decrease your consumption of refined processed foods, your EFA levels will naturally increase. It is also beneficial to increase EFA levels by taking flaxseed or hemp oil (one to two tablespoons per day) and eating cold-water fish, such as salmon, halibut, tuna, cod, mackerel, and trout. Fish is also an excellent protein source. For more information, see the fats and oils section in Basic Guidelines for the Juice Lady's Health and Healing Diet (page 313).

❥ **Eat smaller, more frequent meals.** You will do best eating five or six smaller meals throughout the day rather than two or three larger meals. Eating more frequently, and eating some protein at each meal or snack, helps keep blood sugar at a relatively constant level, as opposed to the big surges in blood sugar that occur after a large meal. One way to accomplish this is to save half a meal and eat it later as a snack. A protein snack before bedtime also helps to keep blood sugar even throughout the night. This is important because low sugar levels can cause you to sleep poorly.

❥ **Cleanse and support your liver.** In hypoglycemia, the liver has been overworked. Support your liver by eating and drinking more liver-support foods; beets and artichokes are especially helpful. Other beneficial foods include peas, parsnips, pumpkin, sweet potatoes, squash, yams, beans, broccoli, Brussels sprouts, cabbage, carrots, cauliflower, celery, chives, cucumber, eggplant, garlic, kale, kohlrabi, mustard greens, okra, onion, and parsley. The Liver Cleanse (page 333) can also support liver function.

❥ **Avoid alcohol.** Hypoglycemia is made worse by alcohol consumption. Alcohol increases insulin secretion, thereby causing a drop in blood sugar. This state often creates a hunger for foods, such as simple carbohydrates, that can quickly raise blood sugar. These types of foods cause a greater craving for alcohol, and a dangerous spiral effect is created. Also, the work of breaking down alcohol puts an additional burden on the liver.

❥ **Eat more seaweeds and microalgae.** These foods, including spirulina, chlorella, and wild blue-green algae, help normalize blood-sugar metabolism. Seaweed, such as kelp and dulse, supply energy and contain high amounts of trace minerals, including iodine, silicon, and phosphorus.

Nutrient Recommendations

❧ **Chromium** is the most essential nutrient for blood-sugar control. It is a key part of glucose tolerance factor (GTF), which increases insulin's effectiveness in getting sugar into the body's cells. A chromium deficiency is thought to be an underlying contributor to both diabetes and hypoglycemia. Brewer's yeast is considered to be the best food source of chromium, and can be added to fresh vegetable juices. Best juice sources of chromium (in order of effectiveness): green peppers, parsnips, spinach, carrots, lettuce, string beans, and cabbage. Chromium picolinate is the preferred form of supplemental chromium.

❧ **Magnesium** may help reduce glucose-induced insulin secretion. Best juice sources of magnesium (in order of effectiveness): beet greens, spinach, parsley, dandelion greens, garlic, beets, broccoli, cauliflower, carrots, and celery.

❧ **Vitamin B$_3$ (niacin)** is another GTF component. Best food sources of vitamin B$_3$ (in order of effectiveness): brewer's yeast, rice and wheat bran, peanuts, turkey, chicken, and fish. It is not available in fruits and vegetables.

Herb Recommendations

❧ **Dandelion root** is a gentle tonic for the liver.

❧ **Licorice** is used to support the adrenal glands. Licorice tea is sweet and can help you if you are having a difficult time cutting sweets out of your diet. Avoid licorice if you have high blood pressure, and do not use it for prolonged periods of time. Use a medicinal form of the herb, not licorice candy.

Juice Ingredient Recommendations

❧ **Beet, celery,** and **dandelion** juices have traditionally been used to cleanse and support the liver.

❧ **Jerusalem artichoke** juice helps support the liver and pancreas, and helps normalize blood-sugar levels.

❧ **Parsley** juice is rich in magnesium. Intake should be limited to a safe, therapeutic dose of $^1/_2$ to 1 cup per day. Parsley can be toxic in overdose, and should be especially avoided by pregnant women.

❧ **String bean** juice is a tonic for the pancreas and helps regulate blood sugar. One cup per meal is recommended along with two cups as snacks; see Jack & The Bean on page 191.

❥ **Tomato** juice, with a pinch of cayenne or a dash of hot sauce, can provide energy, and help to revitalize the liver and adrenal glands.

Juice Recipes

THE MORNING ENERGIZER

5 medium carrots, scrubbed well, green tops removed, ends trimmed

½ small beet with leaves and stems, scrubbed well

½ small or medium lemon, washed, or peeled if not organic

½- to 1-inch piece fresh ginger root, washed

Juice the carrots, beet, lemon, and ginger. Stir the juice, and pour into a glass. Serve at room temperature, or chilled, as desired.

SWEET DREAMS NIGHTCAP

2 romaine lettuce leaves, washed

1 handful parsley, rinsed

4 carrots, scrubbed well, green tops removed, ends trimmed

3 organic celery stalks with leaves, washed

Bunch up the lettuce leaves and parsley, and push through the feed tube with the carrots and celery. Stir the juice, and pour into a glass. Serve at room temperature or chilled, as desired.

LIVER REJUVENATOR

1 handful dandelion greens, washed

5 medium carrots, scrubbed well, green tops removed, ends trimmed

½ small or medium lemon, washed, or peeled if not organic

Bunch up the dandelion greens and juice with the carrots and lemon. Stir the juice, and pour into a glass. Serve at room temperature or chilled, as desired.

WEIGHT-LOSS BUDDY

1 small Jerusalem artichoke, scrubbed well

4–5 carrots, scrubbed well, green tops removed, ends trimmed

½ small beet with no stems and leaves, scrubbed well

Cut the Jerusalem artichoke into sections that fit your juicer's feed tube. Juice the artichoke along with the carrots and beet. Stir the juice, and pour into a glass. Serve at room temperature or chilled, as desired.

JACK & THE BEAN

1 large vine-ripened tomato, washed

2 romaine lettuce leaves, washed

8 organic string beans, washed

3 Brussels sprouts, washed

½ small or medium lemon, washed, or peeled if not organic

Cut the tomato into sections that fit your juicer's feed tube. Bunch up the lettuce leaves, and push through the feed tube with the tomato, string beans, Brussels sprouts, and lemon. Stir the juice, and pour into a glass. Serve at room temperature or chilled, as desired.

SPICY TOMATO ON ICE

2 vine-ripened tomatoes, washed

2 dark green lettuce leaves, such as romaine or green leaf, washed

1 small handful parsley, rinsed

2 radishes with green tops, washed

½ small or medium lime or lemon, washed, or peeled if not organic

Dash hot sauce

Cut the tomato in sections that fit your juicer's feed tube. Bunch up the lettuce leaves and parsley, and push them through the feed tube with the tomatoes, radishes, and lime or lemon. Add a dash of hot sauce, and stir to combine. Pour into tall, ice-filled glasses.

BEAUTIFUL SKIN, HAIR, AND NAIL SOLUTION

1 medium organic cucumber, scrubbed well

1 medium parsnip, scrubbed well

3 carrots, scrubbed well, green tops removed, ends trimmed

½ small or medium lemon, washed, or peeled if not organic

¼ small green bell pepper, washed

Cut the cucumber in half lengthwise, and juice with the parsnip, carrots, lemon, and bell pepper. Stir the juice, and pour into a glass. Serve at room temperature or chilled, as desired.

POPEYE'S POWER

1 handful organic spinach, washed

1 small handful parsley, rinsed

5 medium carrots, scrubbed well, green tops removed, ends trimmed

1 stalk organic celery with leaves, washed

½ beet with leaves, scrubbed well

Bunch up the spinach and parsley, and push them through the feed tube with the carrots, celery, and beet. Stir the juice, and pour into a glass. Serve at room temperature or chilled, as desired.

MAGNESIUM SPECIAL

5 medium carrots, scrubbed well, green tops removed, ends trimmed

2 stalks organic celery with leaves, washed

1/2 small beet with leaves and stems, scrubbed well

2 broccoli florets, washed

1/2 small or medium lemon, washed, or peeled if not organic

Juice the carrots, celery, beet, broccoli, and lemon. Stir the juice, and pour into a glass. Serve at room temperature or chilled, as desired.

MEMORY MENDER

2 medium vine-ripened tomatoes, washed

1/4 small head iceberg lettuce, washed

4 cauliflower florets, washed

1/2 small or medium lemon, washed, or peeled if not organic

Cut the tomatoes and lettuce into sections that will fit your juicer's feed tube. Juice the tomatoes and lettuce along with the cauliflower and lemon. Pour into a glass and serve at room temperature or chilled, as desired.

Indigestion

Often referred to commonly as heartburn, and medically as dyspepsia, indigestion is a catchall term for eating-related discomforts. There are a variety of symptoms associated with this condition, including discomfort in the upper abdomen following meals, burning pain, belching, flatulence, bloating, and a feeling of fullness. Indigestion is an extremely common problem.

The causes of indigestion are as varied as the symptoms themselves. Poor eating habits—eating too fast; not chewing food well; eating high-fat, fried, or spicy foods; eating under stressful conditions—can cause digestive disturbances. Food allergies and sensitivities can also be a root cause. Continually eating foods you are sensitive to can have a buildup effect, and can cause symptoms of indigestion that were not present before. A highly stressful lifestyle will affect how your digestive system functions. Decreased secretion of digestive juices and enzymes, which aid in breaking down food, can cause indigestion. Hydrochloric acid is produced by the cells lining the stomach, and is a key component of digestive juices. A deficiency or excess of this acid can cause indigestion. Bile, a substance made by the liver and stored in the gallbladder, aids in the digestion of fat and fat-soluble vitamins. If there is insufficient production or secretion of bile, indigestion will be worse after a high-fat meal. More serious problems can also cause indigestion, such as hernias and ulcers (*see* **Ulcers**).

Diet Recommendations

❥ **Chew your food well, and sip juices slowly.** This is perhaps the single most important step you can take to improve indigestion. Chewing begins the digestive process in your mouth by mixing food with saliva. Saliva contains the enzyme amylase, which starts the breakdown of starches into smaller molecules. There's a saying in natural medicine that you should juice your food [with your teeth] and chew your juice. This is because thorough chewing allows better assimilation and utilization of the nutrients contained in food. If the starting point of eating is rushed or inadequate, digestion suffers.

❥ **Eat smaller, more frequent meals.** Overindulging in food can directly cause indigestion. Eating smaller meals—ones chewed thoroughly—on a regular basis allows the digestive system to function optimally. Avoid drinking liquids during a meal. Instead, consume plenty of liquids between meals. Also, avoid lying down directly after a meal.

❥ **Eat in a relaxed environment.** Anxiety and stress while eating cause indigestion. Create a peaceful environment around mealtime. Sit down during meals. Don't watch TV while you eat. Focus on the enjoyment of eating, and grant yourself this time to set aside the worries and problems of the day.

❥ **Reduce your intake of foods that irritate the digestive system.** Foods that irritate the lining of the stomach include foods that are fried, spicy, salty, overly sweet, or high in fat. Alcohol and caffeine are irritating to the gastrointestinal tract—coffee can actually cause symptoms that can be mistaken for an ulcer. Therefore, both regular and decaffeinated coffee, as well as alcohol, should be eliminated from your diet. Heartburn, caused by stomach acid splashing into the esophagus, can often be controlled by eliminating these items, and by avoiding chocolate, and peppermint and spearmint oils. In some people, these substances relax the muscle at the top of the stomach, letting stomach acid leak upward. Meals high in animal protein are difficult to digest, and consumption of foods containing chemicals, dyes, and additives can strain the digestive system. That's why you should eat more whole, natural foods, with an emphasis on fresh fruits, vegetables, and juices. There is also some evidence that people who suffer from chronic dyspepsia benefit from a low-carbohydrate diet—one study documented a 70-percent improvement in dyspeptic individuals who went on such a diet. (For more information, see *The Zone* by Barry Sears or *Sugar Busters* by H. Leighton Steward and others; both are available in bookstores.)

❥ **Eat more alkaline foods.** Foods are either alkaline or acid depending on the residue they leave behind after being metabolized by the body. The typical Western diet is high in acid-forming foods, which include meat, sugar, refined flour, fats, oil, dairy, and eggs. Not surprisingly, these are the foods that should be consumed in moderation if you suffer from indigestion or heartburn. Focus on more alkaline foods, which include vegetables, most fruits (except strawberries and cranberries), millet, olive oil, and sea vegetables. Vegetable juices are very beneficial.

❥ **Eat raw almonds.** Carry raw almonds with you to eat during the day or when eating out. Chew them slowly to alleviate heartburn. (Raw almonds can be purchased at most health food stores.) If you tend to put on weight, do not overindulge in almonds, since they are fairly high in calories.

❥ **Go on juice fasts.** Give your digestive system a rest with a short one- to three-day juice fast. You can quickly turn an acidic system around to one with a proper alkaline-acid balance by juice fasting. For more information, see the Juice Fast (page 324).

❥ **Avoid foods that cause allergies and sensitivities.** It is beneficial if you have recurring indigestion to determine if you have food allergies and sensitivities, and then to avoid those foods. *See* **Allergies**; also see the Elimination Diet, page 321.

Nutrient Recommendations

❥ **Vitamin A** and **beta-carotene** should be consumed liberally if you have chronic indigestion. Vitamin A supports the mucus-secreting cells of the mucous membranes, which include the lining of the digestive tract, where the vitamin acts as an anti-inflammatory. When there is a vitamin A deficiency, the intestinal tract is much more susceptible to injury from such strong irritants as caffeine, alcohol, and spicy foods. Beta-carotene is converted to vitamin A in the body as needed and is the only form of vitamin A found in nonanimal foods. Best juice sources of carotenes in general (in order of effectiveness): carrots, kale, parsley, spinach, chard, beet greens, watercress, mangoes, cantaloupes, apricots, broccoli, and romaine lettuce.

Herb Recommendations

❥ **Anise and chamomile** aid digestion through the action of their volatile oils, which relax the bowels. Be sure to use German chamomile, *Matricaria recutita*, and not Roman chamomile, *Chamaemelum nobile*.

❥ **Dandelion, gentian,** and **goldenseal** are bitter herbs that have been used throughout history to aid digestion. Their action comes directly from their bitter taste, which stimulates the central nervous system and eventually causes the release of gastrin, a digestive hormone. Avoid goldenseal if you are pregnant, and do not use it for more than ten days.

❥ **Slippery elm bark** protects and soothes inflamed tissue through the action of the mucilage it contains.

Juice Ingredient Recommendations

❥ **Banana** has been shown in animal studies to protect the stomach from stomach acids. Though bananas do not juice well, they make great additions to smoothies (see Tropical Sunrise).

❥ **Cabbage** juice, with its ulcer-healing factor, works for both indigestion and gastritis.

❥ **Fennel** juice aids digestion and relieves gas.

❥ **Ginger** has been used as a gas-relieving substance for thousands of years.

❥ **Lemon** juice and water, consumed one-half hour before a meal, is a traditional tonic for stimulating salivary and gastric secretions. For a refreshing lemon sparkler, try fresh lemon juice mixed with sparkling water. Or try one of the following lemon-containing recipes.

❥ **Papaya** and **pineapple** juices contain papain and bromelain respectively; they are both protein-digesting enzymes that are helpful in treating indigestion and heartburn. These digestive enzymes increase digestive activity, tone the stomach, and directly soothe heartburn. These juices can be helpful sipped in small quantity with a meal. (Papaya does not juice well, but it makes a great addition to such smoothies as Tropical Surprise.)

❥ **Parsley** juice contains beta-carotene. Intake should be limited to a safe, therapeutic dose of $1/2$ to 1 cup per day. Parsley can be toxic in overdose, and should be especially avoided by pregnant women.

Juice Recipes

TROPICAL SURPRISE

1 three-inch chunk pineapple, scrubbed well or peeled if not organic

1 ripe medium banana, peeled

1/2 medium papaya, peeled and seeded

1/2 cup plain or vanilla soy milk, or lowfat dairy milk

1/4 teaspoon pure vanilla extract

6 ice cubes

Cut the pineapple into strips that fit your juicer's feed tube and juice the strips. Pour the juice into a blender, and add the banana, papaya, milk, vanilla, and ice cubes; blend until smooth. Pour the mixture into two glasses and serve immediately.

TRIPLE C

1/4 small head green cabbage, washed

4 carrots, scrubbed well, green tops removed, and ends trimmed

4 stalks organic celery with leaves, washed

Cut the cabbage into sections that fit your juicer's feed tube. Juice the cabbage along with the carrots and celery. Stir the juice, and pour into a glass. Serve at room temperature or chilled, as desired.

THE FEEL GOOD COCKTAIL

1/2 pear, washed

4 medium carrots, scrubbed well, green tops removed, ends trimmed

3 fennel stalks with leaves and flowers, washed

1 stalk organic celery with leaves, washed

Cut the pear into sections that fit your juicer's feed tube, and juice along with the carrots, fennel, and celery. Stir the juice, and pour into a glass. Serve at room temperature or chilled, as desired.

THE GINGER HOPPER

1/2 organic Red or Golden Delicious apple, washed

5 medium carrots, scrubbed well, green tops removed, ends trimmed

1/2- to 1-inch piece fresh ginger root, washed

Cut the apple into sections, and juice along with the carrots and ginger. Stir the juice, and pour into a glass. Serve at room temperature or chilled, as desired.

SWEET CALCIUM COCKTAIL

1 three-inch chunk fresh pineapple, scrubbed well, or peeled if not organic

1–2 kale leaves, washed

Cut the pineapple into strips that fit your juicer's feed tube. Bunch up the kale, and push through the feed tube with the pineapple. Stir the juice, and pour into a glass. Serve at room temperature or chilled, as desired.

THE MORNING ENERGIZER

1/2 organic Red or Golden Delicious apple, washed

5 medium carrots, scrubbed well, green tops removed, ends trimmed

1/2 small beet with leaves and stems, scrubbed well

1/2 small or medium lemon, washed, or peeled if not organic

1/2- to 1-inch piece fresh ginger root, washed

Cut the apple into sections that will fit your juicer's feed tube. Juice the apple along with the carrots, beet, lemon, and ginger. Stir the juice, and pour into a glass. Serve at room temperature or chilled, as desired.

POPEYE'S POWER

1/2 medium organic apple, any kind, washed

1 handful organic spinach, washed

1 small handful parsley, rinsed

4 medium carrots, scrubbed well, green tops removed, ends trimmed

1 stalk organic celery with leaves, washed

1/2 beet with leaves, scrubbed well

Cut the apple into sections that will fit your juicer's feed tube. Bunch up the spinach and parsley, and push them through the feed tube with the apple, carrots, celery, and beet. Stir the juice, and pour into a glass. Serve at room temperature or chilled, as desired.

GINGER TWIST

1 organic Red or Golden Delicious apple, washed

1 handful parsley, rinsed

4 carrots, scrubbed well, green tops removed, ends trimmed

1-inch piece fresh ginger root, washed

1/4 small or medium lemon, washed, or peeled if not organic

Cut the apple into sections that fit your juicer's feed tube. Bunch up the parsley and push it through the feed tube with the apple, carrots, ginger, and lemon. Stir the juice, and pour into a glass. Serve at room temperature or chilled, as desired.

Inflammation

Inflammation is a natural bodily response to trauma, infection, and other assaults. It helps to rid the body of invading organisms and toxins, and also helps to "mop up" any dead cells and tissues. Without inflammation, injured tissues would not heal and infections would rage out of control.

An injury, such as a sprained ankle, will result in an inflammatory response that includes redness, swelling, heat, and pain. These are protective measures. For example, swelling helps to stabilize the joint, and pain tells you not to walk on that foot. It may be accompanied by a slight fever, headache, loss of appetite, discomfort, and sometimes fatigue. Fever is one way the body gets its defense system to respond rapidly to a physical threat. Fatigue is a result of the body using more energy to fight the infection, and is a signal that you need more rest; your body heals best during deep sleep.

Many ailments are associated with chronic inflammation, such as lupus, rheumatoid arthritis (*see* **Rheumatoid Arthritis**), fibromyalgia (*see* **Fibromyalgia**), atherosclerosis (*see* **Cardiovascular Disease**), inflammatory bowel disease (*see* **Colitis**), chronic pancreatitis, and chronic hepatitis. While inflammation does allow healing to take place, it can also cause discomfort. See the following suggestions for ways to speed the healing process.

Diet Recommendations

❥ **Reduce your intake of red meat, poultry, and dairy products.** Animal products are the primary sources of arachidonic acid, a fatty acid that is converted to hormonelike substances called prostaglandins and leukotrienes—substances that can aggravate the inflammatory response. Instead, eat fish. Fish is a good choice because it contains essential fatty acids (see the Nutrient Recommendations).

❥ **Eat and juice more fresh fruits and vegetables.** In inflammation, the blood vessels become more permeable to allow immune cells and chemicals to enter spaces within the tissues. When the inflammation becomes chronic, this process can destroy healthy tissue surrounding the injured or infected area. Fruits and vegetables are high in bioflavonoids, which improve blood-vessel strength and reduce the tendency of capillaries to leak fluid (see the Nutrient Recommendations).

❥ **Eliminate food allergens.** Food allergies can cause and/or contribute to the inflammatory process. (*See* **Allergies**; also see the Elimination Diet, page 321.)

Nutrient Recommendations

❥ **Antioxidants** are powerful free-radical quenchers. Free radicals, produced as part of the inflammatory process, are unstable molecules that damage cells. Damaged cells then become sources of even more free radicals, and a chain reaction is set in motion. Antioxidant nutrients bind to free radicals, preventing them from injuring healthy tissue and thereby reducing the inflammation process. The following antioxidants are quite helpful:

* *Selenium* is a powerful antioxidant. Best juice sources of selenium (in order of effectiveness): chard, turnips, garlic, oranges, radishes, grapes, carrots, and cabbage.

* *Vitamin A* and *beta-carotene* are potent antioxidants. Beta-carotene is converted to vitamin A in the body as needed. Best juice sources of carotenes in general (in order of effectiveness): carrots, kale, parsley, spinach, chard, beet greens, watercress, mangoes, cantaloupes, apricots, broccoli, and romaine lettuce.

* *Vitamin C* and *bioflavonoids* both inhibit the release of histamine, a substance that is released in response to infections and allergies. In addition, vitamin C stabilizes cell membranes, and bioflavonoids enhance the action of vitamin C. Best juice sources of vitamin C (in order of effectiveness): kale, parsley, broccoli, Brussels sprouts, watercress, cauliflower, cabbage, strawberries, papaya, spinach, citrus fruit, turnips, mangoes, asparagus, and cantaloupes. Best juice sources of bioflavonoids: apricots, bell peppers, berries (blueberry, blackberry, and cranberry), broccoli, cabbage, cantaloupes, cherries, citrus fruit, grapes, plums, parsley, prunes, and tomatoes.

* *Vitamin E* is an anti-inflammatory substance. Best juice sources of vitamin E (in order of effectiveness): spinach, watercress, asparagus, carrots, and tomatoes.

❥ **Copper** has been shown to decrease inflammation in laboratory animals. Best juice sources of copper (in order of effectiveness): ginger root, turnips, parsley, garlic, carrots, grapes, spinach, cabbage, lettuce, cucumbers, and tangerines.

❥ **Essential fatty acids (EFAs),** especially the beneficial omega-3 fatty acids, are found in cold-water fish, such as salmon, tuna, trout, cod, and halibut. These omega-3s, especially eicosapentaenoic acid (EPA) and docosahexaenoic acid (DHA), help decrease inflammation. Other sources of omega-3 EFAs are flaxseeds and flaxseed oil, walnuts, pumpkin seeds, and hemp oil. For more information, see the fats and oils section in Basic Guidelines for the Juice Lady's Health and Healing Diet (page 313).

❥ **Zinc** promotes anti-inflammatory activity. Best juice sources of zinc (in order of effectiveness): ginger root, turnips, parsley, garlic, carrots, grapes, spinach, cabbage, lettuce, cucumbers, and tangerines.

Herb Recommendations

❥ **Curcumin,** a constituent of turmeric, has anti-inflammatory effects. Traditionally, it has been used on wounds, sprains, and inflamed joints to decrease inflammation. It is as effective as some prescription drugs in relieving the swelling and stiffness associated with arthritis. Curcumin is available in supplement form.

❥ **Devil's claw** is similar in its anti-inflammatory effects to cortisone. It also helps relieve pain.

Juice Ingredient Recommendations

❥ **Ginger** juice has anti-inflammatory properties. It can also protect the stomach from the effects of nonsteriodal anti-inflammatory drugs (NSAIDs).

❥ **Parsley** juice contains a wealth of nutrients. Intake should be limited to a safe, therapeutic dose of $1/2$ to 1 cup per day. Parsley can be toxic in overdose, and should be especially avoided by pregnant women.

❥ **Pineapple** juice contains the enzyme bromelain, which has anti-inflammatory properties.

Juice Recipes

THE GINGER HOPPER

$1/2$ organic Red or Golden Delicious apple, washed

5 medium carrots, scrubbed well, green tops removed, ends trimmed

$1/2$- to 1-inch piece fresh ginger root, washed

Cut the apple into sections, and juice along with the carrots and ginger. Stir the juice, and pour into a glass. Serve at room temperature or chilled, as desired.

SWEET CALCIUM COCKTAIL

1 three-inch chunk fresh pineapple, scrubbed well or peeled if not organic

1–2 kale leaves, washed

Cut the pineapple into strips that fit your juicer's feed tube. Bunch up the kale, and push through the feed tube with the pineapple. Stir the juice, and pour into a glass. Serve at room temperature or chilled, as desired.

THE MORNING ENERGIZER

½ organic Red or Golden Delicious apple, washed

5 medium carrots, scrubbed well, green tops removed, ends trimmed

½ small beet with leaves and stems, scrubbed well

½ small or medium lemon, washed, or peeled if not organic

½- to 1-inch piece fresh ginger root, washed

Cut the apple into sections that will fit your juicer's feed tube. Juice the apple along with the carrots, beet, lemon, and ginger. Stir the juice, and pour into a glass. Serve at room temperature or chilled, as desired.

POPEYE'S POWER

½ medium organic apple, any kind, washed

1 handful organic spinach, washed

1 small handful parsley, rinsed

4 medium carrots, scrubbed well, green tops removed, ends trimmed

1 stalk organic celery with leaves, washed

½ beet with leaves, scrubbed well

Cut the apple into sections that will fit your juicer's feed tube. Bunch up the spinach and parsley, and push them through the feed tube with the apple, carrots, celery, and beet. Stir the juice, and pour into a glass. Serve at room temperature or chilled, as desired.

SPRING TONIC

1 medium vine-ripened tomato, washed

1 organic cucumber, scrubbed well

8 asparagus stems, washed

½ small or medium lemon, washed, or peeled if not organic

Cut the tomato into sections that fit your juicer's feed tube. Cut the cucumber in half lengthwise. Juice the tomato, cucumber, asparagus, and lemon. Stir the juice, and pour into a glass. Serve at room temperature or chilled, as desired.

BEAUTIFUL SKIN, HAIR, AND NAIL SOLUTION

1 medium organic cucumber, scrubbed well

1 medium parsnip, scrubbed well

3 carrots, scrubbed well, green tops removed, ends trimmed

$\frac{1}{2}$ small or medium lemon, washed, or peeled if not organic

$\frac{1}{4}$ small green bell pepper, washed

Cut the cucumber in half lengthwise, and juice with the parsnip, carrots, lemon, and bell pepper. Stir the juice, and pour into a glass. Serve at room temperature or chilled, as desired.

THE IMMUNE BUILDER

1 organic Golden or Red Delicious apple, washed

1 turnip, scrubbed well

1 handful watercress, rinsed (optional)

5 carrots, scrubbed well, green tops removed, ends trimmed

1 large garlic clove with peel, washed

Cut the apple and turnip into sections that fit your juicer's feed tube. Bunch up the watercress (if using), and push it through the feed tube with the apple, turnip, carrots, and garlic. Stir the juice, and pour into a glass. Serve at room temperature or chilled, as desired.

RADISH SOLUTION

2 medium vine-ripened tomatoes, washed

4 radishes with green tops, washed

$\frac{1}{4}$ small or medium lime or lemon, washed, or peeled if not organic

Cut the tomato into sections that fit your juicer's feed tube. Juice the tomatoes along with the radishes and lime or lemon. Stir the juice, and pour into a glass. Serve at room temperature or chilled, as desired.

Influenza

Influenza, or the "flu," is a highly contagious viral infection that usually spreads throughout the upper respiratory tract and can go into the lungs. It is transmitted most often through coughing and sneezing. Symptoms may include fever (often higher than that which may accompany a cold), sore throat, dry cough, aching muscles, fatigue, weakness, nasal congestion, sneezing, headache, nausea, and vomiting. Symptoms may appear suddenly after an incubation period of one to three days. Both colds and flu stem from viruses that infect the upper respiratory tract, but flu symptoms are more severe (*see* **Colds**). Flu epidemics, which tend to break out every two or three years, generally occur during the winter months.

Flu vaccinations may help keep you from getting the flu, but only if the vaccine is effective against the specific strain of virus you encounter. Once you have the flu, though, there is no cure—it must run its course. However, following the recommendations noted below can shorten the length of illness by helping to strengthen your immune system. Studies confirm that this approach works. For example, a study in Newfoundland found that consumption of a multivitamin supplement for one year improved people's immune responses to the influenza vaccine.

Diet Recommendations

❥ **Avoid all sugars.** Sweets decrease the functioning of white blood cells, the body's main immune cells. Sugar and vitamin C compete for entry into white cells; if sugar is abundant, the cells' "docking" sites will be filled with sugar molecules and prevent vitamin C from entering. Therefore, avoid eating anything that contains sugar in any form while you are sick. This includes sucrose (table sugar), cane sugar, corn syrup, beet sugar, and such natural sugars as honey, maple syrup, molasses, fruit concentrate, dried fruit, and sugar alcohols like sorbitol and manitol. Avoid aspartame as well. Even fruit juice consumption must be minimized (except for lemon and lime) because of the concentration of fruit sugars. Dilute all fruit juices by half with water, plain mineral water, or vegetable juices.

❥ **Eliminate all alcohol.** Alcohol acts like sugar in the body. Studies show that the consumption of alcohol increases the susceptibility to infection by impairing immune function.

❥ **Eliminate all meat and junk food.** These foods are difficult to digest. Junk food can contain high amounts of toxins. Also, nonfood additives such as dyes, synthetic sweeteners (such as aspartame), flavorings, preservatives, and synthetic oils can toxify the body and stress the mucous membranes. Avoid all artificial foods, such as margarine.

❥ **Eat lightly, and drink plenty of fluids.** Choose primarily vegetable juice recipes. When you are ill, it is best to eat only small amounts of food. A short vegetable juice fast (one to three days) is beneficial (see the Juice Fast, page 324). Give your digestive system a rest, as it takes a lot of energy to digest food. That way your body can concentrate on healing and repair. Water is another good fluid choice, as is green tea (see the Herb Recommendations).

❥ **Eat chicken soup with lots of garlic.** It really does help—Mom was right! But she didn't know that it may be the garlic, which is a natural antibiotic, that has the most powerful effect. Still I must admit, there's something more to garlicky chicken soup than just garlic's action. I have taken just garlic and not received anything close to the powerful effect of my homemade chicken soup. Chicken noodle soup from a can is not what I'd recommend. Make your own, or get someone to make it for you using lots and lots of garlic and vegetables. (I recommend my recipe, Garlicky Chicken Soup with Water Chestnuts, in my cookbook, *The Healthy Gourmet*; see Appendix A.)

Nutrient Recommendations

❥ **Selenium** deficiency may result in reduced antibody protection and a decrease in the microbe-eating ability of white blood cells called phago- cytes. Selenium-deficient phagocytes develop defective membranes, which results in the release of substances that further impair immune function. Selenium deficiency can also lead to reduced activity of hor- mones produced by the thymus gland, a gland important to immune func- tion. Best juice sources of selenium (in order of effectiveness): chard, turnips, garlic, radishes, carrots, and cabbage.

❥ **Vitamin A** and **carotenes** have been shown to enhance activity of immune-system components called natural killer (NK) cells. In one study, immune function was enhanced by 33 percent when participants had sin- gle servings of sweet potato, kale, and tomato juice every day for three weeks. These foods are rich in beta-carotene, lutein, and lycopene—sub- stances that improve the ability of immune cells to multiply. Many carotenes are converted to vitamin A in the body. Best juice sources of carotenes in general (in order of effectiveness): carrots, kale, parsley, spinach, chard, beet greens, watercress, broccoli, and romaine lettuce.

❥ **Vitamin C** and **bioflavonoids** are the first line of defense in neutraliz- ing the attack of toxins called free radicals on immune cells. One study showed that vitamin C enhanced NK cell, and T and B cell, activity up to tenfold in 78 percent of the participants after a single dose of the vitamin. Best juice sources of vitamin C (in order of effectiveness): kale, parsley, broccoli, Brussels sprouts, watercress, cauliflower, cabbage, spinach, citrus fruit, turnips, and asparagus. Best juice sources of bioflavonoids: bell pep- pers, broccoli, cabbage, cherries, citrus fruit, plums, parsley, and tomatoes.

❥ **Vitamin E,** a potent antioxidant, is required for optimal functioning of lymphocytes and mononuclear cells. Best juice sources of vitamin E (in order of effectiveness): spinach, watercress, asparagus, carrots, and tomatoes.

❥ **Zinc** supports the immune system. Studies show zinc deficiency increases susceptibility to infections by impairing immune function. An adequate supply of zinc and other antioxidants will help prevent shrinkage of the thymus gland and will support thymus-hormone activity. Best juice sources of zinc (in order of effectiveness): ginger root, turnips, parsley, garlic, carrots, spinach, cabbage, lettuce, and cucumbers.

Herb Recommendations

❥ **Ginseng** was shown in a recent study to improve the influenza vaccine's effect on NK cell activity by about twice as much as the control group.

❥ **Green tea** has been shown to be effective in rendering the influenza virus inactive.

Juice Ingredient Recommendations

❥ **Apple** juice has antiviral properties. Use only green apples, such as Granny Smiths or Pippins, since they have less sugar than other varieties, and dilute apple juice with $1/2$ cup water.

❥ **Ginger** juice and tea contain anti-inflammatory compounds, and ginger is a traditional remedy for flus and colds.

❥ **Jerusalem artichoke** juice is rich in inulin, which enhances the immune system by activating immunity defense mechanisms.

❥ **Parsley** juice is an excellent source of beta-carotene, vitamin C, and zinc. Intake should be limited to a safe, therapeutic dose of $1/2$ to 1 cup per day. Parsley can be toxic in overdose, and should be especially avoided by pregnant women.

❥ **Wheatgrass** juice is rich in chlorophyll, a blood purifier. Wheatgrass works best taken straight, but if your taste buds need a little help getting started, try the Wheatgrass Light recipe.

Juice Recipes

WALDORF TWIST

1 organic Granny Smith or Pippin apple, washed

3 stalks organic celery with leaves, washed

1/4 small or medium lemon, washed, or peeled if not organic

Cut the apple into sections that will fit your juicer's feed tube, and juice along with the celery and lemon. Stir the juice, and pour into a glass. Serve at room temperature or chilled, as desired.

THE GINGER HOPPER

1/2 organic Granny Smith or Pippin apple, washed

5 medium carrots, scrubbed well, green tops removed, ends trimmed

1/2- to 1-inch piece fresh ginger root, washed

Cut the apple into sections, and juice along with the carrots and ginger. Stir the juice, and pour into a glass. Serve at room temperature or chilled, as desired.

HOT GINGER-LEMON TEA

2-inch piece fresh ginger root, washed

1/2 small or medium lemon, washed, or peeled if not organic

2 cups pure water

1 tablespoon loose licorice tea, or 1 tea bag (optional)

1 stick cinnamon, broken

4–5 whole cloves

Dash nutmeg

Dash cardamom

Juice the ginger and lemon. Pour the juice in a small saucepan with the water; add the licorice (if using), cinnamon stick, and cloves. Bring the mixture to a boil, then reduce the heat and simmer for 5 to 10 minutes. Strain and pour into two mugs, add the nutmeg and cardamom, and serve hot.

WEIGHT-LOSS BUDDY

1 small Jerusalem artichoke, scrubbed well

4–5 carrots, scrubbed well, green tops removed, ends trimmed

1/2 small beet with no stems and leaves, scrubbed well

Cut the Jerusalem artichoke into sections that fit your juicer's feed tube. Juice the artichoke along with the carrots and beet. Stir the juice, and pour into a glass. Serve at room temperature or chilled, as desired.

WHEATGRASS LIGHT

1 organic green apple, washed

1 large handful wheatgrass, rinsed

2–3 sprigs mint, rinsed (optional)

½ small or medium lemon, washed, or peeled if not organic

½ cup water

Cut the apple into sections that will fit your juicer's feed tube. Bunch up the wheatgrass and mint (if using) and push them through the feed tube with the apple and lemon. Stir the juice, and pour into a glass with the water. Serve at room temperature or chilled, as desired.

THE MORNING ENERGIZER

½ organic Granny Smith or Pippin apple, washed

5 medium carrots, scrubbed well, green tops removed, ends trimmed

½ small beet with leaves and stems, scrubbed well

½ small or medium lemon, washed, or peeled if not organic

½- to 1-inch piece fresh ginger root, washed

Cut the apple into sections that will fit your juicer's feed tube. Juice the apple along with the carrots, beet, lemon, and ginger. Stir the juice, and pour into a glass. Serve at room temperature or chilled, as desired.

POPEYE'S POWER

½ medium organic Granny Smith or Pippin apple, washed

1 handful organic spinach, washed

1 small handful parsley, rinsed

4 medium carrots, scrubbed well, green tops removed, ends trimmed

1 stalk organic celery with leaves, washed

½ beet with leaves, scrubbed well

Cut the apple into sections that will fit your juicer's feed tube. Bunch up the spinach and parsley, and push them through the feed tube with the apple, carrots, celery, and beet. Stir the juice, and pour into a glass. Serve at room temperature or chilled, as desired.

TOMATO FLORENTINE

1 vine-ripened tomato, washed

1 handful organic spinach, washed

2–3 fresh basil leaves (optional)

½ small or medium lemon, washed, or peeled if not organic

Cut the tomato into sections that will fit your juicer's feed tube. Bunch up the spinach and basil leaves (if using), and push through the feed tube with the tomato and lemon. Stir the juice, and pour into a glass. Serve at room temperature or chilled, as desired.

SPICY TOMATO ON ICE

2 vine-ripened tomatoes, washed

2 dark green lettuce leaves, such as romaine or green leaf, washed

1 small handful parsley, rinsed

2 radishes with green tops, washed

½ small or medium lime or lemon, washed, or peeled if not organic

Dash hot sauce

Cut the tomato in sections that fit your juicer's feed tube. Bunch up the lettuce leaves and parsley, and push them through the feed tube with the tomatoes, radishes, and lime or lemon. Add a dash of hot sauce, and stir to combine. Pour into tall, ice-filled glasses.

THE COLON CLEANSER

1 bunch organic spinach, washed

1 handful parsley, rinsed

5 medium to large carrots, scrubbed well, green tops removed, ends trimmed

½ small or medium lemon, washed, or peeled if not organic

Bunch up the spinach and parsley, and push them through the feed tube with the carrots and lemon. Stir the juice, and pour into a glass. Serve at room temperature or chilled, as desired.

THE IMMUNE BUILDER

1 organic Granny Smith or Pippin apple, washed

1 turnip, scrubbed well

1 handful watercress, rinsed (optional)

5 carrots, scrubbed well, green tops removed, ends trimmed

1 large garlic clove with peel, washed

Cut the apple and turnip into sections that fit your juicer's feed tube. Bunch up the watercress (if using), and push it through the feed tube with the apple, turnip, carrots, and garlic. Stir the juice, and pour into a glass. Serve at room temperature or chilled, as desired.

Injuries

See **Bruises.**

Insomnia and Jet Lag

Insomnia is defined as a disturbance in normal sleep patterns that has adverse daytime effects. Anyone can have a few sleepless nights, but chronic insomnia persists more than three weeks. Younger people with insomnia typically have more trouble falling asleep, while older adults find it a greater challenge to stay asleep. Insomnia affects about one-third of all Americans, with more women being affected than men.

Psychiatric disorders, such as depression, have been reported as the single greatest cause of insomnia, accounting for 35 percent of all reported cases. Other causes include substance abuse, caffeine intake, poor diet, stress (*see* **Stress**), hypoglycemia (*see* **Hypoglycemia**) and other medical conditions, and abnormal limb movements (such as those caused by restless leg syndrome).

Conventional medical treatment for insomnia uses benzodiazepine tranquilizers. But these drugs have side effects, including addiction, that can be serious for some individuals. Such drugs can cause a person to wake up with a "hangover" and to feel even more tired than before. A natural approach to insomnia that emphasizes proper diet is effective and much easier on the body.

Insomnia induced by jet lag frequently follows travel. Jet lag is characterized by sleeplessness, fatigue, and hunger at odd times. It occurs when the body's natural clock does not have a chance to adjust to time-zone changes.

Diet Recommendations

❥ **Eat a high-complex-carbohydrate, low-fat diet.** One study found that this type of diet produces a significant increase in REM sleep, the sleep that is most refreshing. The researchers suggest that the high-carbohydrate diet leads to increases in levels of serotonin, a sleep-promoting hormone. Complex carbohydrates include vegetables; whole grains such as wheat, rye, barley, oats, and brown rice; and legumes, such as beans, lentils, and split peas. Some specific foods that have been used as traditional sleep remedies include whole wheat, brown rice, oats, mushrooms, and mulberries. The spices dill and basil have an overall calming effect.

❥ **Drink plenty of juice and water when you travel.** To avoid insomnia caused by jet lag, drink plenty of fluids when traveling. Eat such high-water content foods as fruits, vegetables, and sprouts, and drink plenty of fresh juices. People who drink only raw juices and eat fresh fruit and vegetable snacks on the day they travel report feeling energized and free of the effects of jet lag.

❥ **Avoid caffeine, refined sugar, and alcohol.** Caffeine is a stimulant; even a few cups of coffee in the morning can keep you awake at night. Caffeine is found not only in coffee and both green and black tea, but also in chocolate, cola, soft drinks, and aspirin and other painkillers. (Caffeine is also associated with restless leg syndrome.) Sugar can cause a spike and then a sharp drop in blood levels of glucose, and a drop in blood glucose promotes awakening in the night. Alcohol impairs the transport of tryptophan into the brain, which results in insufficient conversion of this amino acid into sleep-promoting serotonin. Alcohol, sugar, and caffeine are also very dehydrating.

❥ **Avoid substances that contain tyramine.** Tyramine is an amino acid that increases levels of norepinephrine, a stimulant brain chemical. The following substances contain tyramine, and should not be eaten close to bedtime: cheese, chocolate, sauerkraut, bacon, ham, sausage, eggplant, potatoes, spinach, and tomatoes. In addition, avoid using tobacco, which also contains tyramine.

Nutrient Recommendations

❥ **Calcium** deficiency will cause you to wake up in the night and then not be able to return to sleep. Low calcium levels also lead to muscles that stay contracted and can't relax. Best juice sources of calcium (in order of effectiveness): kale, parsley, dandelion greens, watercress, beet greens, broccoli, spinach, romaine lettuce, string beans, oranges, celery, and carrots.

❥ **Magnesium** deficiency will cause you to wake up after a few hours of sleep and not be able to drift off again. Magnesium-rich foods such as kelp, wheat bran and germ, almonds, and cashews can help induce sleep. Best juice sources of magnesium (in order of effectiveness): beet greens, spinach, parsley, dandelion greens, garlic, blackberries, beets, broccoli, cauliflower, carrots, and celery.

❥ **Pantothenic acid** deficiency can cause insomnia. Best juice sources of pantothenic acid (in order of effectiveness): broccoli, cauliflower, and kale.

❥ **Tryptophan** is a precursor to both serotonin and melatonin, the body's main sleep hormone, and is considered the best amino acid for inducing sleep. Best food sources of tryptophan: tuna, turkey, and yogurt. Chlorella and blue green algae are also sources of tryptophan. They work best taken at bedtime; the recommended dosage is 0.5 gram.

❧ **Vitamin B$_1$ (thiamine)** deficiency may decrease the availability of serotonin. Best food sources of vitamin B$_1$ (in order of effectiveness): seeds, nuts, beans, split peas, millet, buckwheat, whole wheat, oatmeal, wild rice, lobster, and cornmeal. It can also be found, in lesser quantities, in sunflower and buckwheat sprouts, and in garlic. This nutrient is not available from fruits and vegetables.

Supplement Recommendations

❧ **Melatonin** has been shown in studies to help readjust the sleep/wake cycle and reduce jet lag after traveling across time zones. The best way to use melatonin for jet lag is to take 5 mg in the evening thirty minutes before bedtime for five days **before** traveling to the new destination, and then continue taking it at the new destination. Melatonin can also play an important role in treating insomnia in general, since low levels of this hormone (secreted at night by the pineal gland) can cause sleeplessness. However, melatonin is helpful in promoting sleep only if melatonin levels are low, a condition that is especially common in older people. Melatonin is available at most health food stores (see Appendix A).

Herb Recommendations

❧ **Catnip, chamomile** and **skullcap** soothe the nerves. Be sure to use German chamomile, *Matricaria recutita,* and not Roman chamomile, *Chamaemelum nobile.*

❧ **Chia seeds** and **jujube seeds** have a sedative effect. In Traditional Chinese Medicine, jujube seeds are thought to nourish the heart and calm the spirit.

❧ **Hops** is used in a traditional remedy for insomnia caused by anxiety. To use this herb, fill a small sachet-size pillow with hops and place it near your regular pillow at night.

❧ **Valerian root** has a sedating and tranquilizing effect.

Juice Ingredient Recommendations

❧ **Celery** juice contains silicon. This element strengthens nerve and heart tissue, and has a calming effect.

❧ **Lettuce** juice has a sedative effect.

❧ **Parsley** juice is a good source of both calcium and magnesium. Intake should be limited to a safe, therapeutic dose of $^1/_2$ to 1 cup per day. Parsley can be toxic in overdose, and should be especially avoided by pregnant women.

Juice Recipes

SWEET DREAMS NIGHTCAP

2 romaine lettuce leaves, washed

1 handful parsley, rinsed

4 carrots, scrubbed well, green tops removed, ends trimmed

3 organic celery stalks with leaves, washed

Bunch up the lettuce leaves and parsley, and push through the feed tube with the carrots and celery. Stir the juice, and pour into a glass. Serve at room temperature or chilled, as desired.

THE BEAN & THE CARROT

2 romaine lettuce leaves, washed

4–5 medium carrots, scrubbed well, green tops removed, ends trimmed

8 organic string beans, washed

3 Brussels sprouts, cut in half and washed

$^1/_2$ small or medium lemon, washed, or peeled if not organic

Bunch up the lettuce leaves, and push through the feed tube with the carrots, string beans, Brussels sprouts, and lemon. Stir the juice, and pour into a glass. Serve at room temperature or chilled, as desired.

BEAUTIFUL BONE SOLUTION

1 organic Golden or Red Delicious apple, washed

1–2 kale leaves, washed

1 handful parsley, rinsed

1 stalk organic celery, washed

$^1/_4$ small or medium lemon, washed, or peeled if not organic

$^1/_2$- to 1-inch piece fresh ginger root, washed

Cut the apple into sections that fit your juicer's feed tube. Bunch up the kale and parsley, and push through the feed tube with the apple, celery, lemon, and ginger. Stir the juice, and pour into a glass. Serve at room temperature or chilled, as desired.

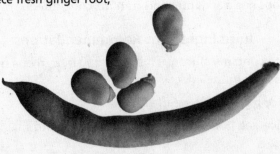

MAGNESIUM SPECIAL

5 medium carrots, scrubbed well, green tops removed, ends trimmed

2 stalks organic celery with leaves, washed

$1/2$ small beet with leaves and stems, scrubbed well

2 broccoli florets, washed

$1/2$ small or medium lemon, washed, or peeled if not organic

Juice the carrots, celery, beet, broccoli, and lemon. Stir the juice, and pour into a glass. Serve at room temperature or chilled, as desired.

THE IMMUNE BUILDER

1 organic Golden or Red Delicious apple, washed

1 turnip, scrubbed well

1 handful watercress, rinsed (optional)

5 carrots, scrubbed well, green tops removed, ends trimmed

1 large garlic clove with peel, washed

Cut the apple and turnip into sections that fit your juicer's feed tube. Bunch up the watercress (if using), and push it through the feed tube with the apple, turnip, carrots, and garlic. Stir the juice, and pour into a glass. Serve at room temperature or chilled, as desired.

SLEEP MENDER

$1/4$ small head iceberg lettuce, washed

5 medium carrots, scrubbed well, green tops removed, ends trimmed

4 cauliflower florets, washed

$1/2$ small or medium lemon, washed, or peeled if not organic

Cut the lettuce into sections that fit your juicer's feed tube, and juice with the carrots, cauliflower, and lemon. Stir the juice, and pour into a glass. Serve at room temperature or chilled, as desired.

Irritable Bowel Syndrome

See **Colitis.**

Jet Lag

See **Insomnia and Jet Lag.**

Low Blood Sugar

See **Hypoglycemia.**

Lupus

See **Rheumatoid Arthritis.**

Macular Degeneration

See **Eye Disorders.**

Menopause

Commonly referred to as "the change of life," menopause is the point at which a woman stops ovulating, and therefore stops menstruating. Some people start early, others late, some start and stop, but most women experience the change around age fifty. During this period, which usually lasts about five years, female hormones do not disappear. Other organs take over for the ovaries. For example, the adrenal glands continue to produce androgens, the hormones responsible for the sex drive. However, levels of estradiol, the most common form of estrogen in the body, drop to one-tenth of their previous levels. It is falling levels of this hormone that is thought to be responsible for such menopausal symptoms as hot flashes, dizziness, night sweats, headache, difficulty in breathing and shortness of breath, heart palpitations, vaginal dryness, nervousness, backache, and depression. If a woman is hypoglycemic (*see* **Hypoglycemia**), the symptoms are more pronounced. The decline in estrogen levels also make a woman more prone to osteoporosis, in which the bones become more fragile, and to the buildup of cholesterol within the arteries, which can lead to heart disease. Synthetic estrogens can help, but they are not without risk. Whether or not you should use hormone replacement therapy (HRT), and what type of therapy would be best, is a decision you and your doctor need to make together.

No matter what you decide about HRT, diet can make a big difference in how you feel during menopause. There are foods that contain natural estrogens, which can be very beneficial. Juicing fresh vegetables and fruits offers a powerhouse of "help in a glass," so plug in your juicer and get going on a change for the better!

Diet Recommendations

❥ **Eat a low-fat, high-fiber diet.** Include plenty of fresh vegetables and fruits, whole grains, legumes (beans, lentils, split peas), seeds, and nuts in your meal plans. Eat animal products sparingly. At least 50 percent of your diet should be made up of raw fruits, vegetables, juices, sprouts, seeds, and nuts.

❥ **Include generous amounts of soy products in your diet.** "Dietary soybean supplementation may be a more acceptable method of estrogen replacement therapy for women," states *Family Practice News*. HRT can protect against atherosclerosis and osteoporosis, but side effects such as moodiness, bloating, weight gain, and increased cancer risk have kept many women from taking estrogens. Soy contains high amounts of phytoestrogens, along with omega-3 and omega-6 essential fatty acids (see the Nutrient Recommendations). In one study it was found that after twelve weeks of eating soy products, the participants found that their hot flashes decreased by 40 percent and their bone mineral content improved. Japanese women eat a diet high in soy-based foods, and their menopausal symptoms are much less frequent and intense than those of Western women. It is wise to incorporate a variety of soy products into your diet, such as soy flour, soy milk, tofu, tempeh, and miso.

❥ **Avoid substances that tend to dry the mucous membranes.** These substances include alcohol, antihistamines, caffeine, and diuretics. Dry membranes contribute to vaginal dryness and irritation. One study also suggests that alcohol may influence the onset of menopause. Eliminate smoking and sugar consumption as well, since they can contribute to adverse menopausal effects.

❧ **Go on periodic juice fasts.** Fasts can help you feel more vibrant and capable of coping with stress. Many people say they experience an improved sense of well-being after a juice fast. For more information, see the Juice Fast (page 324).

Nutrient Recommendations

❧ **Bioflavonoids** and **vitamin C** have been shown in studies to reduce the frequency and intensity of hot flashes. Bioflavonoids (especially hesperidin and rutin) and vitamin C restore the structure of blood-vessel linings. This action helps reduce blood-vessel dilation, which reduces hot flashes. Best juice sources of vitamin C (in order of effectiveness): kale, parsley, broccoli, Brussels sprouts, watercress, cauliflower, cabbage, strawberries, papaya, spinach, citrus fruit, turnips, mangoes, asparagus, and cantaloupes. Best juice sources of bioflavonoids: apricots, bell peppers, berries (blueberry, blackberry, and cranberry), broccoli, cabbage, cantaloupes, cherries, citrus fruit, grapes, parsley, plums, prunes, and tomatoes.

❧ **Essential fatty acids (EFAs)** work with soy products (see the Diet Recommendations) to help ease menopausal symptoms. Studies have found a decrease of 40 percent in hot flashes when women who use soy products incorporate flaxseed oil, which contains EFAs, into their diets. Flaxseed oil not only helps reduced hot flashes, it helps to decrease vaginal dryness. In addition, supplementation with flaxseed oil and evening primrose oil, another EFA-rich oil, has been shown to help the adrenal glands produce more estrogen. High-lignan flaxseed oil is recommended because lignans are particularly helpful in reducing hot flashes. A high-lignan, unrefined organic flaxseed oil can be purchased at most health food stores. For more information, see the fats and oils section in Basic Guidelines for the Juice Lady's Health and Healing Diet (page 313).

❧ **Vitamin E** can help reduce hot flashes and vaginal dryness. Best juice sources of vitamin E (in order of effectiveness): spinach, watercress, asparagus, carrots, and tomatoes.

Herb Recommendations

❧ **Black cohosh** is used to help relieve hot flashes, depression, and vaginal atrophy.

❥ **Dong quai** is a Chinese herb that has been studied for its potential to control hot flashes. Most Chinese herbalists use dong quai in combination with other herbs; you may want to consult an Oriental medicine doctor (OMD) for further recommendations.

❥ **Licorice** contains flavonoids, which have estrogenlike effects, and saponin, which has progesteronelike effects. Avoid licorice if you have high blood pressure, and do not use it for prolonged periods of time. Use a medicinal form of the herb, not licorice candy.

❥ **Motherwort** is used for menopausal symptoms.

❥ **Wild yam,** also known as dioscorea, is used to make an over-the-counter progesterone cream. When applied to the skin, this cream can help ease hot flashes and mood swings (see Appendix A). You may want to use wild yam cream under a doctor's supervision.

Juice Ingredient Recommendations

❥ **Ginger** is a juice ingredient you may want to *avoid*, since it raises body temperature.

❥ **Parsley** juice contains bioflavonoids and vitamin C. Intake should be limited to a safe, therapeutic dose of $1/2$ to 1 cup per day. Parsley can be toxic in overdose, and should be especially avoided by pregnant women.

❥ **Soy milk**-based smoothies can be very beneficial because of the phytoestrogens in soy foods.

Juice Recipes

SO BERRY SMOOTH

$1/2$ organic Golden or Red Delicious apple, washed

1 cup blueberries, raspberries, or blackberries, washed

1 ripe medium to large banana, peeled

$1/2$ cup silken tofu, or $1/2$ cup plain or vanilla soy milk

6 ice cubes

Cut the apple into sections that fit your juicer's feed tube. Juice the apple with the blueberries. Pour the juice into a blender, and add the banana, tofu or soy milk, and ice cubes; blend until smooth. Pour the mixture into one or two glasses and serve immediately.

POPEYE'S POWER

½ medium organic apple, any kind, washed

1 handful organic spinach, washed

1 small handful parsley, rinsed

4 medium carrots, scrubbed well, green tops removed, ends trimmed

1 stalk organic celery with leaves, washed

½ beet with leaves, scrubbed well

Cut the apple into sections that will fit your juicer's feed tube. Bunch up the spinach and parsley, and push them through the feed tube with the apple, carrots, celery, and beet. Stir the juice, and pour into a glass. Serve at room temperature or chilled, as desired.

STRAWBERRY-CANTALOUPE COCKTAIL

½ ripe organic cantaloupe with seeds, washed, or peeled if not organic

1 cup organic strawberries, washed

Cut the cantaloupe into strips that fit your juicer's feed tube. Juice the cantaloupe and strawberries; stir the juice and pour into a glass. Serve at room temperature or chilled, as desired.

SANTA FE SALSA COCKTAIL

1 medium vine-ripened tomato, washed

½ medium organic cucumber, scrubbed well

¼ cup cilantro, rinsed

¼ small or medium lime or lemon, washed, or peeled if not organic

Dash hot sauce (optional)

Cut the tomato into sections that fit your juicer's feed tube. Cut the cucumber in half again lengthwise. Bunch up the cilantro, and push through the feed tube with the tomato, cucumber, and lime or lemon. Pour the juice into a glass, add the hot sauce (if using), and stir. Serve at room temperature or chilled, as desired.

SPRING TONIC

1 medium vine-ripened tomato, washed

1 organic cucumber, scrubbed well

8 asparagus stems, washed

½ small or medium lemon, washed, or peeled if not organic

Cut the tomato into sections that fit your juicer's feed tube. Cut the cucumber in half lengthwise. Juice the tomato, cucumber, asparagus, and lemon. Stir the juice, and pour into a glass. Serve at room temperature or chilled, as desired.

Sweet Dreams Nightcap

2 romaine lettuce leaves, washed

1 handful parsley, rinsed

4 carrots, scrubbed well, green tops removed, ends trimmed

3 organic celery stalks with leaves, washed

Bunch up the lettuce leaves and parsley, and push through the feed tube with the carrots and celery. Stir the juice, and pour into a glass. Serve at room temperature or chilled, as desired.

Beautiful Skin, Hair, and Nail Solution

1 medium organic cucumber, scrubbed well

1 medium parsnip, scrubbed well

3 carrots, scrubbed well, green tops removed, ends trimmed

1/2 small or medium lemon, washed, or peeled if not organic

1/4 small green bell pepper, washed

Cut the cucumber in half lengthwise, and juice with the parsnip, carrots, lemon, and bell pepper. Stir the juice, and pour into a glass. Serve at room temperature or chilled, as desired.

The Feel Good Cocktail

1/2 pear, washed

4 medium carrots, scrubbed well, green tops removed, ends trimmed

3 fennel stalks with leaves and flowers, washed

1 stalk organic celery with leaves, washed

Cut the pear into sections that fit your juicer's feed tube, and juice along with the carrots, fennel, and celery. Stir the juice, and pour into a glass. Serve at room temperature or chilled, as desired.

Menstrual Disorders

Disorders associated with the menstrual cycle are among the most prevalent female health problems. Some women have periods that occur too frequently or not frequently enough, some women don't have periods at all, and others experience bleeding that is not related to the menstrual cycle. However, among the most common menstrual disorders are menorrhagia, or excessive menstrual bleeding, and dysmenorrhea, or painful menstruation. While either condition can arise from a number of distinct physical disorders, such as various types of uterine growths, they often occur for no identifiable reason. Another common problem is premenstrual syndrome (PMS), a term that covers a variety of physical and emotional symptoms that occur from seven to fourteen days prior to the start of menstruation. These symptoms, which include decreased energy, tension, irritability, depression, headache, breast tenderness, bloating, and water retention (*see* **Water Retention**), are related to hormone imbalances.

Many health professionals feel that menstrual disorders are associated with such lifestyle factors as diet (including eating disorders), stress (*see* **Stress**), lack of exercise, and obesity (*see* **Overweight/Obesity**). In one study, women were asked to list up to three treatments they had tried and found most effective for treating PMS. They mentioned taking nutritional supplements, getting more exercise, and making dietary changes.

Lifestyle Recommendations

❥ **Get regular exercise.** Do at least thirty minutes of aerobic exercise three times a week. Walking, swimming, and aerobic dance are all good choices.

Diet Recommendations

❥ **Eat a low-fat, high-complex-carbohydrate diet.** Eating fewer animal products decreases the amount of saturated fat in your body. This can help reduce PMS symptoms by reducing circulating estrogen levels and by removing sources of outside estrogens. Research shows that women with menorrhagia have higher concentrations of an inflammatory substance called arachidonic acid in the uterine lining, which leads to excessive bleeding and cramping during menstruation. A high-fiber diet has been shown to result in a significant reduction in estrogen levels because fiber causes more estrogen to be excreted from the body. For more information, see Basic Guidelines for the Juice Lady's Health and Healing Diet (page 313).

❥ **Increase your consumption of soy products.** Tofu, tempeh, soy milk, and miso should all be a part of your diet. These foods are rich in phytoestrogens, which have a balancing effect on the female reproductive system. For this reason, they are recommended for menstrual disorders caused by either estrogen excess or estrogen deficiency.

❥ **Avoid sugar, caffeine, and alcohol.** Sugar, especially when combined with caffeine, has a detrimental effect on PMS and mood. A high sugar intake impairs estrogen metabolism and is associated with higher estrogen levels. Caffeine—found in coffee, green and black tea, cola, and chocolate—promotes anxiety, depression, and breast tenderness associated with PMS.

❥ **Use juice fasting and liver cleansing.** A short juice fast and a liver cleanse can help improve most menstrual disorders. See the Juice Fast (page 324) and the Liver Cleanse (page 333).

Nutrient Recommendations

❥ **Calcium** and **magnesium** have been shown to improve mood, concentration, and behaviorial symptoms, as well as lessen pain, during the menstrual phase, and to reduce water retention during the premenstrual phase. These minerals work together—studies show that just increasing calcium intake, without increasing magnesium, did not improve mood and pain symptoms during the premenstrual phase. Best juice sources of calcium (in order of effectiveness): kale, parsley, dandelion greens, watercress, beet greens, broccoli, spinach, romaine lettuce, string beans, oranges, celery, and carrots. Best juice sources of magnesium: beet greens, spinach, parsley, dandelion greens, garlic, blackberries, beets, broccoli, cauliflower, carrots, and celery.

❥ **Essential fatty acids (EFAs)** are divided into two groups, omega-3 and omega-6 fatty acids. Studies have shown a correlation between low EFA levels and menstrual discomfort. EFAs are found in cold-water fish, such as salmon, tuna, trout, halibut, cod, and mackerel, and in unrefined oils, such as hemp and flaxseed oil. One tablespoon of oil per day is recommended. For more information, see the fats and oils section in Basic Guidelines for the Juice Lady's Health and Healing Diet (page 313).

❥ **Vitamin C** and **bioflavonoids** work together to lessen excessive bleeding. The capillaries in a woman's body weaken briefly just after ovulation and again for a few days before menstruation. Women who have heavy periods have considerably weaker capillaries than women whose flows are normal. Bioflavonoids taken with vitamin C over a period of several months can strengthen capillaries and reduce excessive bleeding. Studies show that pure ascorbic acid (vitamin C) is not as effective in treating capillary fragility as fruits and vegetables that contain both this vitamin and an abundance of bioflavonoids, which improve vitamin C storage in the body. Also, vitamin C enhances iron absorption, which is especially important since iron is lost during menstruation. Best juice sources of vitamin C (in order of effectiveness): kale, parsley, broccoli, Brussels sprouts, watercress, cauliflower, cabbage, strawberries, papaya, spinach, citrus fruit, turnips, mangoes, asparagus, and cantaloupes. Best juice sources of bioflavonoids: apricots, bell peppers, berries (blueberry, blackberry, and cranberry), broccoli, cabbage, cantaloupes, cherries, citrus fruit, grapes, parsley, plums, prunes, and tomatoes.

Herb Recommendations

❥ **American cranesbill** is helpful in preventing excessive blood loss through menorrhagia.

❥ **Black cohosh** is a relaxant and normalizer of the female reproductive system. It is helpful for painful or delayed menstruation.

❥ **Black haw bark** relaxes the uterus.

❥ **Cramp bark** relaxes the uterus and relieves painful cramps associated with menstruation.

❥ **Motherwort** stimulates delayed or suppressed menstruation, particularly when anxiety or tension is involved.

Juice Ingredient Recommendations

❥ **Fennel** juice is a uterine tonic.

❥ **Dark, leafy greens,** which are rich in chlorophyll and iron, help relieve excessive menstrual flow. Mustard greens are specifically recommended for PMS. Mustard greens are very strong tasting and should be mixed with generous amounts of such mild-flavored juices as carrot and apple.

❥ **Parsley** juice contains bioflavonoids and vitamin C. Intake should be limited to a safe, therapeutic dose of $1/2$ to 1 cup per day. Parsley can be toxic in overdose, and should be especially avoided by pregnant women.

❥ **Soy products,** such as tofu and soy milk, are rich in phytoestrogens. They are delicious when used in smoothies.

Juice Recipes

THE FEEL GOOD COCKTAIL

$1/2$ pear, washed

4 medium carrots, scrubbed well, green tops removed, ends trimmed

3 fennel stalks with leaves and flowers, washed

1 stalk organic celery with leaves, washed

Cut the pear into sections that fit your juicer's feed tube, and juice along with the carrots, fennel, and celery. Stir the juice, and pour into a glass. Serve at room temperature or chilled, as desired.

POPEYE'S POWER

1/2 medium organic apple, any kind, washed

1 handful organic spinach, washed

1 small handful parsley, rinsed

4 medium carrots, scrubbed well, green tops removed, ends trimmed

1 stalk organic celery with leaves, washed

1/2 beet with leaves, scrubbed well

Cut the apple into sections that will fit your juicer's feed tube. Bunch up the spinach and parsley, and push them through the feed tube with the apple, carrots, celery, and beet. Stir the juice, and pour into a glass. Serve at room temperature or chilled, as desired.

SO BERRY SMOOTH

1/2 organic Golden or Red Delicious apple, washed

1 cup blueberries, raspberries, or blackberries, washed

1 ripe medium to large banana, peeled

1/2 cup silken tofu, or 1/2 cup plain or vanilla soy milk

6 ice cubes

Cut the apple into sections that fit your juicer's feed tube. Juice the apple with the blueberries. Pour the juice into a blender, and add the banana, tofu or soy milk, and ice cubes; blend until smooth. Pour the mixture into one or two glasses and serve immediately.

THE CALCIUM CHAMP

1/2 organic Golden or Red Delicious apple, washed

1 handful organic spinach with stems, washed

1 small handful parsley, rinsed

1 ripe medium banana, peeled

1/2 cup plain or vanilla soy milk

1 tablespoon tahini (sesame butter)

6 ice cubes

Cut the apple in sections that fit your juicer's feed tube. Bunch up the spinach and parsley, and push through the feed tube with the apple. Pour the juice into a blender, and add the banana, soy milk, tahini, and ice; blend until smooth. Pour into one or two glasses and serve immediately.

SWEET CALCIUM COCKTAIL

1 three-inch chunk fresh pineapple, scrubbed well or peeled if not organic

1–2 kale leaves, washed

Cut the pineapple into strips that fit your juicer's feed tube. Bunch up the kale, and push through the feed tube with the pineapple. Stir the juice, and pour into a glass. Serve at room temperature or chilled, as desired.

BEAUTIFUL BONE SOLUTION

1 organic **Golden** or **Red Delicious** apple, **washed**

1–2 kale leaves, washed

1 handful parsley, rinsed

1 stalk organic celery, washed

¼ small or medium lemon, washed, or peeled if not organic

½- to 1-inch piece fresh ginger root, washed

Cut the apple into sections that fit your juicer's feed tube. Bunch up the kale and parsley, and push through the feed tube with the apple, celery, lemon, and ginger. Stir the juice, and pour into a glass. Serve at room temperature or chilled, as desired.

ANTIAGING COCKTAIL

1 small bunch organic purple grapes (about 1 cup) with small stems* and seeds, washed

½ cup blueberries, blackberries, or raspberries, washed

¼ small or medium lemon, washed, or peeled if not organic

½-inch piece fresh ginger root, washed

*Large stems can dull your juicer's blade.

Juice the grapes, berries, lemon, and ginger. Stir the juice, and pour into a glass. Serve at room temperature or chilled, as desired.

TANGERINE SQUEEZE

¼ ripe pineapple, scrubbed well or peeled if not organic

2–3 tangerines, peeled

¼ lime, washed or peeled if not organic

Cut the pineapple into strips, and divide the tangerines into sections that fit your juicer's feed tube, and juice them with the lime. Stir the juice, and pour into a glass. Serve at room temperature or chilled, as desired.

Migraine

There are estimates that as many as eight million people suffer from migraines in the United States. Migraine attacks, which can last anywhere from two hours to three days, cause severe, throbbing pain on one or both sides of the head, and may be accompanied by nausea and vomiting. Other symptoms include sensitivity to light, tingling, dizziness, ringing in the ears, chills, sweating, and drowsiness. Migraine can be debilitating— sufferers can sometimes do nothing but lie down in a darkened room until the symptoms abate. Symptoms are believed to start in childhood, but often do not show themselves directly as headaches. Rather, a child may experience colic, periodic abdominal pains, vomiting, and dizziness.

It has yet to be determined exactly what triggers a migraine headache, but researchers believe that, in addition to nerve disorders and biochemical imbalances, there is an underlying blood-vessel instability that causes excessive vessel constriction followed by excessive dilation. Some migraine patients show severe restriction in blood flow to the brain just prior to the onset of a headache. Another suspected mechanism involves blood components called platelets, which cause the blood to clot. The platelets of migraine sufferers clump together much more readily than those of other people. Serotonin, a substance stored in platelets and released when they stick together, is a strong blood-vessel constrictor, and in this case a contributor to migraines. The pattern seen prior to the onset of a headache is blood-vessel constriction with higher than normal levels of plasma serotonin, followed by blood-vessel dilation with low levels of serotonin.

Diet Recommendations

❥ **Eat more vegetables and other complex carbohydrates.** Whole grains, such as brown rice and millet, and legumes, such as beans, lentils, and split peas, are good choices. Complex carbohydrates appear to help reduce migraines by normalizing serotonin levels. For more information, see Basic Guidelines for the Juice Lady's Health and Healing Diet (page 313).

❥ **Eliminate all food allergies and intolerances.** Various food allergies, sensitivities, and intolerances are thought to underlie many migraine headaches. It is vital to determine which foods trigger an attack. In one study, eleven of the sixteen patients who followed an elimination diet had a significant decrease in headaches, and six became headache-free. In another study, seventy-eight of eighty-three children became headache-free when food allergens were eliminated. Some of the most common migraine-triggering foods are those that contain tyramine. This amino acid is found in alcoholic beverages, especially red wine and beer; yeast products (breads, rolls, crackers) and yeast concentrates found in prepared boullions and gravies; sour cream; aged cheese, especially Stilton,

cheddar, and blue; red plums; figs; aged game; liver; canned and pre-
served meats and fish; Italian broad beans; string beans; eggplant; and soy
sauce. Other foods that commonly trigger migraines include shellfish and
fish; citrus fruit, especially oranges; wheat; tea; coffee; meat, especially
pork and beef; tomatoes; milk; rye; rice; oats; cane sugar; grapes; corn;
nuts, especially walnuts; onions; and food additives, especially benzoic
acid, sodium nitrate, and tartrazine. For more information, *see* **Allergies**
and the Elimination Diet, page 321.

❡ **Go on a juice fast before identifying your allergens.** Before going on
the Elimination Diet, follow a one- to three-day juice fast. (See the Juice
Fast, page 324.) During a juice fast there may be some initial worsening of
symptoms, but by the end there is usually a great measure of relief.

❡ **Eliminate all sources of monosodium glutamate (MSG).** This food
additive causes headaches in susceptible individuals. Added as a flavor
enhancer, it is often found in packaged processed foods, Chinese restaurant dishes, and frozen foods.

❡ **Avoid all foods containing aspartame.** This artificial sweetener has
been shown to cause severe headaches in some individuals.

❡ **Decrease your intake of animal fats.** Saturated fats contribute to
platelet stickiness. Meats and fatty foods are often reported as triggers of
migraine headaches.

❡ **Increase your intake of liver-supporting foods.** Traditional Oriental
medicine looks at migraines as a result of liver problems, a condition
known as *liver heat.* Liver heat is said to be generated by a strained liver,
generally due to overindulgence in rich foods. Overconsumption of meats,
cheese, fats, eggs, alcohol, and sweets cause "liver stagnation," and
migraines are among the conditions that result from this type of diet. Rye
is a grain that Oriental medicine says is especially beneficial for the liver.
Rye broth, or a watery rye cereal called congee can be very helpful, unless
you are allergic to rye. Celery is another food that helps relieve liver heat.
If you suffer from migraines, drink celery juice often.

Nutrient Recommendations

❡ **Essential fatty acids (EFAs),** specifically the omega-3 fatty acids, have
shown a significant ability to alleviate severe migraines. One study saw
both migraine intensity and frequency decrease when individuals were
given fish oils rich in omega-3s, which decrease platelet clumping. The

best sources of omega-3 fatty acids include cold-water fish, such as salmon, tuna, halibut, cod, trout, and mackerel; flaxseed, hemp, and soybean oils; walnuts; wheat germ; and tofu and other soybean products. For more information on omega-3 oils, see the fats and oils section in Basic Guidelines for the Juice Lady's Health and Healing Diet (page 313).

❥ **Magnesium** plays a role in headaches of all types, and people who suffer migraines often have low blood levels of this mineral. Low levels of magnesium can cause blood-vessel constriction in the head and reduce blood flow to the brain. One study showed that intravenous magnesium sulfate brought considerable relief to migraine patients. Best juice sources of magnesium (in order of effectiveness): beet greens, spinach, parsley, dandelion greens, garlic, blackberries, beets, broccoli, cauliflower, carrots, and celery.

❥ **Vitamin B$_3$ (niacin)** causes blood-vessel dilation, and so is clearly useful in treating migraine headaches. Studies found that intramuscular injections of vitamin B$_3$ help relieve migraine headaches. The current recommendation is 500 mg of B$_3$ (taken orally) at the onset of a headache. Best food sources of this vitamin (in order of effectiveness): brewer's yeast, rice and wheat bran, peanuts, turkey, chicken, and fish. Vitamin B$_3$ is not available in fruits and vegetables.

Herb Recommendations

❥ **Cayenne pepper** contains capsaicin, which inhibits platelet clumping and controls pain. This herb may be most effective in preventing, rather than alleviating, migraine attacks.

❥ **Feverfew** is the herb most widely recommended for migraine headaches. One study showed that patients who ate fresh feverfew leaves, and who were then taken off feverfew and given an inactive placebo, had a significant increase in the frequency and severity of migraines. It may take up to one month for feverfew to bring relief.

❥ **Valerian** is a sedative herb that is helpful in treating migraines brought on by stress. This herb will not alleviate the headache, but will lessen the pain.

Juice Ingredient Recommendations

❥ **Cantaloupe, garlic,** and **ginger** juices have all been shown to reduce platelet stickiness.

❥ **Celery** juice mixed with a little lemon is recommended for headaches (see Waldorf Twist).

❥ **Parsley** juice contains magnesium. Intake should be limited to a safe, therapeutic dose of $1/2$ to 1 cup per day. Parsley can be toxic in overdose, and should be especially avoided by pregnant women.

Juice Recipes

STRAWBERRY-CANTALOUPE COCKTAIL

$1/2$ ripe organic cantaloupe with seeds, washed, or peeled if not organic

1 cup organic strawberries, washed

Cut the cantaloupe into strips that fit your juicer's feed tube. Juice the cantaloupe and strawberries; stir the juice and pour into a glass. Serve at room temperature or chilled, as desired.

THE IMMUNE BUILDER

1 organic Golden or Red Delicious apple, washed

1 turnip, scrubbed well

1 handful watercress, rinsed (optional)

5 carrots, scrubbed well, green tops removed, ends trimmed

1 large garlic clove with peel, washed

Cut the apple and turnip into sections that fit your juicer's feed tube. Bunch up the watercress (if using), and push it through the feed tube with the apple, turnip, carrots, and garlic. Stir the juice, and pour into a glass. Serve at room temperature or chilled, as desired.

GINGER TWIST

1 organic Red or Golden Delicious apple, washed

1 handful parsley, rinsed

4 carrots, scrubbed well, green tops removed, ends trimmed

1-inch piece fresh ginger root, washed

$1/4$ small or medium lemon, washed, or peeled if not organic

Cut the apple into sections that fit your juicer's feed tube. Bunch up the parsley and push it through the feed tube with the apple, carrots, ginger, and lemon. Stir the juice, and pour into a glass. Serve at room temperature or chilled, as desired.

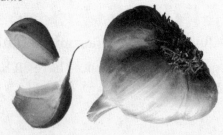

WALDORF TWIST

1 organic Red or Golden Delicious apple, washed

3 stalks organic celery with leaves, washed

¼ small or medium lemon, washed, or peeled if not organic

Cut the apple into sections that will fit your juicer's feed tube, and juice along with the celery and lemon. Stir the juice, and pour into a glass. Serve at room temperature or chilled, as desired.

MAGNESIUM SPECIAL

5 medium carrots, scrubbed well, green tops removed, ends trimmed

2 stalks organic celery with leaves, washed

½ small beet with leaves and stems, scrubbed well

2 broccoli florets, washed

½ small or medium lemon, washed, or peeled if not organic

Juice the carrots, celery, beet, broccoli, and lemon. Stir the juice, and pour into a glass. Serve at room temperature or chilled, as desired.

POPEYE'S POWER

½ medium organic apple, any kind, washed

1 handful organic spinach, washed

1 small handful parsley, rinsed

4 medium carrots, scrubbed well, green tops removed, ends trimmed

1 stalk organic celery with leaves, washed

½ beet with leaves, scrubbed well

Cut the apple into sections that will fit your juicer's feed tube. Bunch up the spinach and parsley, and push them through the feed tube with the apple, carrots, celery, and beet. Stir the juice, and pour into a glass. Serve at room temperature or chilled, as desired.

Multiple Sclerosis

Multiple sclerosis (MS) is a chronic neurological disease that usually appears in people between the ages of twenty and fifty. Symptoms include tingling, loss of sensation, numbness, loss of balance, visual impairment, muscle weakness or stiffness, bladder and/or bowel problems, paralysis, depression, difficulty in concentrating, memory loss, and fatigue.

The cause of MS is not completely known, although it appears to be an autoimmune reaction in which the body's white blood cells, which normally fight infection, attack the myelin sheaths that covers nerves in the spinal cord and brain. This action scars scattered nerve segments, which slows down the electrical impulses that travel along those nerves. This autoimmune reaction may occur as the result of an inborn hereditary abnormality being set off by a viral infection, or by an environmental or psychological trigger.

To some extent, the myelin can regenerate, allowing partial or complete recovery. Thus attacks may happen frequently, or they may occur years apart. Conversely, an apparently mild case of MS can turn chronic and progressive, resisting all attempts at treatment.

Studies show a strong association between MS and a lack of winter sunshine—the disease becomes more prevalent as one moves away from the equator. High meat, gluten (the protein found in bread), and dairy consumption, and a lower intake of fruits and vegetables, are also associated with MS. Dairy states, such as Wisconsin, Iowa, and Oregon, have up to 50-percent more MS cases than such states as Georgia and Tennessee, where vegetable oils are used more commonly than butter. Dairy states also tend to be at a greater latitude than other states, which means that either diet or latitude could be the bigger factor.

Currently there is no cure for MS, but flareups can be tamed or halted. Diet can play an important role in an overall treatment plan.

Diet Recommendations

❥ **Go on the low-saturated-fat Swank Diet.** The most compelling evidence for the role of diet in MS comes from the studies of Dr. Roy Swank. Beginning in 1948, Dr. Swank followed 144 MS patients. One group ate a diet very low in saturated fat—17 grams or less—while the rest ate more than 20 grams of saturated fat per day. The low-fat Swank diet eliminated butter, margarine, hydrogenated oils, coconut and palm oil, hydrogenated peanut butter, and shortening. Patients were allowed 10 to 40 grams of vegetable oils and 5 grams of cod-liver oil. During his thirty-four years of study, Dr. Swank observed that the patients who ate 10 to 15 grams or less of saturated fat a day showed the least fatigue and the least progression toward disability. Saturated fats are known to cause blood cells to stick together in clumps. This action may block small blood vessels in the central nervous system, starving some areas for oxygen and resulting in damage to myelin. To follow the Swank diet, avoid most animal products—no meat, poultry, eggs, or dairy. The only animal food you should eat is cold-water fish, which provides essential fatty acids (see the Nutrient Recommendations). Choose whole grains, vegetables, fruit, and fresh juices, and eat or drink at least one serving of dark green vegetables every day.

❥ **Use fresh juice and juice fasting in your treatment plan.** Dr. Norman Walker, one of the great pioneers in juicing, recommended three quarts of fresh juice each day for MS. He observed that the juices, along with frequent colonics, slowly helped MS patients to recover. He specifically recommended carrot, celery, parsley, and spinach juices. Periodic juice fasts lasting from one to three days may also be beneficial (see the Juice Fast, page 324).

Nutrient Recommendations

❥ **Essential fatty acids (EFAs)** can arrest or slow the deterioration of myelin. In parts of the world where EFA consumption is high, MS is rare. The best oils are fresh, unrefined sunflower and flaxseed or hemp oil; unrefined sunflower, safflower, and sesame oils are also helpful. In addition, evening primrose oil has been used in the treatment of MS, and octacosanol, present in wheat germ oil, may help nerves to regenerate. Buy small amounts of oil at a time, and keep them refrigerated at all times. These oils can go rancid quickly, which will do you more harm than good. Cold-water fish is another good source of EFAs, especially the anti-inflammatory eicosapentaenoic acid (EPA) and docosahexaenoic acid (DHA). Best choices are salmon, tuna, trout, mackerel, herring, sardines, and kippers. Another EFA, gamma-linolenic acid (GLA), can be found in black and red currant juices, but is most readily obtainable in capsule form. For more information on omega-3 oils, see the fats and oils section in Basic Guidelines for the Juice Lady's Health and Healing Diet (page 313).

❥ **Vitamin D** appears to protect the body against MS. It has been observed that people in temperate latitudes may be more prone to MS because of a vitamin D deficiency. Insufficient exposure to sunlight may not allow the body to make enough vitamin D_3, the hormonal form of vitamin D. (Studies show that administering vitamin D_3 completely prevents an MS-like disease in mice.) The relative scarcity of MS in Japan and coastal Norway, and among Eskimo populations, could be explained by local diets rich in fish, an excellent source of vitamin D_3. (Sunlight exposure also inhibits secretion of the hormone melatonin. Melatonin may overstimulate the thymus gland, which can produce the autoimmune reaction that is believed to occur in MS.) Best food sources of vitamin D (in order of effectiveness): cold-water fish, sunflower seeds, sunflower sprouts, and mushrooms. This vitamin is not found in appreciable amounts in fruits or vegetables.

🍐 **Vitamin E** helps prevent lipid peroxidation, or free radical-damage to fats in cells. Best juice sources of vitamin E (in order of effectiveness): spinach, watercress, asparagus, carrots, and tomatoes.

Herb Recommendations

🍐 **Dandelion** and **echinacea** are used as detoxification herbs.

🍐 **Valerian** is used for its calming effect.

Juice Ingredient Recommendations

🍐 **Parsley** juice was used by Dr. Norman Walker for MS. Intake should be limited to a safe, therapeutic dose of $^1/_2$ to 1 cup per day. Parsley can be toxic in overdose, and should be especially avoided by pregnant women.

Juice Recipes

PURE GREEN SPROUT DRINK

1 organic cucumber, scrubbed well

1 large handful sunflower sprouts, rinsed

1 small handful buckwheat sprouts, rinsed

1 small handful clover sprouts, rinsed

Cut the cucumber in half lengthwise. Bunch up the sprouts, and push through the feed tube with the cucumber. Stir the juice, and pour into a glass. Serve at room temperature or chilled, as desired.

POPEYE'S POWER

$^1/_2$ medium organic apple, any kind, washed

1 handful organic spinach, washed

1 small handful parsley, rinsed

4 medium carrots, scrubbed well, green tops removed, ends trimmed

1 stalk organic celery with leaves, washed

$^1/_2$ beet with leaves, scrubbed well

Cut the apple into sections that will fit your juicer's feed tube. Bunch up the spinach and parsley, and push them through the feed tube with the apple, carrots, celery, and beet. Stir the juice, and pour into a glass. Serve at room temperature or chilled, as desired.

SPRING TONIC

1 medium vine-ripened tomato, washed

1 organic cucumber, scrubbed well

8 asparagus stems, washed

½ small or medium lemon, washed, or peeled if not organic

Cut the tomato into sections that fit your juicer's feed tube. Cut the cucumber in half lengthwise. Juice the tomato, cucumber, asparagus, and lemon. Stir the juice, and pour into a glass. Serve at room temperature or chilled, as desired.

THE MORNING ENERGIZER

½ organic Red or Golden Delicious apple, washed

5 medium carrots, scrubbed well, green tops removed, ends trimmed

½ small beet with leaves and stems, scrubbed well

½ small or medium lemon, washed, or peeled if not organic

½- to 1-inch piece fresh ginger root, washed

Cut the apple into sections that will fit your juicer's feed tube. Juice the apple along with the carrots, beet, lemon, and ginger. Stir the juice, and pour into a glass. Serve at room temperature or chilled, as desired.

SANTA FE SALSA COCKTAIL

1 medium vine-ripened tomato, washed

½ medium organic cucumber, scrubbed well

¼ cup cilantro, rinsed

¼ small or medium lime or lemon, washed, or peeled if not organic

Dash hot sauce (optional)

Cut the tomato into sections that fit your juicer's feed tube. Cut the cucumber in half again lengthwise. Bunch up the cilantro, and push through the feed tube with the tomato, cucumber, and lime or lemon. Pour the juice into a glass, add the hot sauce (if using), and stir. Serve at room temperature or chilled, as desired.

Obesity

See **Overweight/Obesity.**

Osteoarthritis

Osetoarthritis, the most common form of arthritis, afflicts more than 40 million Americans (*see also* **Rheumatoid Arthritis**), with women outnumbering men after the age of forty-five. A significant percentage of all osteoarthritis cases begin in the knees; the hips, hands, and spine are other common sites. Osteoarthritis can begin as early as age thirty, and the number of people affected increases dramatically with age, with 80 percent of all persons over age fifty showing some signs of the disorder. Mild early-morning stiffness, stiffness following periods of rest, pain that gets worse on joint use, and loss of joint function are often the first symptoms. As the disease progresses, more joints may be affected, and the bone can become deformed.

Osetoarthritis causes the joints, especially the cartilage that lines the joints, to degenerate. Primary osteoarthritis is caused by wear and tear that occurs as a person ages. Secondary osteoarthritis is associated with such predisposing factors as bone or joint abnormalities, injury, or inflammatory disease. This disease can be halted and even reversed through dietary and lifestyle changes.

Lifestyle Recommendations

❥ **Get physical therapy and regular exercise.** The Arthritis Foundation states that physical therapy may be the single most valuable treatment for arthritis—see your doctor for referral to a qualified therapist. In addition, you should engage in regular, low-impact exercise. Walking and swimming are excellent.

❥ **Reduce or eliminate the use of nonsteriodal anti-inflammatory drugs (NSAIDs) and aspirin.** These drugs not only have gastrointestinal side effects, but they also inhibit the creation of collagen, the main protein found in cartilage, and increase joint destruction.

Diet Recommendations

❥ **Eat a low-fat, high-fiber diet.** Include more raw foods—fruits, vegetables, juices, sprouts, nuts, and seeds—in your meal plans. Strive for a diet in which 50 percent of what you eat and drink consists of raw foods and juices. Following a low-fat, high-fiber diet will also help you maintain a normal weight, especially if you exercise regularly. The Arthritis Center of Boston University says that being overweight is the most potent risk factor for osteoarthritis, especially of the knee and probably of the hips and hands as well. For more information, see Basic Guidelines for the Juice Lady's Health and Healing Diet (page 313).

❥ Do not ingest plants from the nightshade family. Tomatoes, potatoes, eggplants, and bell peppers fall into this category, as does tobacco. Some researchers believe that substances in these plants either inhibit normal collagen repair in the joints or promote inflammatory degeneration. You may notice some improvement by eliminating this group of foods, and by not using tobacco.

❥ Avoid citrus fruits. Some people with arthritis benefit when they stop eating citrus fruits. Try avoiding oranges, grapefruits, tangerines, lemons, and limes, and see if you notice an improvement.

❥ Use cleansing programs, including juice fasting and liver cleansing. The removal of noxious substances from the joints through the lymphatic system can help reduce cartilage damage. For more information, see the Juice Fast (page 324) and the cleansing programs (pages 323 through 339).

Nutrient Recommendations

❥ B vitamins, specifically vitamin B_{12} (cobalamin), folic acid, and pantothenic acid, are important in treating osteoarthritis. Folic acid and vitamin B_{12} have been shown in several studies to help arthritic hand joints, and pantothenic acid has provided relief from symptoms when as little as 12.5 mg was taken. Vitamin B_{12} is not found in foods than can be juiced. The best food sources are meat, poultry, and fish; it is also available in some fermented soy-based foods, such as tofu and tempeh. Best juice sources of folic acid (in order of effectiveness): asparagus, spinach, kale, broccoli, cabbage, and blackberries. Best juice sources of pantothenic acid: broccoli, cauliflower, and kale.

❥ Glucosamine is a naturally occurring substance found in joint structures that stimulates cartilage regeneration, protects against joint destruction, and alleviates the symptoms of osteoarthritis. As some people age, they lose the ability to manufacture sufficient levels of glucosamine. The result is that cartilage loses its gel-like consistency and its ability to act as a shock absorber. Numerous studies have proven the effectiveness of glucosamine supplementation and the longer it is used, the more therapeutic benefits it provides. The recommended dosage is 1,500 mg daily of glucosamine sulfate (best divided into three doses of 500 mg each).

❥ Phytoestrogens are estrogenlike factors found in plants that can help protect cartilage. The higher incidence of osteoarthritis among women suggests that estrogens may play a role in the development of this condition. Phytoestrogens are capable of binding to estrogen receptors on cells, keeping estrogen itself from binding to the cells and thus decreasing cartilage erosion. Best juice sources of phytoestrogens: apples, celery, fennel, and parsley. Soy foods are rich in phytoestrogens—use soy milk in place of dairy milk or creamers and eat more tofu, soy cheese, and miso.

❥ **Vitamin C** can affect collagen synthesis and repair. Best juice sources of vitamin C (in order of effectiveness): kale, parsley, broccoli, Brussels sprouts, watercress, cauliflower, cabbage, strawberries, papaya, spinach, turnips, mangoes, asparagus, and cantaloupes.

❥ **Vitamin D** is needed for joint health. Studies show that low blood levels of vitamin D are associated with both the loss of cartilage and the development of bony outgrowths called osteophytes. In addition, low vitamin D levels present a risk factor for disease progression in osteoarthritic knees. Vitamin D in its active form is a hormone, and our bodies make it from sunlight. People who live in primarily overcast climates, such as the Pacific Northwest, should supplement their diets with vitamin D. This vitamin is not found in fruits and vegetables. Best food sources of vitamin D (in order of effectiveness): cold-water fish, sunflower seeds, sunflower sprouts (can be juiced), and mushrooms.

❥ **Vitamin E** has been shown to help fight osteoarthritis, possibly because of its membrane-stabilizing effect and its ability to stimulate increased deposits of proteoglycans, substances that form part of the joint structure. Best juice sources of vitamin E (in order of effectiveness): spinach, watercress, asparagus, and carrots.

Herb Recommendations

❥ **Boswellia serrata** has antiarthritic effects.

❥ **Devil's claw** has anti-inflammatory and pain-relieving effects.

❥ **Yucca** has shown positive therapeutic effects in a double-blind study.

Juice Ingredient Recommendations

❥ **Cherry** and **blueberry** juices contain anthocyanidins and proanthocyanidins, compounds that are beneficial in enhancing collagen strength and structure.

❥ **Dandelion** juice, half a cup morning and evening, has been used as a traditional remedy for osteoarthritis. Dandelion juice is very strong tasting, so it helps to mix it with carrot or other mild-tasting juices, as in Liver Life Tonic.

❥ **Ginger** has been used in Ayurvedic (traditional Indian) medicine to ease inflammation. In one study with osteoarthritic patients, over 75 percent found varying degrees of relief from pain and swelling after using ginger.

❥ **Parsley** juice is an excellent source of phytoestrogens and vitamin C. Intake should be limited to a safe, therapeutic dose of $^1/_2$ to 1 cup per day. Parsley can be toxic in overdose, and should be especially avoided by pregnant women.

❥ **Watermelon** juice is a traditional remedy for osteoarthritis.

Juice Recipes

ANTIAGING COCKTAIL

1 small bunch organic purple grapes (about 1 cup) with small stems* and seeds, washed

$^1/_2$ cup blueberries, blackberries, or raspberries, washed

$^1/_2$-inch piece fresh ginger root, washed

*Large stems can dull your juicer's blade.

Juice the grapes, berries, and ginger. Stir the juice, and pour into a glass. Serve at room temperature or chilled, as desired.

CHERRY JUBILEE

1 three-inch chunk fresh pineapple, scrubbed well, or peeled if not organic

$^1/_2$ organic Golden or Red Delicious apple, washed

6–8 organic Bing cherries, washed, pits removed

Cut the pineapple into strips, and the apple into sections, that fit your juicer's feed tube, and juice them with the cherries. Stir the juice, and pour it into a glass. Serve at room temperature or chilled, as desired.

WATERMELON REFRESHER

1-inch slice watermelon, with seeds and well-scrubbed rind

Cut the watermelon into strips that fit your juicer's feed tube. Juice the watermelon, and pour into a glass. Serve at room temperature or chilled, as desired.

LIVER LIFE TONIC

1 organic green apple such as Granny Smith or Pippin, washed

1 handful dandelion greens, washed

5 carrots, scrubbed well, green tops removed, ends trimmed

Cut the apple into wedges that will fit your juicer's feed tube. Bunch up the dandelion greens, and push through the feed tube with the apple, carrots, and lemon. Stir the juice, and pour into a glass. Serve at room temperature or chilled, as desired.

THE GINGER HOPPER

½ organic Red or Golden Delicious apple, washed

5 medium carrots, scrubbed well, green tops removed, ends trimmed

½- to 1-inch piece fresh ginger root, washed

Cut the apple into sections, and juice along with the carrots and ginger. Stir the juice, and pour into a glass. Serve at room temperature or chilled, as desired.

GINGER TWIST

1 organic Red or Golden Delicious apple, washed

1 handful parsley, rinsed

4 carrots, scrubbed well, green tops removed, ends trimmed

1-inch piece fresh ginger root, washed

¼ small or medium lemon, washed, or peeled if not organic

Cut the apple into sections that fit your juicer's feed tube. Bunch up the parsley and push it through the feed tube with the apple, carrots, ginger, and lemon. Stir the juice, and pour into a glass. Serve at room temperature or chilled, as desired.

BEAUTIFUL BONE SOLUTION

1 organic Golden or Red Delicious apple, washed

1–2 kale leaves, washed

1 handful parsley, rinsed

1 stalk organic celery, washed

¼ small or medium lemon, washed, or peeled if not organic

½- to 1-inch piece fresh ginger root, washed

Cut the apple into sections that fit your juicer's feed tube. Bunch up the kale and parsley, and push through the feed tube with the apple, celery, lemon, and ginger. Stir the juice, and pour into a glass. Serve at room temperature or chilled, as desired.

PURE GREEN SPROUT DRINK

1 organic cucumber, scrubbed well

1 large handful sunflower sprouts, rinsed

1 small handful buckwheat sprouts, rinsed

1 small handful clover sprouts, rinsed

Cut the cucumber in half lengthwise. Bunch up the sprouts, and push through the feed tube with the cucumber. Stir the juice, and pour into a glass. Serve at room temperature or chilled, as desired.

SWEET CALCIUM COCKTAIL

1 three-inch chunk fresh pineapple, scrubbed well, or peeled if not organic

1–2 kale leaves, washed

Cut the pineapple into strips that fit your juicer's feed tube. Bunch up the kale, and push through the feed tube with the pineapple. Stir the juice, and pour into a glass. Serve at room temperature or chilled, as desired.

MAGNESIUM SPECIAL

5 medium carrots, scrubbed well, green tops removed, ends trimmed

2 stalks organic celery with leaves, washed

1/2 small beet with leaves and stems, scrubbed well

2 broccoli florets, washed

1/2 small or medium lemon, washed, or peeled if not organic

Juice the carrots, celery, beet, broccoli, and lemon. Stir the juice, and pour into a glass. Serve at room temperature or chilled, as desired.

STRAWBERRY-CANTALOUPE COCKTAIL

1/2 ripe organic cantaloupe with seeds, washed, or peeled if not organic

1 cup organic strawberries, washed

Cut the cantaloupe into strips that fit your juicer's feed tube. Juice the cantaloupe and strawberries; stir the juice and pour into a glass. Serve at room temperature or chilled, as desired.

The Feel Good Cocktail

½ pear, washed

4 medium carrots, scrubbed well, green tops removed, ends trimmed

3 fennel stalks with leaves and flowers, washed

1 stalk organic celery with leaves, washed

Cut the pear into sections that fit your juicer's feed tube, and juice along with the carrots, fennel, and celery. Stir the juice, and pour into a glass. Serve at room temperature or chilled, as desired.

So Berry Smooth

½ organic Golden or Red Delicious apple, washed

1 cup blueberries, raspberries, or blackberries, washed

1 ripe medium to large banana, peeled

½ cup silken tofu, or ½ cup plain or vanilla soy milk

6 ice cubes

Cut the apple into sections that fit your juicer's feed tube. Juice the apple with the blueberries. Pour the juice into a blender, and add the banana, tofu or soy milk, and ice cubes; blend until smooth. Pour the mixture into one or two glasses and serve immediately.

Osteoporosis

Osteoporosis means "porous bone." It is normal for bones to lose density after age forty at a rate of about 2 percent per year. But in osteoporosis, the rate of bone loss exceeds that of bone creation. As a result, bone is lost gradually from the spine, hips, and ribs, which become more fragile and prone to fracture.

Osteoporosis affects more than twenty million people in the United States, most of them over the age of fifty. More than 1.5 million Americans have fractures related to osteoporosis each year. Nearly one-third of all women and one-sixth of all men will fracture their hips at some time in their lives. The reason women are more prone to osteoporosis is that their bodies produce much less estrogen after menopause, and estrogen helps control the use of calcium in bone creation.

A fracture, often after just a minor injury, may be the first sign that a person has osteoporosis. Back pain can occur when weakened vertebrae collapse. When a fracture does occur, it tends to heal very slowly. Risk factors for developing this condition include smoking, low calcium intake, lack of weight-bearing exercise, family history, and the use of certain medications, including steroids and barbiturates.

Diet Recommendations

❥ **Eat a low-fat, high-complex-carbohydrate diet; lower your protein intake.** Diets high in animal proteins (which are high in phosphates) have been linked to increased loss of calcium. The best diet is one based on whole grains, vegetables, and fruits. For more information on the healthy diet plan, see Basic Guidelines for the Juice Lady's Health and Healing Diet (page 313).

❥ **Eat more soy products.** Tofu, tempeh, soy cheese, soy milk, and miso are all good choices. Soy foods contain phytoestrogens, which for menopausal women may provide a suitable alternative to synthetic estrogens in the prevention of osteoporosis. You can substitute soy milk or silken tofu in smoothie recipes for a delicious dose of soy every day. Use soy milk on cereal and in hot beverages instead of creamers.

❥ **Drink fresh green juices.** Green vegetables—such as kale, collards, parsley, and lettuce—are rich in the vitamins and minerals—such as vitamin K, calcium, magnesium, and boron—needed to support healthy joints and bones. Freely drink juices made with these vegetables.

❥ **Avoid alcohol, tobacco, caffeine, aluminum, and carbonated beverages.** Studies show that bone loss is directly correlated with smoking and excessive alcohol use. In addition, studies have shown that even moderate coffee consumption, on the order of two to three cups daily, will cause calcium loss. Aluminum—which is used in baking powder, salt, cookware, antacids, processed cheese, and deodorant, to name a few culprits—can interfere with calcium absorption. Be sure to choose only aluminum-free products. Soft drinks contain phosphates; when phosphate levels are high and calcium levels are low, calcium is leached out of the bones. Sodas may be a major factor in osteoporosis because Americans consume such large quantities of them—about three quarts per week for every person in the country.

Nutrient Recommendations

❥ **Boron** can help prevent urinary loss of calcium. Boron is widely available in fruits and vegetables.

❥ **Calcium,** when taken in adequate amounts, can slow the rate of post-menopausal bone loss by between 30 and 50 percent. Adequate calcium intake has been shown to produce significant improvements in bone density more than five years after menopause. You should take between 1,000 and 1,500 mg daily. Best juice sources of calcium (in order of effectiveness): kale, parsley, dandelion greens, watercress, beet greens, broccoli, spinach, romaine lettuce, string beans, oranges, celery, and carrots.

❥ **Copper** deficiency can result in fragile bones. Copper is essential for the effectiveness of an enzyme that is involved in the creation of collagen, the major structural component of bone. Best juice sources of copper (in order of effectiveness): carrots, garlic, ginger root, and turnips.

❥ **Magnesium** helps calcium get in and out of cells. A recent Israeli study revealed that women who consumed from 250 to 750 mg of magnesium daily experienced bone density increases of between 1 and 8 percent. Reduced amounts of magnesium can negatively affect the body's use of estrogen, which in turn affects the bones. Best juice sources of magnesium (in order of effectiveness): beet greens, spinach, parsley, dandelion greens, garlic, blackberries, beets, broccoli, cauliflower, carrots, and celery.

❥ **Manganese** is required for the creation of connective tissue, especially cartilage, and is generally deficient in the standard American diet. Best juice sources of manganese (in order of effectiveness): spinach, beet greens, Brussels sprouts, carrots, broccoli, cabbage, peaches, tangerines, beets, apples, oranges, and pears.

❥ **Silicon** promotes the formation of bones and teeth. The best juice sources of silicon are bell pepper, cucumber, and root vegetables.

❥ **Vitamin C** is important in the production of collagen. Best juice sources of vitamin C (in order of effectiveness): kale, parsley, broccoli, Brussels sprouts, watercress, cauliflower, cabbage, strawberries, papaya, spinach, citrus fruit, turnips, mangoes, asparagus, and cantaloupes.

❥ **Vitamin D** is associated with a significant reduction in the number of hip fractures among postmenopausal women. Low-dose vitamin D supplementation can help prevent bone loss and osteoarthritis that occurs as the result of problems with the parathyroid glands located in the neck. Take between 400 and 800 IU daily. Vitamin D is not available in fruits and vegetables. Best food sources of vitamin D (in order of effectiveness): cold-water fish, sunflower seeds, sunflower sprouts (can be juiced), and mushrooms.

❥ **Vitamin K_1** is found in plants, especially green leafy vegetables. It is important for converting a substance called osteocalcin to its active form, which anchors calcium in bone. Best juice sources of vitamin K_1 (in order of effectiveness): kale, collard and turnip greens, broccoli, parsley, lettuce, cabbage, spinach, watercress, asparagus, and string beans.

❥ **Zinc** can stimulate protein synthesis in bone. Best juice sources of zinc (in order of effectiveness): ginger root, turnips, parsley, garlic, carrots, grapes, spinach, cabbage, lettuce, cucumbers, and tangerines.

Herb Recommendations

❥ **Alfalfa, dong quai,** and **licorice** all contain phytoestrogens that may be suitable alternatives to synthetic estrogen; your doctor can help you decide on the hormone replacement regimen that's best for you (*see* **Menopause**). Avoid licorice if you have high blood pressure, do not use it for prolonged periods of time, and use a medicinal form of the herb, not licorice candy.

Juice Ingredient Recommendations

❥ **Kale** is a good source of both calcium and vitamins C and K, nutrients needed for good bone health.

❥ **Parsley** juice is rich in calcium, magnesium, vitamin K, and zinc. Intake should be limited to a safe, therapeutic dose of $1/2$ to 1 cup per day. Parsley can be toxic in overdose, and should be especially avoided by pregnant women.

Juice Recipes

BEAUTIFUL BONE SOLUTION

1 organic Golden or Red Delicious apple, washed

1–2 kale leaves, washed

1 handful parsley, rinsed

1 stalk organic celery, washed

$1/4$ small or medium lemon, washed, or peeled if not organic

$1/2$- to 1-inch piece fresh ginger root, washed

Cut the apple into sections that fit your juicer's feed tube. Bunch up the kale and parsley, and push through the feed tube with the apple, celery, lemon, and ginger. Stir the juice, and pour into a glass. Serve at room temperature or chilled, as desired.

SWEET CALCIUM COCKTAIL

1 three-inch chunk fresh pineapple, scrubbed well, or peeled if not organic

1–2 kale leaves, washed

Cut the pineapple into strips that fit your juicer's feed tube. Bunch up the kale, and push through the feed tube with the pineapple. Stir the juice, and pour into a glass. Serve at room temperature or chilled, as desired.

MORNING EXPRESS

1 orange, peeled

4–5 carrots, well scrubbed, green tops removed, ends trimmed

Divide the orange into segments that fit your juicer's feed tube, and juice with the carrots. Stir the juice, and pour into a glass. Serve at room temperature or chilled, as desired.

MORNING SUNRISE

1 pink, red, or white grapefruit, peeled

1 orange, peeled

Divide the grapefruit and orange into segments that fit your juicer's feed tube. Juice the grapefruit and orange, and stir the juice. Pour into a glass, and serve at room temperature or chilled, as desired.

SWEET DREAMS NIGHTCAP

2 romaine lettuce leaves, washed

1 handful parsley, rinsed

4 carrots, scrubbed well, green tops removed, ends trimmed

3 organic celery stalks with leaves, washed

Bunch up the lettuce leaves and parsley, and push through the feed tube with the carrots and celery. Stir the juice, and pour into a glass. Serve at room temperature or chilled, as desired.

MEMORY MENDER

2 medium vine-ripened tomatoes, washed

$1/4$ small head iceberg lettuce, washed

4 cauliflower florets, washed

$1/2$ small or medium lemon, washed, or peeled if not organic

Cut the tomatoes and lettuce into sections that will fit your juicer's feed tube. Juice the tomatoes and lettuce along with the cauliflower and lemon. Pour into a glass and serve at room temperature or chilled, as desired.

PURE GREEN SPROUT DRINK

1 organic cucumber, scrubbed well

1 large handful sunflower sprouts, rinsed

1 small handful buckwheat sprouts, rinsed

1 small handful clover sprouts, rinsed

Cut the cucumber in half lengthwise. Bunch up the sprouts, and push through the feed tube with the cucumber. Stir the juice, and pour into a glass. Serve at room temperature or chilled, as desired.

THE GINGER HOPPER

½ organic Red or Golden Delicious apple, washed

5 medium carrots, scrubbed well, green tops removed, ends trimmed

½- to 1-inch piece fresh ginger root, washed

Cut the apple into sections, and juice along with the carrots and ginger. Stir the juice, and pour into a glass. Serve at room temperature or chilled, as desired.

THE IMMUNE BUILDER

1 organic Golden or Red Delicious apple, washed

1 turnip, scrubbed well

1 handful watercress, rinsed (optional)

5 carrots, scrubbed well, green tops removed, ends trimmed

1 large garlic clove with peel, washed

Cut the apple and turnip into sections that fit your juicer's feed tube. Bunch up the watercress (if using), and push it through the feed tube with the apple, turnip, carrots, and garlic. Stir the juice, and pour into a glass. Serve at room temperature or chilled, as desired.

MAGNESIUM SPECIAL

5 medium carrots, scrubbed well, green tops removed, ends trimmed

2 stalks organic celery with leaves, washed

½ small beet with leaves and stems, scrubbed well

2 broccoli florets, washed

½ small or medium lemon, washed, or peeled if not organic

Juice the carrots, celery, beet, broccoli, and lemon. Stir the juice, and pour into a glass. Serve at room temperature or chilled, as desired.

JACK & THE BEAN

1 large vine-ripened tomato, washed

2 romaine lettuce leaves, washed

8 organic string beans, washed

3 Brussels sprouts, washed

½ small or medium lemon, washed, or peeled if not organic

Cut the tomato into sections that fit your juicer's feed tube. Bunch up the lettuce leaves, and push through the feed tube with the tomato, string beans, Brussels sprouts, and lemon. Stir the juice, and pour into a glass. Serve at room temperature or chilled, as desired.

SO BERRY SMOOTH

½ organic Golden or Red Delicious apple, washed

1 cup blueberries, raspberries, or blackberries, washed

1 ripe medium to large banana, peeled

½ cup silken tofu, or ½ cup plain or vanilla soy milk

6 ice cubes

Cut the apple into sections that fit your juicer's feed tube. Juice the apple with the blueberries. Pour the juice into a blender, and add the banana, tofu or soy milk, and ice cubes; blend until smooth. Pour the mixture into one or two glasses and serve immediately.

THE CALCIUM CHAMP

½ organic Golden or Red Delicious apple, washed

1 handful organic spinach with stems, washed

1 small handful parsley, rinsed

1 ripe medium banana, peeled

½ cup plain or vanilla soy milk

1 tablespoon tahini (sesame butter)

6 ice cubes

Cut the apple in sections that fit your juicer's feed tube. Bunch up the spinach and parsley, and push through the feed tube with the apple. Pour the juice into a blender, and add the banana, soy milk, tahini, and ice; blend until smooth. Pour into one or two glasses and serve immediately.

Overweight/Obesity

Being overweight is generally defined as exceeding the recommended weight for one's height and build. Under revised guidelines set by the federal government, 55 percent of all Americans are too heavy. These guidelines are based on the Body Mass Index (BMI), a measurement that uses height and weight to determine the amount of body fat. The panel that set the revised standards defined overweight as having a BMI of 25.0 to 29.9 and obesity as having a BMI of 30.0 and above. (The National Institutes of Health publishes a BMI table; see Appendix B.)

A high BMI is especially troublesome for people who carry their weight around their middles. Waist circumference is associated with abdominal fat, which in turn is associated with an increased risk for such disorders as heart disease and diabetes. A waist circumference of more than forty inches in men and thirty-five inches in women signifies a problem in persons with a BMI of 25 or over.

With all the low-fat foods available and so many diet programs, why are so many Americans overweight? Although there are many contributing factors—including, in some people, a genetic tendency to gain weight—the most obvious cause of weight gain is a sedentary lifestyle and excessive consumption of high-fat, high-sugar foods. This pattern of little exercise and poor diet often starts in childhood; that explains why the number of overweight children in the United States has doubled over a thirty-year span. And obesity in older children is an increasingly important predictor of adult obesity.

No matter how old you are, you *can* lose weight. Diet and lifestyle changes can make all the difference.

Lifestyle Recommendations

❦ **Get out and exercise.** To lose one pound per week, you need to take in 500 fewer calories a day than you burn off. That means eating less and/or exercising more. As an example, taking a brisk walk for one hour and fifteen minutes will burn 500 calories. But if you eat 250 fewer calories a day, you can take a shorter walk and still lose that pound. Strength training to build your muscles is also important. Because muscle tissue burns more calories per pound than fat tissue, more muscle means more fat-burning potential, even when you are at rest.

Dietary Recommendations

❦ **Increase the fiber in your diet.** Eat more high-fiber foods, such as whole grains, vegetables, fruits, and legumes (beans, lentils, split peas). One study has shown that eating more whole grains may make insulin activity more effective, which supports weight loss (see chromium in the Nutrient Recommendations list). In addition to choosing high-fiber foods, add a fiber supplement to your diet, such as psyllium, guar gum, or pectin. (Avoid fiber products that contain sugar or other sweeteners.) When taken with juice or water before a meal, these supplements form a gelatinous mass in the digestive tract that creates a feeling of fullness. As a result, you will be more likely to eat less food. An added bonus is that fiber supplements have been shown to enhance blood-sugar control and insulin sensitivity, and to actually reduce the number of calories your body absorbs. A high-fiber diet also supports good colon function and helps eliminate the toxins released during weight loss.

❥ **Reduce the amount of fat you eat.** Make sure that the total number of fat calories you consume each day is less than 25 percent of your total calorie intake. There are nine calories in one fat gram versus four calories in one gram of protein or carbohydrate. Fat is stored more efficiently than carbohydrates or protein because it enters the body in a ready-to-store form. Also, eating a high-fat diet makes it easy to consume far too many calories before you feel full. One recent study found that people in one group who ate a low-fat, high-carbohydrate diet consumed an average of 680 calories a meal, while it took 1,350 calories of high-fat food before those in the other group felt full.

❥ **Avoid sugars and artificial sweeteners.** Sweets stimulate the appetite. They also contain empty calories that tend to be stored as fat rather than used for energy. Artificial sweeteners aren't better for weight loss or your health; in fact, they may be worse. A recent study followed fourteen dieting women and found that those drinking a beverage sweetened with aspartame ate significantly more food than those drinking a beverage sweetened with sucrose (refined sugar). Neither sweetener is a good choice, but the artificial sweetener is even less desirable.

❥ **Drink two to three glasses of fresh fruit and vegetable juices daily, and use juice fasting.** Vegetables in particular are wise juice choices because your body can make virtually every calorie count for metabolism, rather than storage. Fruit juice contains sugar, so always dilute fruit juice by half with water to lower the calorie count and prevent appetite stimulation. (This applies to the fruit juices listed under the Nutrient Recommendations.) A great weight loss and maintenance program is to juice fast one day, or at least a half day, a week (see the Juice Fast, page 324). *On a personal note:* I have received scores of letters and calls from people who have lost 10, 20, 70, 150 pounds by following my weight-loss program, which includes two to three glasses of fresh juice each day in addition to replacing one meal with one glass of juice. Personally, I have found that juice fasts provide a great jump start for any weight-loss program. They help you not only to lose a pound or two, but to feel energized and renewed as well. I followed this program for nearly two decades and have maintained about the same weight (and a size 6) year after year.

❥ **Drink at least eight glasses of water daily.** Drinking a glass of water before a meal can help you feel full more quickly, so you'll eat less. Water also helps your body use its stored fat, promotes good colon function, and flushes away the toxins released during weight loss.

Nutrient Recommendations

❥ **Chromium,** a trace mineral, can significantly improve your body's sensitivity to insulin, the main sugar-control hormone. Proper insulin function is the key to maintaining normal blood-sugar levels and to promoting thermogenesis, or the burning of calories by raising body heat. When chromium is deficient in the diet, insulin activity is blocked, blood-sugar levels become elevated, thermogenesis diminishes, and cravings for sweet foods develop. Several studies using chromium combined with exercise training have shown significant weight loss, increased muscle mass, and improved insulin response in the participants. Best juice sources of chromium (in order of effectiveness): green peppers, apples, parsnips, spinach, carrots, lettuce, string beans, and cabbage.

❥ **Magnesium** is involved in energy regulation. In one study, a deficiency of this mineral was associated with higher levels of body fat. Best juice sources of magnesium (in order of effectiveness): beet greens, spinach, parsley, dandelion greens, garlic, blackberries, beets, broccoli, cauliflower, carrots, and celery.

❥ **Pantothenic acid,** a B vitamin, plays a role in fat metabolism. This vitamin was shown to facilitate weight loss in one study. Best juice sources of pantothenic acid (in order of effectiveness): broccoli, cauliflower, and kale.

❥ **Vitamins C** and **E** play an important role in fat metabolism. Deficiencies of these vitamins have been associated with higher body fat levels. Best juice sources of vitamin C (in order of effectiveness): kale, parsley, broccoli, Brussels sprouts, watercress, cauliflower, cabbage, strawberries, papaya, spinach, citrus fruit, turnips, mangoes, asparagus, and cantaloupes. Best juice sources of vitamin E: spinach, watercress, asparagus, carrots, and tomatoes.

❥ **Zinc** deficiency has been associated with higher body fat levels in a recent study. Best juice sources of zinc (in order of effectiveness): ginger root, turnips, parsley, garlic, carrots, grapes, spinach, cabbage, lettuce, cucumbers, and tangerines.

Herbal Recommendations

❥ **Bladderwrack** and **hawthorn** are used to stimulate the adrenal glands and improve thyroid function. Bladderwrack is a species of kelp, a sea-weed that contains significant amounts of iodine. Limit consumption to once a week, in order to avoid ingesting too much iodine.

❥ **Chickweed** is a traditional herbal remedy that has been used to suppress the appetite.

❥ **Juniper berries** act as a diuretic that also facilitates detoxification. To avoid kidney irritation, do not take juniper berries for long periods of time.

Juice Ingredient Recommendations

❥ **Alfalfa, asparagus, cucumber, dandelion, lemon, parsley,** and **watermelon** juices are good diuretics; in addition, alfalfa and dandelion are good detoxification agents. Cantaloupe (with seeds) and kiwi fruit juices also have diuretic properties. Parsley juice intake should be limited to a safe, therapeutic dose of $1/2$ to 1 cup per day. Parsley can be toxic in overdose, and should be especially avoided by pregnant women.

❥ **Daikon radish** has been used in Traditional Chinese Medicine to help eliminate excess fat.

❥ **Ginger** juice can stimulate thermogenesis.

❥ **Jerusalem artichoke** and **parsnip** are traditional remedies that help curb cravings for sweets and junk food. The key is to sip the juice slowly when you have a craving for high-fat or high-sugar food.

❥ **Radish** has been used as a traditional remedy to help promote healthy thyroid function. A healthy thyroid gland is important in weight loss and maintenance.

Juice Recipes

SKINNY SIP

½ small or medium lemon, washed, or peeled if not organic
1 cup unsweetened mineral water

Juice the lemon, and pour the juice in an ice-filled glass. Add the mineral water, and stir to combine.

WEIGHT-LOSS EXPRESS

½ organic cucumber, scrubbed well

½ small organic green apple, such as Granny Smith or Pippin, washed

1 small handful parsley, rinsed

5 medium carrots, scrubbed well, green tops removed, ends trimmed

¼ small or medium lemon, washed, or peeled if not organic

1-inch piece fresh ginger root, washed

Cut the cucumber in half lengthwise and the apple into sections that fit your juicer's feed tube. Bunch up the parsley, and push through the feed tube with the cucumber, apple, carrots, lemon, and ginger. Stir the juice, and pour into a glass. Serve at room temperature or chilled, as desired.

ORIENT EXPRESS

2-inch chunk jicama, scrubbed, or peeled if not organic (optional)

5 carrots, scrubbed well, green tops removed, ends trimmed

2-inch piece daikon radish, scrubbed well, without green top or end

½-inch piece fresh ginger root, washed

Cut the jicama into strips (if using) that fit your juicer's feed tube. Juice the jicama with the carrots, radish, and ginger. Stir the juice, and pour into a glass. Serve at room temperature. This is a very hot-tasting drink because of the radish and ginger, so you may want to dilute it by half with water.

WEIGHT-LOSS BUDDY

1 small Jerusalem artichoke, scrubbed well

4–5 carrots, scrubbed well, green tops removed, ends trimmed

½ small beet with no stems and leaves, scrubbed well

Cut the Jerusalem artichoke into sections that fit your juicer's feed tube. Juice the artichoke along with the carrots and beet. Stir the juice, and pour into a glass. Serve at room temperature or chilled, as desired.

SPRING TONIC

1 medium vine-ripened tomato, washed

1 organic cucumber, washed

8 asparagus stems, washed

½ small or medium lemon, washed, or peeled if not organic

Cut the tomato into sections that fit your juicer's feed tube. Cut the cucumber in half lengthwise and remove the tips of the asparagus (steam or grill the tips). Juice the tomato, cucumber, asparagus, and lemon. Stir the juice and pour into a glass. Serve at room temperature or chilled, as desired.

LIVER LIFE TONIC

½ organic green apple such as
Granny Smith or Pippin, washed

1 handful dandelion greens, washed

5 carrots, scrubbed well, green tops
removed, ends trimmed

½ small lemon, washed, or peeled if
not organic

Cut the apple into wedges that will fit your juicer's feed tube. Bunch up the dandelion greens, and push through the feed tube with the apple, carrots, and lemon. Stir the juice, and pour into a glass. Serve at room temperature or chilled, as desired.

RADISH CARE

5 carrots, scrubbed well, green tops
removed, ends trimmed

5–6 radishes (green tops removed),
washed well

½ small or medium lemon, washed,
or peeled if not organic

Juice the carrots, radishes, and lemon. Stir the juice and pour into a glass. Serve at room temperature or chilled, as desired.

MAGNESIUM SPECIAL

5 medium carrots, scrubbed well,
green tops removed, ends trimmed

2 stalks organic celery with leaves,
washed

½ small beet with leaves and stems,
scrubbed well

2 broccoli florets, washed

½ small or medium lemon, washed,
or peeled if not organic

Juice the carrots, celery, beet, broccoli, and lemon. Stir the juice, and pour into a glass. Serve at room temperature or chilled, as desired.

PURE GREEN SPROUT DRINK

1 organic cucumber, scrubbed well

1 large handful sunflower sprouts,
rinsed

1 small handful buckwheat sprouts,
rinsed

1 small handful alfalfa sprouts, rinsed

Cut the cucumber in half lengthwise. Bunch up the sprouts, and push through the feed tube with the cucumber. Stir the juice, and pour into a glass. Serve at room temperature or chilled, as desired.

GINGER TWIST

1 organic Red or Golden Delicious apple, washed

1 handful parsley, rinsed

4 carrots, scrubbed well, green tops removed, ends trimmed

1-inch piece fresh ginger root, washed

1/4 small or medium lemon, washed, or peeled if not organic

Cut the apple into sections that fit your juicer's feed tube. Bunch up the parsley and push it through the feed tube with the apple, carrots, ginger, and lemon. Stir the juice, and pour into a glass. Serve at room temperature or chilled, as desired.

AFTERNOON REFRESHER

1 medium to large organic cucumber, scrubbed well

1/2 small or medium lemon, washed, or peeled if not organic

Cut the cucumber in half lengthwise, and juice with the lemon. (For an especially cooling version, let the juice splash over a few ice cubes in the juice pitcher.) Stir the juice, and pour into a glass. Serve at room temperature or chilled, as desired.

BEAUTIFUL SKIN, HAIR, AND NAIL SOLUTION

1 medium organic cucumber, scrubbed well

1 medium parsnip, scrubbed well

3 carrots, scrubbed well, green tops removed, ends trimmed

1/2 small or medium lemon, washed, or peeled if not organic

1/4 small green bell pepper, washed

Cut the cucumber in half lengthwise, and juice with the parsnip, carrots, lemon, and bell pepper. Stir the juice, and pour into a glass. Serve at room temperature or chilled, as desired.

Panic Attacks

See **Anxiety and Panic Attacks.**

Parasitic Infections

Parasites are creatures that feed off a host organism, and in our bodies they can cause harm. Protozoa (single-cell organisms), such as *Cryptosporidia, Giardia lamblia, Entamoeba histolytica, Blastocystis hominis,* and *Dientamoeba fragilis;* helminths or worms, such as pinworms, roundworms, tapeworms, and hookworms; and flukes, such as blood and liver flukes, are a major cause of illness in the United States. And the problem is getting worse; research suggests that three out of every five Americans will be infected by parasites at some point in their lives. Parasitic infections are often misdiagnosed, since health care professionals, like most people, think these infections only occur in developing countries. This is simply not true.

Symptoms include such digestive problems as bloating, flatulence, abdominal pain, chronic constipation or diarrhea, anal itching, and mucus in the stool. But other parts of the body can also be affected. Allergies, vaginal irritation, joint and muscle aches, brain or nervous system damage, immune dysfunction, night sweats, and chronic fatigue can all result from parasitic infection. Just as varied are the points of contamination: international travel, infected food handlers, contaminated water, household pets, day care centers, and sexual partners. Another factor is the overuse of antibiotics that kill both good and bad bacteria, which disrupts the digestive tract.

Parasitic infection can cause nutritional deficiencies by impairing nutrient absorption and/or causing increased nutrient loss through the stool. Different organisms can cause malabsorption of different nutrients. For example, the tapeworm *Diphyllobothrium lathum* interferes with the absorption of vitamin B_{12}, which can cause pernicious anemia, and roundworm infection may interfere with the absorption of vitamin A. When an infection causes diarrhea, there may be serious nutrient losses that result in impaired immune function.

Lifestyle Recommendations

❥ **Follow safe food-preparation practices.** Knowing how to head off parasites before they reach the dinner table is vital, and especially so if you are subject to parasitic infections. Wash your hands often, especially after handling raw meat, fish, or eggs. Disinfect cutting boards and utensils by soaking them in a gallon of water to which a teaspoon of chlorine bleach has been added. Cook animal protein thoroughly: meat and poultry until it is no longer pink inside, fish until it is flaky and white, and eggs until the yolks are set.

Diet Recommendations

❥ **Cleanse the colon.** Parasites tend to become embedded in a mucus-encrusted intestinal wall. No treatment can dislodge them until the waste matter is removed. Mucus layers form as a result of eating devitalized or spoiled food; taking prescription or recreational drugs; and ingesting toxic or irritating substances, such as coffee, alcohol, and candy and other sweets. The body produces mucus to protect the intestinal tract from irritants. But when we consume irritating or toxic substances on a regular basis, the body's colon-cleansing processes are overwhelmed, and mucus layers build up. See the Intestinal Cleanse (page 332).

❥ **Eat a diet rich in complex carbohydrates, especially vegetables.** This food group should make up about half of your daily diet. Vegetables contain a lot of the nutrients you may be deficient in, and they promote the growth of beneficial intestinal bacteria. Choose vegetables rich in carotenes (see the Nutrient Recommendations). Eat plenty of vegetable-rich soups and stews, as well.

❥ **Eat lean, well-cooked protein.** Fish, white-meat turkey, chicken, eggs, and lamb are all good choices, especially if they are organically raised (no hormones, antibiotics, or pesticides). This food group should make up about a quarter of your daily diet. These foods provide the amino-acid building blocks necessary to rebuild tissues and strengthen the immune system. The other quarter of your diet should come from nuts, seeds, and legumes (lentils, split peas, and beans), dairy products, and whole grains (wheat, rye, oats, brown rice, and barley). However, do not eat too much of any one of these food groups. These foods can cause flatulence and irritate the gastrointestinal tract when parasites are present, which prevents the absorption of nutrients. The goal is to eat foods that will promote healing of the digestive system.

❥ **Drink vegetable juices and pure water.** Vegetable juices can heal the intestinal tract because of their high vitamin and mineral content. Minimize your use of fruit juices, which contain too much sugar. Drink no more than four to six ounces of fruit juice daily, and always dilute it by half with pure water. Use a water filter fine enough to catch extremely tiny parasites, such as *Cryptosporidia*.

❥ **Include plenty of healthy oils in your diet.** Flaxseed oil, hemp oil, evening primrose oil, and black currant seed oil help lubricate the intestinal tract and serve as carriers of such fat-soluble vitamins as A and E. For more information, see the fats and oils section in Basic Guidelines for the Juice Lady's Health and Healing Diet (page 313).

❥ **Completely eliminate sugars from your diet.** That means no sucrose (white sugar), brown sugar, corn syrup, fructose, dehydrated cane juice, fruit concentrate, honey, molasses, maple syrup, and brown rice syrup. Avoid not only all sweets and desserts, but also all dried fruit and full-strength fruit juices, and eat fresh fruit sparingly. Parasites love to dine on sugars, their favorite form of food. Sugars also suppress the immune system, your much-needed ally in the battle with parasites.

❥ **Choose foods with antiparasitic properties.** Pumpkin and pumpkin seeds, garlic, onions, radishes, kelp, raw cabbage, ground almonds, and sauerkraut all act directly against parasites.

Nutrient Recommendations

❥ **Vitamin A** and **carotenes** are especially important nutrients, since they help increase resistance to the penetration of parasitic larvae into tissues. Vitamin A is only present in fruits and vegetables as carotenes, which the body can convert to vitamin A as needed. Best juice sources of carotenes (in order of effectiveness): carrots, kale, parsley, spinach, chard, beet greens, watercress, broccoli, and romaine lettuce.

Supplement Recommendations

❥ **Hydrochloric acid,** a digestive fluid normally found in the stomach, can destroy many parasites. After age forty, hydrochloric acid secretion diminishes, which lowers resistance to parasites. Some people are genetically prone to low acid levels. Supplemental HCl betaine can be helpful; take one to three 10-mg tablets or capsules with meals.

❥ **Proteases** are digestive enzymes that break down protein. They are responsible, along with other digestive secretions, for keeping the small intestine free of parasites. Use undiluted pancreatic extract (8-10X USP), 750 to 1,000 mg ten to twenty minutes before meals. Bromelain (pineapple enzymes) and papain (papaya enzymes) are digestive aids that can also act against parasites. Because of the sugars in the fruits themselves, use these enzymes in supplement form.

❥ **Thymus extract** improves thymus gland activity. The thymus gland is responsible for many immune functions, including production of T cells. These white blood cells responsible for what is called cell-mediated immunity, an immune function that is very important for parasite resistance. If you suffer from parasites, it is a good indicator that your cell-mediated immunity is not functioning well. Use predigested calf thymus extract in a recommended dose of 750 mg per day.

Herb Recommendations

❦ **Barberry, goldenseal,** and **Oregon grape root** can be effective against different types of parasites (see Appendix A). Do not use any of these herbs if you are pregnant, and do not use them for more than ten days at a time.

❦ **Black walnut** works against tapeworms.

❦ **Citrus seed extract** is highly effective against bacteria, protozoa, yeast, and viruses.

❦ **Pinkroot** is especially effective against roundworms.

Juice Ingredient Recommendations

❦ **Cabbage** and **radish** juices are antiparasitic.

❦ **Garlic** juice is effective against roundworm, pinworm, tapeworm, and hookworm.

❦ **Parsley** juice is a rich source of beta-carotene. Intake should be limited to a safe, therapeutic dose of $1/2$ to 1 cup per day. Parsley can be toxic in overdose, and should be especially avoided by pregnant women.

Juice Recipes

ORIENT EXPRESS

2-inch chunk jicama, scrubbed, or peeled if not organic (optional)

5 carrots, scrubbed well, green tops removed, ends trimmed

2-inch piece daikon radish, scrubbed well, without green top or end

$1/2$-inch piece fresh ginger root, washed

Cut the jicama into strips (if using) that fit your juicer's feed tube. Juice the jicama with the carrots, radish, and ginger. Stir the juice, and pour into a glass. Serve at room temperature. This is a very hot-tasting drink because of the radish and ginger, so you may want to dilute it by half with water.

TRIPLE C

¼ small head green cabbage, washed

4 carrots, scrubbed well, green tops removed, and ends trimmed

4 stalks organic celery with leaves, washed

Cut the cabbage into sections that fit your juicer's feed tube. Juice the cabbage along with the carrots and celery. Stir the juice, and pour into a glass. Serve at room temperature or chilled, as desired.

TURNIP TIME

1 turnip, scrubbed well

2-inch piece jicama, scrubbed well or peeled if not organic (optional)

1 handful watercress, rinsed

4 carrots, scrubbed well, green tops removed, ends trimmed

1 garlic clove with peel, washed

½ small or medium lemon, washed, or peeled if not organic

Cut the turnip and jicama (if using) into strips that fit your juicer's feed tube. Bunch up the watercress, and push through the feed tube with the turnip, jicama, carrots, garlic, and lemon. Stir the juice, and pour into a glass. Serve at room temperature or chilled, as desired.

THE MORNING ENERGIZER

5 medium carrots, scrubbed well, green tops removed, ends trimmed

½ small beet with leaves and stems, scrubbed well

½ small or medium lemon, washed, or peeled if not organic

½- to 1-inch piece fresh ginger root, washed

Juice the carrots, beet, lemon, and ginger. Stir the juice, and pour into a glass. Serve at room temperature or chilled, as desired.

THE IMMUNE BUILDER

1 turnip, scrubbed well

1 handful watercress, rinsed (optional)

5 carrots, scrubbed well, green tops removed, ends trimmed

1 large garlic clove with peel, washed

½ small or medium lemon, washed, or peeled if not organic

Cut the turnip into sections that fit your juicer's feed tube. Bunch up the watercress (if using), and push it through the feed tube with the turnip, carrots, garlic, and lemon. Stir the juice, and pour into a glass. Serve at room temperature or chilled, as desired.

POPEYE'S POWER

1 handful organic spinach, washed

1 small handful parsley, rinsed

5 medium carrots, scrubbed well, green tops removed, ends trimmed

1 stalk organic celery with leaves, washed

½ beet with leaves, scrubbed well

Bunch up the spinach and parsley, and push them through the feed tube with the carrots, celery, and beet. Stir the juice, and pour into a glass. Serve at room temperature or chilled, as desired.

AFTERNOON REFRESHER

1 medium to large organic cucumber, scrubbed well

½ small or medium lemon, washed, or peeled if not organic

Cut the cucumber in half lengthwise, and juice with the lemon. (For an especially cooling version, let the juice splash over a few ice cubes in the juice pitcher.) Stir the juice, and pour into a glass. Serve at room temperature or chilled, as desired.

SANTA FE SALSA COCKTAIL

1 medium vine-ripened tomato, washed

½ medium organic cucumber, scrubbed well

¼ cup cilantro, rinsed

¼ small or medium lime or lemon, washed, or peeled if not organic

Dash hot sauce (optional)

Cut the tomato into sections that fit your juicer's feed tube. Cut the cucumber in half again lengthwise. Bunch up the cilantro, and push through the feed tube with the tomato, cucumber, and lime or lemon. Pour the juice into a glass, add the hot sauce (if using), and stir. Serve at room temperature or chilled, as desired.

SINUS SOLUTION

2 medium vine-ripened tomatoes, washed

4 radishes with green tops, washed

¼ small or medium lime or lemon, washed, or peeled if not organic

Cut the tomato into sections that fit your juicer's feed tube. Juice the tomatoes along with the radishes and lime or lemon. Stir the juice, and pour into a glass. Serve at room temperature or chilled, as desired.

PURE GREEN SPROUT DRINK

1 organic cucumber, scrubbed well

1 large handful sunflower sprouts, rinsed

1 small handful buckwheat sprouts, rinsed

1 small handful clover sprouts, rinsed

Cut the cucumber in half lengthwise. Bunch up the sprouts, and push through the feed tube with the cucumber. Stir the juice, and pour into a glass. Serve at room temperature or chilled, as desired.

THE COLON CLEANSER

1 bunch organic spinach, washed

1 handful parsley, rinsed

5 medium to large carrots, scrubbed well, green tops removed, ends trimmed

1/2 small or medium lemon, washed, or peeled if not organic

Bunch up the spinach and parsley, and push them through the feed tube with the carrots and lemon. Stir the juice, and pour into a glass. Serve at room temperature or chilled, as desired.

Pneumonia

See **Respiratory Disorders.**

Premenstrual Syndrome (PMS)

See **Menstrual Disorders.**

Prostate Enlargement, Benign

The prostate is a chestnut-sized gland that surrounds the urethra, the narrow tube through which both sperm and urine flow. This gland secretes the milky white fluid that transports and protects sperm. As a man ages, the prostate can start to enlarge, creating a condition known medically as benign prostatic hyperplasia (BPH). The early stages of BPH may be symptomless. But symptoms generally develop as the enlargement continues, and include increased need to urinate, nighttime awakening to urinate, and reduced force of urine flow. Urination can become painful. If left untreated, BPH can eventually obstruct the bladder outlet. This causes retention of urine, which can lead to bladder infection and possibly kidney damage.

BPH is very common, and affects over 50 percent of all men at some time in their lives. It is primarily the result of hormonal changes associated with aging. Levels of testosterone decrease, but levels of other hormones, including estrogen and prolactin, increase. The ultimate effect is an increased concentration of testosterone within the prostate gland, which is mainly caused by an increase in an enzyme called 5-alpha-reductase. The extra testosterone stimulates tissue growth in the prostate, which causes the enlargement of the gland and eventual narrowing of the urethra.

Because diet plays an important role in prostate health, the following suggestions should help you prevent or correct BPH. This condition is *not* malignant. But its symptoms are similar to those of prostate cancer, so see your doctor if you are having urinary difficulties.

Diet Recommendations

❥ **Eat a low-saturated-fat, low-cholesterol diet.** Lipid peroxidation, or free-radical damage to cholesterol and other fats, is particularly toxic and carcinogenic to the prostate gland. Damaged forms of cholesterol are believed to play a role in abnormal cell growth and can contribute to BPH. Lower your intake of cholesterol and saturated fats by reducing consumption of fatty meats, dairy products, and fried foods. Also, follow the Basic Guidelines for the Juice Lady's Health and Healing Diet (page 313).

❥ **Choose organically grown fruits, vegetables, grains, lean meat, and poultry.** Pesticides and other contaminants increase the actions of 5-alpha-reductase. See page 14 for more information.

❥ **Avoid alcohol, caffeine, and sugar.** Consumption of these substances is associated with BPH. Beer, in particular, raises prolactin levels.

Nutrient Recommendations

❥ **Bioflavonoids** are among the phytonutrients used as the first-line BPH treatment in Germany and Austria. A review of the scientific literature shows that these compounds have provided significant benefits in 70 percent of the BPH patients who took it. Best juice sources of bioflavonoids: apricots, bell peppers, berries (blueberry, blackberry, and cranberry), broccoli, cabbage, cantaloupes, cherries, citrus fruit, grapes, parsley, plums, prunes, and tomatoes.

❥ **Essential fatty acids (EFAs)** are divided into two main categories, omega-3s and omega-6s. Boosting EFA levels has led to significant improvements for many people with BPH. Gamma-linolenic acid (GLA), derived from evening primrose and borage oils, is particularly beneficial; this fatty acid appears to be a powerful inhibitor of 5-alpha-reductase. For more information on EFAs, see the fats and oils section in Basic Guidelines for the Juice Lady's Health and Healing Diet (page 313).

❥ **Vitamin B_6 (pyridoxine)** is important to hormone metabolism and works with zinc to reduce prolactin levels. Best juice sources of vitamin B_6 (in order of effectiveness): kale, spinach, turnip greens, bell peppers, and prunes.

❥ **Zinc** has been shown to reduce the size of the prostate and to lessen symptoms for most BPH patients. Zinc inhibits the activity of 5-alpha-reductase. Best juice sources of zinc (in order of effectiveness): ginger root, turnips, parsley, garlic, carrots, grapes, spinach, cabbage, lettuce, cucumbers, and tangerines.

Herb Recommendations

❥ **Saw palmetto** has been shown in double-blind studies to be as effective in treating prostate enlargement as conventional drugs.

Juice Ingredient Recommendations

❥ **Asparagus** juice was used by juicing pioneer Dr. Norman Walker for prostate problems. Walker combined asparagus juice with carrot and lettuce or carrot, cucumber, and beet juices.

❥ **Parsley** juice is a rich source of both bioflavonoids and zinc. Intake should be limited to a safe, therapeutic dose of $1/2$ to 1 cup per day. Parsley can be toxic in overdose, and should be especially avoided by pregnant women.

Juice Recipes

THE GINGER HOPPER

½ organic Red or Golden Delicious apple, washed

5 medium carrots, scrubbed well, green tops removed, ends trimmed

½- to 1-inch piece fresh ginger root, washed

Cut the apple into sections, and juice along with the carrots and ginger. Stir the juice, and pour into a glass. Serve at room temperature or chilled, as desired.

KIDNEY TONIC

1 organic cucumber, scrubbed well

8 asparagus stems, washed

5 medium carrots, scrubbed well, green tops removed, ends trimmed

½ small beet with leaves and stems, scrubbed well

½ small or medium lemon, washed, or peeled if not organic

Cut the cucumber in half lengthwise, and juice it with the asparagus, carrots, beet, and lemon. Stir the juice, and pour it into a glass. Serve at room temperature or chilled, as desired.

MORNING SUNRISE

1 pink, red, or white grapefruit, peeled

1 orange, peeled

Divide the grapefruit and orange into segments that fit your juicer's feed tube. Juice the grapefruit and orange, and stir the juice. Pour into a glass and serve at room temperature or chilled, as desired.

BEAUTIFUL BONE SOLUTION

1 organic Golden or Red Delicious apple, washed

1–2 kale leaves, washed

1 handful parsley, rinsed

1 stalk organic celery, washed

¼ small or medium lemon, washed, or peeled if not organic

½- to 1-inch piece fresh ginger root, washed

Cut the apple into sections that fit your juicer's feed tube. Bunch up the kale and parsley, and push through the feed tube with the apple, celery, lemon, and ginger. Stir the juice, and pour into a glass. Serve at room temperature or chilled, as desired.

CHERIE'S QUICK ENERGY SOUP

1¼ cups fresh carrot juice (5–7 medium, or approx. 1 pound, yield about 1 cup)

1 avocado, peeled and seed removed

½ teaspoon ground cumin

Place the carrot juice, avocado, and cumin in a blender, and purée until smooth. Pour the mixture into a single soup bowl, and chill until ready to serve. You may add any of the following, as desired: chopped basil; grated zucchini, carrot, or beet; or fresh corn cut off the cob.

ANTIAGING COCKTAIL

1 small bunch organic purple grapes (about 1 cup) with small stems* and seeds, washed

½ cup blueberries, blackberries, or raspberries, washed

¼ small or medium lemon, washed, or peeled if not organic

½-inch piece fresh ginger root, washed

*Large stems can dull your juicer's blade.

Juice the grapes, berries, lemon, and ginger. Stir the juice, and pour into a glass. Serve at room temperature or chilled, as desired.

SWEET DREAMS NIGHTCAP

2 romaine lettuce leaves, washed

1 handful parsley, rinsed

4 carrots, scrubbed well, green tops removed, ends trimmed

3 organic celery stalks with leaves, washed

Bunch up the lettuce leaves and parsley, and push through the feed tube with the carrots and celery. Stir the juice, and pour into a glass. Serve at room temperature or chilled, as desired.

MEMORY MENDER

2 medium vine-ripened tomatoes, washed

¼ small head iceberg lettuce, washed

4 cauliflower florets, washed

½ small or medium lemon, washed, or peeled if not organic

Cut the tomatoes and lettuce into sections that will fit your juicer's feed tube. Juice the tomatoes and lettuce along with the cauliflower and lemon. Pour into a glass and serve at room temperature or chilled, as desired.

THE CALCIUM CHAMP

½ organic Golden or Red Delicious apple, washed

1 handful organic spinach with stems, washed

1 small handful parsley, rinsed

1 ripe medium banana, peeled

½ cup plain or vanilla soy milk

1 tablespoon tahini (sesame butter)

6 ice cubes

Cut the apple in sections that fit your juicer's feed tube. Bunch up the spinach and parsley, and push through the feed tube with the apple. Pour the juice into a blender, and add the banana, soy milk, tahini, and ice; blend until smooth. Pour into one or two glasses and serve immediately.

Psoriasis

Psoriasis is a common skin disorder that occurs when skin cells divide at a rate at up to ten times faster than in normal skin. As a result, there are too many dead cells for the skin to shed. This cell accumulation results in the formation of red plaques with silvery scales, along with slightly elevated papules and patches, and mild to extreme itchiness. The lesions appear most often on the knees, elbows, and scalp, and nail pitting is common. Psoriasis can also affect the joints (psoriatic arthritis). Psoriasis tends to occur in cycles, with flareups followed by periods of remission.

Family history plays a role in psoriasis, and fair-skinned people are particularly susceptible. A number of other factors appear to cause or contribute to this condition, including streptococcal infection, bowel toxins, poor protein digestion, poor liver function, alcohol and animal-fat consumption, and nutritional imbalances. Stress seems to worsen the eruptions (*see* **Stress**)—up to 80 percent of patients report an emotional trauma prior to a flareup. Obesity (*see* **Overweight/Obesity**), skin injuries, and some drugs can aggravate the condition.

Psoriasis is caused by a basic defect in cell division. This process is controlled by a balance between two substances, cyclic adenosine monophosphate (AMP) and cyclic guanidine 5-monophosphate (GMP). Higher levels of GMP increase the rate of cell division, while higher levels of AMP decrease it. AMP and GMP levels can be rebalanced through dietary changes.

Diet Recommendations

❥ **Eat a high-fiber, low-fat diet.** At least 50 percent of your diet should consist of raw fruits, vegetables, sprouts, and juices, and another 25 percent from whole grains and legumes. One study documented a decrease in psoriasis symptoms with an increase in fruit and vegetable consumption. A low-fiber diet contributes to an increase in intestinal toxins, which include bacteria and yeast overgrowths (*see* **Candidiasis**) and parasites (*see* **Parasitic Infections**). These microbes can promote an increase in cyclic GMP levels within skin cells. For more information on healthy eating, see Basic Guidelines for the Juice Lady's Health and Healing Diet (page 313).

❥ **Avoid alcohol.** Alcohol consumption worsens psoriasis. It must be completely eliminated.

❥ **Use cleansing programs to aid the healing process.** A connection has been made between a sluggish liver and psoriasis. This is not surprising, since a poorly functioning liver cannot easily clear toxins from the body. The Liver Cleanse (page 333) can promote healing, as can other cleansing programs, such as the Intestinal Cleanse (page 332) and the Skin Cleanse (page 338).

❥ **Use juice fasting to remove toxins.** Going on juice fasts from one to three days several times a year can be very beneficial in clearing toxins from the body. This can help heal psoriasis. Fasting and a vegetarian diet has helped some people with psoriasis, according to one study. Some people have also benefited from eliminating gluten (the protein in wheat) and other food allergens from the diet. See the Juice Fast (page 324) and **Allergies**.

Nutrient Recommendations

❥ **Beta-carotene** has been shown in studies to benefit people with psoriasis. Vitamin A, created from beta-carotene within the body, is of primary importance for healthy skin. Best juice sources of carotenes in general (in order of effectiveness): carrots, kale, parsley, spinach, chard, beet greens, watercress, mangoes, cantaloupes, apricots, broccoli, and romaine lettuce.

❥ **Essential fatty acids (EFAs),** especially the omega-3 fatty acids, are important in the treatment of psoriasis. In this disorder there is excessive production of inflammatory compounds (leukotrienes) formed from a fat component called arachidonic acid, which is found only in meat and other animal fats. Reduce arachidonic acid levels by limiting meat, poultry, and dairy intake, and increase omega-3 levels by eating more cold-water fish, such as salmon, tuna, trout, mackerel, halibut, cod, and sardines. Flaxseed and hemp oils are also rich in omega-3s; take at least one tablespoon per day. For more information, see the fats and oils section in Basic Guidelines for the Juice Lady's Health and Healing Diet (page 313).

❥ **Lecithin** helps clear cholesterol from tissues. Psoriasis-affected skin typically contains abnormally high levels of cholesterol. Out of 155 psoriasis patients in one study, 118 either controlled or improved their symptoms by taking lecithin. Lecithin can be purchased at most health food stores; add lecithin granules to juice or smoothies, or take lecithin in capsule form.

❥ **Zinc** can help people with psoriasis. A zinc-copper imbalance has been observed in psoriasis patients—too little zinc, too much copper. Best juice sources of zinc (in order of effectiveness): ginger root, turnips, parsley, garlic, carrots, grapes, spinach, cabbage, lettuce, cucumbers, and tangerines.

Herb Recommendations

❥ **Milk thistle (silymarin)** is used in the treatment of psoriasis. This herb can help improve liver function, inhibit inflammation, and reduce excessive skin-cell proliferation.

Juice Ingredient Recommendations

❥ **Carrot** juice provides both beta-carotene and zinc.

Juice Recipes

THE MORNING ENERGIZER

½ organic Red or Golden Delicious apple, washed

5 medium carrots, scrubbed well, green tops removed, ends trimmed

½ small beet with leaves and stems, scrubbed well

½ small or medium lemon, washed, or peeled if not organic

½- to 1-inch piece fresh ginger root, washed

Cut the apple into sections that will fit your juicer's feed tube. Juice the apple along with the carrots, beet, lemon, and ginger. Stir the juice, and pour into a glass. Serve at room temperature or chilled, as desired.

REFRESHING COMPLEXION COCKTAIL

½ organic Golden or Red Delicious
   apple, washed

2-inch chunk pineapple, washed
   (peeled if not organic)

1 medium organic cucumber, washed

*Cut the apple into sections, and the
pineapple into strips, that will fit your
juicer's feed tube. Cut the cucumber
lengthwise. Juice the apple, pineapple,
and cucumber. Stir the juice, and pour
into a glass. Serve at room temperature
or chilled, as desired.*

BEAUTIFUL SKIN, HAIR, AND NAIL SOLUTION

1 medium organic cucumber,
   scrubbed well

1 medium parsnip, scrubbed well

3 carrots, scrubbed well, green tops
   removed, ends trimmed

½ small or medium lemon, washed,
   or peeled if not organic

¼ small green bell pepper, washed

*Cut the cucumber in half lengthwise,
and juice with the parsnip, carrots,
lemon, and bell pepper. Stir the juice,
and pour into a glass. Serve at room
temperature or chilled, as desired.*

THE COLON CLEANSER

2 organic Granny Smith, McIntosh, or
   Golden Delicious apples, washed

1 bunch organic spinach, washed

1 handful parsley, rinsed

¼ small or medium lemon, washed,
   or peeled if not organic

*Cut the apples into sections that fit
your juicer's feed tube. Bunch up the
spinach and parsley, and push them
through the feed tube with the apples
and lemon. Stir the juice, and pour
into a glass. Serve at room temperature
or chilled, as desired.*

LIVER LIFE TONIC

½ organic green apple such as
   Granny Smith or Pippin, washed

1 handful dandelion greens, washed

5 carrots, scrubbed well, green tops
   removed, ends trimmed

½ small lemon, washed, or peeled if
   not organic

*Cut the apple into wedges that will fit
your juicer's feed tube. Bunch up the
dandelion greens, and push through
the feed tube with the apple, carrots,
and lemon. Stir the juice, and pour
into a glass. Serve at room temperature
or chilled, as desired.*

THE GINGER HOPPER

½ organic Red or Golden Delicious apple, washed

5 medium carrots, scrubbed well, green tops removed, ends trimmed

½- to 1-inch piece fresh ginger root, washed

Cut the apple into sections, and juice along with the carrots and ginger. Stir the juice, and pour into a glass. Serve at room temperature or chilled, as desired.

SPRING TONIC

1 medium vine-ripened tomato, washed

1 organic cucumber, scrubbed well

8 asparagus stems, washed

½ small or medium lemon, washed, or peeled if not organic

Cut the tomato into sections that fit your juicer's feed tube. Cut the cucumber in half lengthwise. Juice the tomato, cucumber, asparagus, and lemon. Stir the juice, and pour into a glass. Serve at room temperature or chilled, as desired.

Respiratory Disorders

The respiratory tract, from the nose to the lungs, is subject to a number of disorders. Colds and flu are two of the more common respiratory problems (*see* **Colds** and **Influenza**), but inflammation can occur anywhere in the tract.

Sinusitis is an inflammation of the sinuses, the open spaces in the facial bones. The most common cause of acute sinusitis is infection, whether viral, bacterial, or fungal in nature. When a sinus is blocked for any length of time, it fills with a thin fluid that becomes a host to microbial growth. Chronic sinusitis can occur as the result of food allergies (*see* **Allergies**) or dental infections. Symptoms include nasal congestion, profuse discharge (usually yellow or green), fever, chills, a foul smell, and frontal headaches that worsen when lying down or bending over.

Laryngitis, an inflammation of the larynx, is usually caused by respiratory infection or such irritants as cigarette smoke. It is marked by hoarseness or loss of voice.

Bronchitis is an inflammation of the bronchial tubes. This condition is often preceded by an upper respiratory infection. It can arise from exposure to extreme cold or to noxious agents, such as ammonia, smoke, or chlorine. A dry cough is the first symptom, followed by sore throat, fatigue, nasal discharge, and muscle aches. After several days, the cough brings up yellow or green mucus. Wheezing is common.

Pneumonia is an acute infection or inflammation of the lungs. The air sacs in the lungs fill up with fluid and dead white blood cells, reducing the amount of air space. The most common cause of pneumonia is bacterial, viral, or fungal infection. The symptoms are fever and chills, followed by cough with lots of phlegm, chest pain, difficulty in breathing, and shortness of breath.

Diet Recommendations

❥ **Drink plenty of fluids.** For all respiratory tract conditions, it is very important to drink plenty of fluids. Fluid keeps the mucous membranes moist and better able to repel viral infections. Drink only nutritious liquids, such as vegetable juices and broths, herbal tea, and pure water. Do not drink soda; the chemicals and sugar or artificial sweeteners can weaken your immune system. Even fruit juice, with its fruit sugar, is not recommended (see the sugar item on this list). Going on a vegetable juice fast for between one and three days can be very beneficial—see the Juice Fast (page 324).

❥ **Eat lightly, and include plenty of vegetables in your diet.** A very light diet is recommended for the days you don't juice fast. Vegetable soups, stews, juices, and broths are recommended. Vegetables rich in beta-carotene and vitamin C are particularly helpful (see the Nutrient Recommendations).

❥ **Avoid foods that contain sugar.** Simple sugars, including such natural sugars as honey and fruit sugar, impair immune functioning. That's because sugar competes with vitamin C for the same route of transportation into white blood cells, the body's main infection fighters. Consuming too much sugar decreases vitamin C levels in these cells, which impairs their effectiveness. Therefore, avoid all sugary foods. Eat whole fruit in moderation, and avoid fruit juice (except for lemon and lime) entirely. Or drink fruit juice in small quantities, diluted by half with pure water.

❥ **Reduce your intake of dairy products, refined flour products, and eggs.** These foods, along with sugar, contribute to mucus production. Ridding the body of excess mucus is part of the healing process for all respiratory conditions.

❥ **Increase your consumption of spicy foods.** Hot and spicy foods—

cayenne pepper, chili pepper, horseradish, mustard—can help ease respiratory symptoms. For instance, spicy foods help to open air passages and bring some relief for bronchitis sufferers. Cayenne pepper is often used to increase circulation and to help produce a clearing effect in the mucous membranes. Cayenne also acts as an antibiotic.

Nutrient Recommendations

❥ **Vitamin A** and **beta-carotene** are recommended for combating respiratory illnesses. Vitamin A contributes to the health of the epithelial cells that coat the respiratory tract. It is also capable of stimulating various immune processes, including natural killer cell activity and antibody response. Beta-carotene and other carotenes are the only form of vitamin A found in fruits and vegetables, and are converted into vitamin A within the body as needed. Best juice sources of carotenes in general (in order of effectiveness): carrots, kale, parsley, spinach, chard, beet greens, watercress, broccoli, and romaine lettuce.

❥ **Vitamin C** and **bioflavonoids** are important immune-system stimulators. Vitamin C is found in great quantities in white blood cells, and the supply needs to be constantly replenished when the body is fighting infection or inflammation. One study showed that if vitamin C levels were low, the individual was more likely to develop bronchitis. Bioflavonoids make vitamin C more effective. Best juice sources of vitamin C (in order of effectiveness): kale, parsley, broccoli, Brussels sprouts, watercress, cauliflower, cabbage, spinach, citrus fruit, turnips, and asparagus. Best juice sources of bioflavonoids: bell peppers, broccoli, cabbage, parsley, and tomatoes.

❥ **Vitamin E** is another strong ally in supporting the immune system. It plays a role in a broad range of defense mechanisms on the cellular level. Best juice sources of vitamin E (in order of effectiveness): spinach, watercress, asparagus, carrots, and tomatoes.

❥ **Zinc** is an important immune-stimulating mineral. Studies have shown that zinc lozenges can soothe sore throat and reduce a cold's duration. Best juice sources of zinc (in order of effectiveness): ginger root, turnips, parsley, garlic, carrots, spinach, cabbage, lettuce, and cucumbers.

Supplement Recommendations

❥ **Bromelain,** a digestive enzyme found in pineapple, has been shown to alleviate symptoms and lessen mucous membrane inflammation, especially in acute and chronic sinusitis. It makes bronchial secretions more fluid and helps to decrease the amount of secretions. One study showed an improvement in nasal inflammation and breathing difficulties in 87 percent of the patients taking bromelain. Because pineapple juice has a lot of fruit sugar, it is best to take a bromelain supplement when fighting a respiratory infection.

Herb Recommendations

❥ **Echinacea** contains several compounds that make it a good immune-system support herb. For example, inulin directly affects important cellular processes involved in fighting infection and inflammation. Caffeic acid is antibacterial and contains compounds that help to keep mucous membranes strong.

❥ **Goldenseal** contains a compound that is an effective antibiotic. This herb also enhances the immune system by increasing blood flow to the spleen, the organ responsible for releasing many important immune-stimulating compounds. Avoid goldenseal if you are pregnant, and do not use it for more than ten days.

❥ **Lobelia** is an herbal expectorant that propels mucus from the lungs. It does this while also relaxing the muscles of the respiratory system, which reduces wheezing and chest discomfort. It is especially helpful for bronchitis.

❥ **Yarrow** promotes sweating, thereby helping the body deal with fevers.

Juice Ingredient Recommendations

❥ **Celery** juice will help you sleep better.

❥ **Garlic** juice is a strong immune-system stimulant, and is both antibacterial and antiviral. It also helps reduce bronchial secretions.

❥ **Lemon** juice with a little horseradish is helpful for the sinuses.

❥ **Parsley** juice contains beta-carotene, bioflavonoids, vitamin C, and zinc. Intake should be limited to a safe, therapeutic dose of $1/2$ to 1 cup per day. Parsley can be toxic in overdose, and should be especially avoided by pregnant women.

❥ **Pear** juice, diluted by half with water and served at room temperature, helps loosen congestion in the lungs.

❥ **Radish** juice is a traditional remedy for sinus disorders.

❥ **Watercress** and **turnip** juices help ease bronchitis and pneumonia.

Juice Recipes

SWEET DREAMS NIGHTCAP

2 romaine lettuce leaves, washed

1 handful parsley, rinsed

4 carrots, scrubbed well, green tops removed, ends trimmed

3 organic celery stalks with leaves, washed

Bunch up the lettuce leaves and parsley, and push through the feed tube with the carrots and celery. Stir the juice, and pour into a glass. Serve at room temperature.

ANTIVIRAL COCKTAIL

1 organic Granny Smith or Pippin apple, washed

1 turnip, scrubbed well

1 handful watercress, rinsed

5 carrots, scrubbed well, green tops removed, ends trimmed

1 large garlic clove with peel, washed

Cut the apple and turnip into sections that fit your juicer's feed tube. Bunch up the watercress, and juice it with the apple, turnip, carrots, and garlic. Stir the juice, and pour into a glass. Serve at room temperature.

THE FEEL GOOD COCKTAIL

4 medium carrots, scrubbed well, green tops removed, ends trimmed

3 fennel stalks with leaves and flowers, washed

1 stalk organic celery with leaves, washed

½ small or medium lemon, washed, or peeled if not organic

Juice the carrots, fennel, celery, and lemon. Stir the juice, and pour into a glass. Serve at room temperature or chilled, as desired.

THE MORNING ENERGIZER

5 medium carrots, scrubbed well, green tops removed, ends trimmed

½ small beet with leaves and stems, scrubbed well

½ small or medium lemon, washed, or peeled if not organic

½- to 1-inch piece fresh ginger root, washed

Juice the carrots, beet, lemon, and ginger. Stir the juice, and pour into a glass. Serve at room temperature.

SINUS SOLUTION

2 medium vine-ripened tomatoes, washed

4 radishes with green tops, washed

1/4 small or medium lime or lemon, washed, or peeled if not organic

Cut the tomato into sections that fit your juicer's feed tube. Juice the tomatoes along with the radishes and lime or lemon. Stir the juice, and pour into a glass. Serve at room temperature.

GINGER TWIST

1 handful parsley, rinsed

5 carrots, scrubbed well, green tops removed, ends trimmed

1-inch piece fresh ginger root, washed

1/2 small or medium lemon, washed, or peeled if not organic

Bunch up the parsley and push it through the feed tube with the carrots, ginger, and lemon. Stir the juice, and pour into a glass. Serve at room temperature.

AFTERNOON REFRESHER

1 medium to large organic cucumber, scrubbed well

1/2 small or medium lemon, washed, or peeled if not organic

Cut the cucumber in half lengthwise, and juice with the lemon. Stir the juice, and pour into a glass. Serve at room temperature.

POPEYE'S POWER

1 handful organic spinach, washed

1 small handful parsley, rinsed

5 medium carrots, scrubbed well, green tops removed, ends trimmed

1 stalk organic celery with leaves, washed

1/2 beet with leaves, scrubbed well

Bunch up the spinach and parsley, and push them through the feed tube with the carrots, celery, and beet. Stir the juice, and pour into a glass. Serve at room temperature.

TOMATO FLORENTINE

1 vine-ripened tomato, washed

1 handful organic spinach, washed

2–3 fresh basil leaves (optional)

1/2 small or medium lemon, washed, or peeled if not organic

Cut the tomato into sections that will fit your juicer's feed tube. Bunch up the spinach and basil leaves (if using), and push through the feed tube with the tomato and lemon. Stir the juice, and pour into a glass. Serve at room temperature.

RADISH CARE

5 carrots, scrubbed well, green tops removed, ends trimmed

5–6 radishes (green tops removed), washed well

½ small or medium lemon, washed, or peeled if not organic

Juice the carrots, radishes, and lemon. Stir the juice and pour into a glass. Serve at room temperature or chilled, as desired.

TURNIP TIME

1 turnip, scrubbed well

2-inch piece jicama, scrubbed well or peeled if not organic (optional)

1 handful watercress, rinsed

4 carrots, scrubbed well, green tops removed, ends trimmed

1 garlic clove with peel, washed

½ small or medium lemon, washed, or peeled if not organic

Cut the turnip and jicama (if using) into strips that fit your juicer's feed tube. Bunch up the watercress, and push through the feed tube with the turnip, jicama, carrots, garlic, and lemon. Stir the juice, and pour into a glass. Serve at room temperature.

BEAUTIFUL BONE SOLUTION

1 organic Granny Smith or Pippin apple, washed

1–2 kale leaves, washed

1 handful parsley, rinsed

1 stalk organic celery, washed

½ small or medium lemon, washed, or peeled if not organic

½- to 1-inch piece fresh ginger root, washed

Cut the apple into sections that fit your juicer's feed tube. Bunch up the kale and parsley, and push through the feed tube with the apple, celery, lemon, and ginger. Stir the juice, and pour into a glass. Serve at room temperature.

LIVER LIFE TONIC

½ organic green apple such as Granny Smith or Pippin, washed

1 handful dandelion greens, washed

5 carrots, scrubbed well, green tops removed, ends trimmed

½ small lemon, washed, or peeled if not organic

Cut the apple into wedges that will fit your juicer's feed tube. Bunch up the dandelion greens, and push through the feed tube with the apple, carrots, and lemon. Stir the juice, and pour into a glass. Serve at room temperature.

Rheumatoid Arthritis

Rheumatoid arthritis (RA) is a chronic inflammatory condition that affects the entire body, especially the joints. Symptoms include fatigue, low-grade fever, weakness, sleeplessness, and joint stiffness. There is often severe joint pain, with increasing inflammation beginning in the small joints and progressively affecting all the joints. Eventually, deformities can develop that limit range of motion in joints, with the ends of bones becoming enlarged. More women are affected by RA than men.

Unlike arthritis caused by wear and tear (*see* **Osteoarthritis**), there is evidence that RA is an autoimmune reaction in which the body's own immune system produces antibodies that attack joint tissue components. Another theory is that RA is an immune reaction to a viral infection somewhere in the body. What causes these possible reactions is unknown, but investigation has centered on lifestyle and nutritional factors, food allergies, abnormal bowel permeability, and genetic factors. There are several studies that point to diet therapy as a promising way to ease symptoms and possibly reverse the progression of this disease.

In addition to RA, there are several other autoimmune diseases that affect connective tissue, including lupus, ankylosing spondylitis, and scleroderma. From a nutritional perspective, the treatment for any of these autoimmune diseases is the same as the one used for RA.

Lifestyle Recommendations

❥ **Avoid or reduce nonsteriodal anti-inflammatory drug (NSAID) use.** These agents, including aspirin and ibuprofen, can damage the intestines, allowing allergy-causing particles to leak into the system and thereby contribute to RA.

❥ **Eliminate any small intestine bacterial and yeast overgrowth.** Many patients with RA have bacterial and yeast overgrowth in the small intestine. This condition has been shown to be connected with both severity of symptoms and disease activity. There are numerous reports that treatment of Candida yeast infections has eased rheumatic symptoms. For more information, *see* **Candidiasis** and the Intestinal Cleanse (page 332).

Dietary and Recommendations

❥ **Eat a predominantly vegetarian diet.** Switching to a meatless diet has been shown to produce significant benefits for RA patients. Exclude all animal products from your diet, with the exception of fish. Consume at least 50 percent of your diet in the form of raw foods—fruits, vegetables, juices, sprouts, nuts, and seeds. For more information on raw foods and juices, see the raw foods section in Basic Guidelines for the Juice Lady's Health and Healing Diet (page 313).

❥ **Go on juice fasts.** Studies have shown that juice fasts decrease joint pain and reverse RA. In one scientific review, the authors concluded that fasting may be the most rapid means of inducing relief of arthritic pain and swelling for persons with RA. See the Juice Fast (page 324).

❥ **Eliminate food allergies that may contribute to RA.** Foods most likely to cause intolerance in RA suffers are, in descending order, wheat, bacon/pork, oranges, milk, oats, rye, eggs, beef, coffee, malt (beer), cheese, grapefruits, tomatoes, peanuts, sugar, butter, lamb, lemons, and soy. If you are allergic to citrus fruits, do not use them as sources of nutrients (see Nutrient Recommendations), and omit them from the recipes. (*See* **Allergies**; also see the Elimination Diet, page 321.)

Nutrient Recommendations

❥ **Antioxidants** are substances that fight the actions of toxins called free radicals. Several studies have indicated that the risk of RA is highest among people with the lowest levels of antioxidants, among them vitamins C and E, beta-carotene, and selenium:

- *Beta-carotene* and *vitamin A* help fight RA. Consumption of foods rich in beta-carotene is associated with a lowered risk of this disorder. Beta-carotene, or provitamin A, is the only form of vitamin A found in fruits and vegetables, and is converted by the body to vitamin A as needed. Best juice sources of carotenes in general (in order of effectiveness): carrots, kale, parsley, spinach, chard, beet greens, watercress, mangoes, cantaloupes, apricots, broccoli, and romaine lettuce.

- *Vitamin C* and *bioflavonoids* play a vital role in fighting RA. Vitamin C promotes anti-inflammatory activity, and people with RA have low levels of vitamin C in their blood. Bioflavonoids help make vitamin C more effective. Best juice sources of vitamin C (in order of effectiveness): kale, parsley, broccoli, Brussels sprouts, watercress, cauliflower, cabbage, strawberries, papaya, spinach, citrus fruit, turnips, mangoes, asparagus, and cantaloupes. Best juice sources of bioflavonoids: apricots, bell peppers, berries (blueberry, blackberry, and cranberry), broccoli, cabbage, cantaloupes, cherries, citrus fruit, grapes, parsley, plums, prunes, and tomatoes.

- *Vitamin E* and *selenium* have provided some benefits for people with RA. Best juice sources of vitamin E (in order of effectiveness): spinach, watercress, asparagus, carrots, and tomatoes. Best juice sources of selenium: chard, turnips, garlic, oranges, radishes, grapes, carrots, and cabbage.

❥ **Essential fatty acids (EFAs),** especially the omega-3 fatty acids, can reduce production of inflammation-stimulating compounds. Fish oils are rich in two omega-3 oils, eicosapentaenoic acid (EPA) and docosahexaenoic acid (DHA). These oils are found most abundantly in such cold-water fish as salmon, tuna, trout, sardines, mackerel, and halibut. The body can also produce EPA and DHA from flaxseed and hemp oils. In addition, studies show that supplementation with gamma-linolenic acid (GLA), found in borage and evening primrose oils, produces statistically significant reductions in RA symptoms. For more information, see the fats and oils section in Basic Guidelines for the Juice Lady's Health and Healing Diet (page 313).

❥ **Pantothenic acid** may be helpful, as deficiencies of this nutrient have been found to be directly related to RA symptoms. Best juice sources of pantothenic acid (in order of effectiveness): broccoli, cauliflower, and kale.

❥ **Vitamin K** may stabilize cell membranes in rheumatoid tissue. Best juice sources of vitamin K (in order of effectiveness): turnip greens, broccoli, lettuce, cabbage, spinach, watercress, asparagus, and string beans.

Herb Recommendations

❥ **Chinese thoroughwax, ginseng,** and **licorice** are traditional remedies for inflammatory ailments. Use Korean or red ginseng (*Panax ginseng*), not Siberian ginseng (*Eleutherococcus senticosus*). Avoid licorice if you have high blood pressure, do not use it for prolonged periods of time, and use a medicinal form of the herb, not licorice candy.

Juice Ingredient Recommendations

❥ **Blackberry, blueberry,** and **cherry** juices, all rich in anthocyanidins and proanthocyanidins, have been shown to be effective in reducing inflammation associated with arthritis.

❥ **Dandelion** juice is a traditional remedy for healing RA. My recommendation is to take one-half cup mornings and evenings. Dandelion juice is very strong tasting; you may want to dilute it with water or other juices. Or you can try Liver Life Tonic.

❥ **Ginger,** which contains anti-inflammatory compounds, relieved pain and swelling in 75 percent of the arthritis patients in one study. All patients who had muscular discomfort found relief.

❥ **Parsley** juice is rich in beta-carotene, bioflavonoids, and vitamin C. Intake should be limited to a safe, therapeutic dose of $1/2$ to 1 cup per day. Parsley can be toxic in overdose, and should be especially avoided by pregnant women.

Juice Recipes

ANTIAGING COCKTAIL

1 small bunch organic purple grapes (about 1 cup) with small stems* and seeds, washed

$1/2$ cup blueberries, blackberries, or raspberries, washed

$1/4$ small or medium lemon, washed, or peeled if not organic

$1/2$-inch piece fresh ginger root, washed

*Large stems can dull your juicer's blade.

Juice the grapes, berries, lemon, and ginger. Stir the juice, and pour into a glass. Serve at room temperature or chilled, as desired.

CHERRY JUBILEE

1 three-inch chunk fresh pineapple, scrubbed well, or peeled if not organic

$1/2$ organic Golden or Red Delicious apple, washed

6–8 organic Bing cherries, washed, pits removed

Cut the pineapple into strips, and the apple into sections, that fit your juicer's feed tube, and juice them with the cherries. Stir the juice, and pour it into a glass. Serve at room temperature or chilled, as desired.

LIVER LIFE TONIC

$1/2$ organic green apple such as Granny Smith or Pippin, washed

1 handful dandelion greens, washed

5 carrots, scrubbed well, green tops removed, ends trimmed

$1/2$ small lemon, washed, or peeled if not organic

Cut the apple into wedges that will fit your juicer's feed tube. Bunch up the dandelion greens, and push through the feed tube with the apple, carrots, and lemon. Stir the juice, and pour into a glass. Serve at room temperature or chilled, as desired.

THE GINGER HOPPER

½ organic Red or Golden Delicious apple, washed

5 medium carrots, scrubbed well, green tops removed, ends trimmed

½- to 1-inch piece fresh ginger root, washed

Cut the apple into sections, and juice along with the carrots and ginger. Stir the juice, and pour into a glass. Serve at room temperature or chilled, as desired.

MAGNESIUM SPECIAL

5 medium carrots, scrubbed well, green tops removed, ends trimmed

2 stalks organic celery with leaves, washed

½ small beet with leaves and stems, scrubbed well

2 broccoli florets, washed

½ small or medium lemon, washed, or peeled if not organic

Juice the carrots, celery, beet, broccoli, and lemon. Stir the juice, and pour into a glass. Serve at room temperature or chilled, as desired.

CHERIE'S QUICK ENERGY SOUP

1¼ cups fresh carrot juice (5–7 medium, or approx. 1 pound, yield about 1 cup)

1 avocado, peeled and seed removed

½ teaspoon ground cumin

Place the carrot juice, avocado, and cumin in a blender, and purée until smooth. Pour the mixture into a single soup bowl, and chill until ready to serve. You may add any of the following, as desired: chopped basil; grated zucchini, carrot, or beet; or fresh corn cut off the cob.

TRIPLE C

¼ small head green cabbage, washed

4 carrots, scrubbed well, green tops removed, and ends trimmed

4 stalks organic celery with leaves, washed

Cut the cabbage into sections that fit your juicer's feed tube. Juice the cabbage along with the carrots and celery. Stir the juice, and pour into a glass. Serve at room temperature or chilled, as desired.

POPEYE'S POWER

½ medium organic apple, any kind, washed

1 handful organic spinach, washed

1 small handful parsley, rinsed

4 medium carrots, scrubbed well, green tops removed, ends trimmed

1 stalk organic celery with leaves, washed

½ beet with leaves, scrubbed well

Cut the apple into sections that will fit your juicer's feed tube. Bunch up the spinach and parsley, and push them through the feed tube with the apple, carrots, celery, and beet. Stir the juice, and pour into a glass. Serve at room temperature or chilled, as desired.

Scleroderma

See **Rheumatoid Arthritis.**

Seizures

See **Epilepsy and Seizures.**

Sinusitis

See **Respiratory Disorders.**

Stress

Modern life is filled with stressors—job pressures, relationship problems, financial worries. Actually, a stressor is almost anything that creates a bodily disturbance. Stressors include environmental or microbial toxins, physical trauma, exposure to heat or cold, and strong emotional reactions. Physical symptoms can include headache, fatigue, insomnia, digestive disturbances, neck and back pain, and either loss of appetite or overeating.

There are three stages of the stress response, called the General Adaptation Syndrome. The first is the alarm stage. This "fight or flight" response triggers the adrenal glands to release adrenaline and other hormones that prepare the body to either fight a perceived danger or run away from it. The second stage is the resistance stage. The body begins to adapt to the stessors by releasing adrenal hormones that convert protein into energy, which elevates blood-sugar levels. There may be depression of the immune system, decreased bone strength, poor memory, and decreased energy at this point. Coping abilities can diminish, causing feelings of insecurity and inadequacy. The third and final stage is exhaustion. The body is depleted of energy by loss of both potassium and such adrenal hormones as cortisol. When adrenal hormones become depleted, hypoglycemia can result because cells are not receiving enough fuel. There is a complete loss of resistance, and the exhaustion will affect any inherently weak organ or system, such as the heart, blood vessels, adrenal glands, or immune system. If the stress continues, there is an increased risk of diabetes, high blood pressure, and cancer.

Negative coping behaviors—substance abuse, overeating, excessive television viewing, inappropriate sexual activity, and so forth—offer only temporary diversion and can create more stress than they relieve. To fight stress, you need to recognize and eliminate such coping behaviors, and instead come up with your own stress-management program. Nutrition plays an important role, as a variety of nutrients and herbs can help support the overworked adrenal glands.

Lifestyle Recommendations

❥ **Develop a comprehensive approach to stress management.** This involves: (1) learning ways to calm your body and mind, such as meditation, prayer, relaxation, and breathing techniques; (2) dealing with such lifestyle factors as time management and relationship issues; (3) exercising on a regular basis; (4) eating a healthy diet; and (5) using nutritional supplements that support the body during stress. The effects of stress on your body are to some extent affected by your perception of the stress. If you can let go of the "self" that says "I want my life to turn out this way," you can use stress creatively. Christopher Hobbs, in his book *Stress & Natural Healing,* says, "we can use stress to grow beyond our self-imposed limits to a point where what was once unimaginable was possible."

Diet Recommendations

❧ **Eat a low-saturated-fat, high-complex-carbohydrate diet that includes adequate protein.** When faced with stressful situations, get the best nutrition possible. This means eating less red meat and refined foods, and eating more whole grains, vegetables, fruits, sprouts, nuts, seeds, and fish. For more information, see Basic Guidelines for the Juice Lady's Health and Healing Diet (page 313).

❧ **Drink plenty of fresh juice, and go on juice fasts.** Your body needs extra nutrition during times of stress, and juice provides a concentration of nutrients in an easily digestible, easily assimilated form. Juicing foods with high concentrations of vitamins (especially C and the B complex) and minerals will help protect you against the negative effects of stress. In addition, studies show that fasting may be helpful during times of stress (see the Juice Fast, page 324).

❧ **Identify food allergies.** Controlling food allergies and intolerances can be helpful in managing stress, because anxiety and fatigue are signs of food allergies. (*See* **Allergies**; also see the Elimination Diet, page 321.)

❧ **Avoid coffee, cigarettes, alcohol, and sugary foods.** These substances offer a quick boost of emotional and physical energy, but leave your body more stressed out and energy depleted in the long term. Caffeine can damage the adrenal glands and/or kidneys. Caffeinism, a condition caused by excess caffeine consumption, is characterized by depression, nervousness, irritability, recurrent headaches, heart palpitations, and insomnia. Tobacco's harmful effects on the body are well known. Alcohol damages the immune system and interferes with normal sleep patterns. Drinking alcohol to wind down from the effects of stress actually puts more stress on your body. Eating refined carbohydrates, such as sweets and white-flour products, affects blood sugar and can lead to hypoglycemia, a blood-sugar dysfunction that results in irritability and depression (*see* **Hypoglycemia**).

Nutrient Recommendations

❧ **Amino acids** that can help protect the body against the ravages of stress include GABA, glycine, leucine, and tryptophan. Gamma-aminobutyric acid (GABA) can help reduce sugar and carbohydrate cravings, and can be taken to calm the body in much the same way as tranquilizers. Take 750 mg of GABA in supplement form twice daily. Glycine acts as a sedative. The best food sources of glycine: almonds, turkey, and wheat germ; best juice sources: carrots and celery. Leucine promotes protein creation, lowers elevated blood-sugar levels, and slows the effects of stress. Best food sources of leucine: almonds, avocado, cheese, chicken, walnuts, wheat germ, and yogurt. Tryptophan is used by the body to create serotonin, a hormone that elevates mood and helps promote restful sleep. Best food sources of tryptophan: tuna, turkey, and yogurt.

❥ **Magnesium** is needed during times of stress. A deficiency can interfere with nerve and muscle impulses, causing irritability and nervousness. Low levels of this mineral are associated with behavioral problems. Best juice sources of magnesium (in order of effectiveness): beet greens, spinach, parsley, dandelion greens, garlic, blackberries, beets, broccoli, cauliflower, carrots, and celery.

❥ **Pantothenic acid** is known as the antistress vitamin. A deficiency results in adrenal atrophy, characterized by fatigue, headache, sleep disturbances, nausea, and abdominal discomfort. Best juice sources of pantothenic acid (in order of effectiveness): broccoli, cauliflower, and kale.

❥ **Potassium** intake should be increased during times of stress to support the adrenal glands. Every effort should be made to maintain adequate potassium levels, and drinking fresh juices is one of *the best* ways to get potassium. Best juice sources of potassium (in order of effectiveness): parsley, chard, garlic, spinach, broccoli, carrots, celery, radishes, cauliflower, watercress, asparagus, and cabbage.

❥ **Selenium** may help protect the body against infections during times of stress. Best juice sources of selenium (in order of effectiveness): chard, turnips, garlic, oranges, radishes, grapes, carrots, and cabbage.

❥ **Vitamin C** and **bioflavonoids** are important for both adrenal gland and immune system functioning. Vitamin C levels can drop during times of stress. Bioflavonoids work with vitamin C, allowing the body to absorb this vitamin more effectively. Best juice sources of vitamin C (in order of effectiveness): kale, parsley, broccoli, Brussels sprouts, watercress, cauliflower, cabbage, strawberries, papaya, spinach, citrus fruit, turnips, mangoes, asparagus, and cantaloupes. Best juice sources of bioflavonoids: apricots, bell peppers, berries (blueberry, blackberry, and cranberry), broccoli, cabbage, cantaloupes, cherries, citrus fruit, grapes, parsley, plums, prunes, and tomatoes.

Herb Recommendations

❥ **California poppy, kava-kava, lavender,** and **valerian** all have a sedative effect. California poppy, kava-kava, and valerian also help fight insomnia.

❥ **Catnip, hops,** and **mugwort** help you fall asleep faster, wake up less often, and go into a deeper sleep.

❥ **Chamomile** and **St. John's wort** reduce nerve or muscle pain. St. John's wort is also effective against depression and insomnia. Be sure to use German chamomile, *Matricaria recutita*, and not Roman chamomile, *Chamaemelum nobile*.

❥ **Ginseng** exerts beneficial effects on adrenal functioning and enhances stress resistance. Both Korean or red ginseng (*Panax ginseng*) and Siberian ginseng (*Eleutherococcus senticosus*) are effective. Avoid Siberian ginseng if you have an autoimmune disease such as rheumatoid arthritis.

Juice Ingredient Recommendations

❥ **Celery** juice has a calming effect and supports the nervous system.

❥ **Fennel** juice helps promote the release of endorphins, the "feel good" brain chemicals.

❥ **Garlic** juice helps prevent infections.

❥ **Lettuce** juice calms digestion.

❥ **Oats** and **wheat germ,** when added to any of the juices in the next section, can help you relax even more.

❥ **Parsley** juice is a source of a number of important nturients, including bioflavonoids, magnesium, potassium, and vitamin C. Intake should be limited to a safe, therapeutic dose of $1/2$ to 1 cup per day. Parsley can be toxic in overdose, and should be especially avoided by pregnant women.

Juice Recipes

SWEET DREAMS NIGHTCAP

2 romaine lettuce leaves, washed

1 handful parsley, rinsed

4 carrots, scrubbed well, green tops removed, ends trimmed

3 organic celery stalks with leaves, washed

Bunch up the lettuce leaves and parsley, and push through the feed tube with the carrots and celery. Stir the juice, and pour into a glass. Serve at room temperature or chilled, as desired.

THE FEEL GOOD COCKTAIL

½ pear, washed

4 medium carrots, scrubbed well, green tops removed, ends trimmed

3 fennel stalks with leaves and flowers, washed

1 stalk organic celery with leaves, washed

Cut the pear into sections that fit your juicer's feed tube, and juice along with the carrots, fennel, and celery. Stir the juice, and pour into a glass. Serve at room temperature or chilled, as desired.

WALDORF TWIST

1 organic Red or Golden Delicious apple, washed

3 stalks organic celery with leaves, washed

¼ small or medium lemon, washed, or peeled if not organic

Cut the apple into sections that will fit your juicer's feed tube, and juice along with the celery and lemon. Stir the juice, and pour into a glass. Serve at room temperature or chilled, as desired.

THE IMMUNE BUILDER

1 organic Golden or Red Delicious apple, washed

1 turnip, scrubbed well

1 handful watercress, rinsed (optional)

5 carrots, scrubbed well, green tops removed, ends trimmed

1 large garlic clove with peel, washed

Cut the apple and turnip into sections that fit your juicer's feed tube. Bunch up the watercress (if using), and push it through the feed tube with the apple, turnip, carrots, and garlic. Stir the juice, and pour into a glass. Serve at room temperature or chilled, as desired.

GINGER TWIST

1 organic Red or Golden Delicious apple, washed

1 handful parsley, rinsed

4 carrots, scrubbed well, green tops removed, ends trimmed

1-inch piece fresh ginger root, washed

¼ small or medium lemon, washed, or peeled if not organic

Cut the apple into sections that fit your juicer's feed tube. Bunch up the parsley and push it through the feed tube with the apple, carrots, ginger, and lemon. Stir the juice, and pour into a glass. Serve at room temperature or chilled, as desired.

TANGERINE SQUEEZE

¼ ripe pineapple, scrubbed well or peeled if not organic

2–3 tangerines, peeled

¼ lime, washed or peeled if not organic

Cut the pineapple into strips, and divide the tangerines into sections, that fit your juicer's feed tube, and juice them with the lime. Stir the juice, and pour into a glass. Serve at room temperature or chilled, as desired.

GRAPE EXPECTATIONS

3 plums, washed, stones removed

½ pound organic purple grapes with small stems* and seeds, washed

8 organic strawberries with caps, washed

¼ small or medium lemon, washed, or peeled if not organic

*Large stems can dull your juicer's blade.

Cut the plums in half, and juice with the grapes, strawberries, and lemon. Stir the juice, and pour into a glass. Serve at room temperature or chilled, as desired.

BEAUTIFUL BONE SOLUTION

1 organic Golden or Red Delicious apple, washed

1–2 kale leaves, washed

1 handful parsley, rinsed

1 stalk organic celery, washed

¼ small or medium lemon, washed, or peeled if not organic

½- to 1-inch piece fresh ginger root, washed

Cut the apple into sections that fit your juicer's feed tube. Bunch up the kale and parsley, and push through the feed tube with the apple, celery, lemon, and ginger. Stir the juice, and pour into a glass. Serve at room temperature or chilled, as desired.

POPEYE'S POWER

½ medium organic apple, any kind, washed

1 handful organic spinach, washed

1 small handful parsley, rinsed

4 medium carrots, scrubbed well, green tops removed, ends trimmed

1 stalk organic celery with leaves, washed

½ beet with leaves, scrubbed well

Cut the apple into sections that will fit your juicer's feed tube. Bunch up the spinach and parsley, and push them through the feed tube with the apple, carrots, celery, and beet. Stir the juice, and pour into a glass. Serve at room temperature or chilled, as desired.

LIVER LIFE TONIC

½ organic green apple such as Granny Smith or Pippin, washed

1 handful dandelion greens, washed

5 carrots, scrubbed well, green tops removed, ends trimmed

½ small lemon, washed, or peeled if not organic

Cut the apple into wedges that will fit your juicer's feed tube. Bunch up the dandelion greens, and push through the feed tube with the apple, carrots, and lemon. Stir the juice, and pour into a glass. Serve at room temperature or chilled, as desired.

TURNIP TIME

1 turnip, scrubbed well

2-inch piece jicama, scrubbed well or peeled if not organic (optional)

1 handful watercress, rinsed

4 carrots, scrubbed well, green tops removed, ends trimmed

1 garlic clove with peel, washed

½ small or medium lemon, washed, or peeled if not organic

Cut the turnip and jicama (if using) into strips that fit your juicer's feed tube. Bunch up the watercress, and push through the feed tube with the turnip, jicama, carrots, garlic, and lemon. Stir the juice, and pour into a glass. Serve at room temperature or chilled, as desired.

CHERIE'S QUICK ENERGY SOUP

1¼ cups fresh carrot juice (5–7 medium, or approx. 1 pound, yield about 1 cup)

1 avocado, peeled and seed removed

½ teaspoon ground cumin

Place the carrot juice, avocado, and cumin in a blender, and purée until smooth. Pour the mixture into a single soup bowl, and chill until ready to serve. You may add any of the following, as desired: chopped basil; grated zucchini, carrot, or beet; or fresh corn cut off the cob.

Stroke

See **Cardiovascular Disease.**

Tendinitis

See **Bursitis and Tendinitis.**

Tuberculosis

Tuberculosis (TB) is an infection caused by *Mycobacterium tuberculosis*. It most commonly affects the respiratory system but can spread to other areas of the body, such as the gastrointestinal and genitourinary tracts, bones, joints, nervous system, lymph nodes, spleen, and liver. TB symptoms include coughing (usually an early-morning cough) and flulike symptoms with chest pain, difficulty in breathing, coughing up blood, decreased appetite, fever, sweats that worsen at night, and weight loss. Sometimes symptoms do not appear for up to two years after the initial infection occurs.

In the United States, 20,000 new cases of TB are now reported each year, after many decades of falling infection rates. TB rates have risen as the AIDS epidemic has spread. People infected with the HIV virus, especially those who are homeless, are at greater risk of developing this disease. More international travel to areas where TB is rampant and increased immigration from these areas have also contributed to the increase in TB. Unfortunately, a form of TB that is resistant to drugs has appeared, making this disease more difficult to treat.

Diet can work miracles when it comes to healing TB. However, it is still important to follow your doctor's advice and include the following recommendations as an adjunct to your prescribed treatment.

Diet Recommendations

❥ **From 50 to 75 percent of your diet should consist of raw food.** Vegetables, fruit, juice, sprouts, seeds, nuts: it is whole, unprocessed, and largely uncooked food that will give your body the nutrients it needs to heal. Raw foods are "alive" with nutrients in their most effective state. You need adequate protein as well, such as fish, white-meat poultry, and legumes (beans, lentils, and split peas). You may benefit from unsweetened yogurt, eggs, and whole grains. Also, include plenty of garlic and onions in your meal plans. For more information, see Basic Guidelines for the Juice Lady's Health and Healing Diet (page 313).

❥ **Drink plenty of fresh juices.** You may find trying to chew plateful after plateful of raw vegetables to be exhausting and impossible. But fresh, raw juice is already broken down and easy to digest. You can drink these life-giving juices throughout the day and your digestive system will not be overtaxed, while at the same time you'll receive a concentration of nutrients. Just be sure to drink your juices at room temperature—chilled juices, or any chilled foods, are hard on weakened lungs.

Nutrient Recommendations

❥ **Antioxidants** both fight free radicals that damage cells and support the immune system. It is very important that you build your immunity by consuming the following antioxidant nutrients:

- *Selenium* plays a key role in the activity of a vital enzyme, glutathione peroxidase, that affects a wide variety of immune-system components. Best juice sources of selenium (in order of effectiveness): chard, turnips, garlic, oranges, radishes, grapes, carrots, and cabbage.

- *Vitamin A* and *beta-carotene* are vital for the development and maintenance of immune cells. The body uses beta-carotene to create vitamin A. Best juice sources of carotenes in general (in order of effectiveness): carrots, kale, parsley, spinach, chard, beet greens, watercress, mangoes, cantaloupes, apricots, broccoli, and romaine lettuce.

- *Vitamin C* and *bioflavonoids* work together to support the immune system. Vitamin C helps stimulate immune-cell activity, particularly that of the germ-eating neutrophils, and increases production of white blood cells. Bioflavonoids act against viruses and have the ability to increase levels of vitamin C within cells. Best juice sources of vitamin C (in order of effectiveness): kale, parsley, broccoli, Brussels sprouts, watercress, cauliflower, cabbage, strawberries, papaya, spinach, citrus fruit, turnips, mangoes, asparagus, and cantaloupes. Best juice sources of bioflavonoids: grapes, prunes, citrus fruit, cherries, plums, parsley, cabbage, apricots, bell peppers, cantaloupes, tomatoes, broccoli, and berries (blueberry, blackberry, and cranberry).

- *Vitamin E* is found in especially high concentrations in immune-cell membranes. This vitamin is essential for normal immune functioning, as it can help prevent the free-radical damage to immune cells that weakens the cells' ability to perform. Best juice sources of vitamin E (in order of effectiveness): spinach, watercress, asparagus, carrots, and tomatoes.

❥ **Essential fatty acids (EFAs),** especially the anti-inflammatory omega-3s, are needed for a strong immune system. I recommend flaxseed or hemp oils, which are good sources of omega-3 fatty acids, as well as such cold-water fish as salmon, tuna, trout, sardines, mackerel, and halibut. For more information, see the fats and oils section in Basic Guidelines for the Juice Lady's Health and Healing Diet (page 313).

Herb Recommendations

❥ **Echinacea** is an immune-system builder.

❥ **Elecampagne, horehound, marshmallow,** and **mullein** are expectorants and decongestants.

Juice Ingredient Recommendations

❥ **Dandelion leaf** juice contains various phytochemicals that are believed to deactivate the TB bacterium.

❥ **Fenugreek** and **alfalfa sprout** juices help heal the lungs.

❥ **Garlic** juice has antiviral properties.

❥ **Parsley** juice contains a wealth of nutrients. Intake should be limited to a safe, therapeutic dose of $^1/_2$ to 1 cup per day. Parsley can be toxic in overdose, and should be especially avoided by pregnant women.

❥ **Pear** juice can help heal the lungs.

❥ **Potato** juice is a traditional remedy for TB.

❥ **Turnips** have been used as a traditional remedy for lung diseases, especially TB. Combine with watercress and garlic for best results; see The Immune Builder Cocktail.

❥ **Wheatgrass** juice is rich in enzymes and blood-purifying chlorophyll. You must have an abundance of enzymes for your body to heal. Wheatgrass juice works best taken straight, but if you need a little help getting it down to start with, try Wheatgrass Light.

Juice Recipes

LIVER LIFE TONIC

½ organic green apple such as
   Granny Smith or Pippin, washed
1 handful dandelion greens, washed
5 carrots, scrubbed well, green tops
   removed, ends trimmed
½ small lemon, washed, or peeled if
   not organic

*Cut the apple into wedges that will fit
your juicer's feed tube. Bunch up the
dandelion greens, and push through
the feed tube with the apple, carrots,
and lemon. Stir the juice, and pour
into a glass. Serve at room
temperature.*

PURE GREEN SPROUT DRINK

1 organic cucumber, scrubbed well
1 large handful sunflower sprouts,
   rinsed
1 small handful buckwheat sprouts,
   rinsed
1 small handful fenugreek sprouts,
   rinsed
1 small handful alfalfa sprouts, rinsed

*Cut the cucumber in half lengthwise.
Bunch up the sprouts, and push
through the feed tube with the
cucumber. Stir the juice, and pour into
a glass. Serve at room temperature.*

THE IMMUNE BUILDER

1 organic Golden or Red Delicious
   apple, washed
1 turnip, scrubbed well
1 handful watercress, rinsed
   (optional)
5 carrots, scrubbed well, green tops
   removed, ends trimmed
1 large garlic clove with peel, washed

*Cut the apple and turnip into sections
that fit your juicer's feed tube. Bunch
up the watercress (if using), and push
it through the feed tube with the apple,
turnip, carrots, and garlic. Stir the
juice, and pour into a glass. Serve at
room temperature.*

THE FEEL GOOD COCKTAIL

½ pear, washed
4 medium carrots, scrubbed well,
   green tops removed, ends trimmed
3 fennel stalks with leaves and
   flowers, washed
1 stalk organic celery with leaves,
   washed

*Cut the pear into sections that fit your
juicer's feed tube, and juice along with
the carrots, fennel, and celery. Stir the
juice, and pour into a glass. Serve at
room temperature.*

THE TB CARE COCKTAIL

1 potato, well scrubbed
2–3 carrots (to make ½ cup juice)
1 teaspoon olive or almond oil
½ teaspoon honey

Juice the potato and allow the starch to settle; pour off the juice and discard the starch. Juice the carrots and combine with the potato juice. Stir in the olive or almond oil and honey, and mix well. Drink three glasses daily.

TURNIP TIME

1 turnip, scrubbed well
2-inch piece jicama, scrubbed well or peeled if not organic (optional)
1 handful watercress, rinsed
4 carrots, scrubbed well, green tops removed, ends trimmed
1 garlic clove with peel, washed
½ small or medium lemon, washed, or peeled if not organic

Cut the turnip and jicama (if using) into strips that fit your juicer's feed tube. Bunch up the watercress, and push through the feed tube with the turnip, jicama, carrots, garlic, and lemon. Stir the juice, and pour into a glass. Serve at room temperature.

WHEATGRASS LIGHT

1 organic Golden or Red Delicious apple, washed
1 small handful wheatgrass, rinsed
2–3 sprigs mint, rinsed (optional)
¼ small or medium lemon, washed, or peeled if not organic

Cut the apple into sections that fit your juicer's feed tube. Bunch up the wheatgrass and mint (if using) and push them through the feed tube with the apple and lemon. Stir the juice, and pour into a glass. Serve at room temperature.

POPEYE'S POWER

½ medium organic apple, any kind, washed
1 handful organic spinach, washed
1 small handful parsley, rinsed
4 medium carrots, scrubbed well, green tops removed, ends trimmed
1 stalk organic celery with leaves, washed
½ beet with leaves, scrubbed well

Cut the apple into sections that will fit your juicer's feed tube. Bunch up the spinach and parsley, and push them through the feed tube with the apple, carrots, celery, and beet. Stir the juice, and pour into a glass. Serve at room temperature.

THE MORNING ENERGIZER

½ organic Red or Golden Delicious apple, washed

5 medium carrots, scrubbed well, green tops removed, ends trimmed

½ small beet with leaves and stems, scrubbed well

½ small or medium lemon, washed, or peeled if not organic

½- to 1-inch piece fresh ginger root, washed

Cut the apple into sections that will fit your juicer's feed tube. Juice the apple along with the carrots, beet, lemon, and ginger. Stir the juice, and pour into a glass. Serve at room temperature.

TOMATO FLORENTINE

1 vine-ripened tomato, washed

1 handful organic spinach, washed

2–3 fresh basil leaves (optional)

½ small or medium lemon, washed, or peeled if not organic

Cut the tomato into sections that will fit your juicer's feed tube. Bunch up the spinach and basil leaves (if using), and push through the feed tube with the tomato and lemon. Stir the juice, and pour into a glass. Serve at room temperature.

SWEET DREAMS NIGHTCAP

2 romaine lettuce leaves, washed

1 handful parsley, rinsed

4 carrots, scrubbed well, green tops removed, ends trimmed

3 organic celery stalks with leaves, washed

Bunch up the lettuce leaves and parsley, and push through the feed tube with the carrots and celery. Stir the juice, and pour into a glass. Serve at room temperature.

Ulcerative Colitis

See **Colitis.**

Ulcers

A peptic ulcer is an erosion of tissue that leaves an open wound in the gastrointestinal tract. Peptic ulcers can develop anywhere in the tract, but generally are found in the stomach (gastric ulcer) or the first part of the small intestine (duodenal ulcer). Duodenal ulcers are more common and affect about 10 percent of Americans, with more men suffering from ulcers than women.

The most noticeable ulcer symptom is a chronic burning or stomach discomfort that occurs between forty-five and sixty minutes after eating, or at night. The pain is usually relieved by eating, taking antacids, drinking water, or vomiting.

Gastric or duodenal ulcers result when the protective mucus that lines the stomach and small intestine is damaged. This lining keeps stomach acids from digesting the body's own tissues. There are many elements that can increase the production of stomach acid, including stress and anxiety, taking aspirin or nonsteriodal anti-inflammatory drugs (NSAIDs) over a long period of time, steroid use, smoking, or drinking too much coffee or alcohol. Research has also found that a bacteria called *Helicobacter pylori* may be responsible for ulcers; this bacteria is almost always present in people who have them.

Diet Recommendations

❥ **Eat a high-fiber, complex-carbohydrate diet.** A high-fiber diet has been associated with a reduced rate of ulcers. A study of 47,806 men found that consumption of the fiber found in fruits, vegetables, and legumes (beans, lentils, and split peas) was associated with a reduced risk of duodenal ulcer. The researchers found that soluble fibers, such as the pectins found in fruits and vegetables (and in fruit and vegetable juices), are more strongly associated with this reduction in risk than insoluble fiber, such as bran. In fact, such fiber was associated with an *increased* ulcer risk. The researchers also found that diets which contained a lot of refined foods, such as white flour and white rice, were associated with a higher rate of duodenal ulcers. Therefore, eat only brown rice and whole-grain breads. Add plain yogurt to your diet; it has been shown to protect the stomach against irritants. For more information, see Basic Guidelines for the Juice Lady's Health and Healing Diet (page 313).

❥ **Eat small meals frequently throughout the day.** This helps reduce stress on your digestive system.

❥ **Eat more unripe bananas.** One study found that substances called protease inhibitors, which are concentrated in unripe bananas, protect against such bacterial infections as those caused by *H. pylori*. Researchers believe this may be why unripened bananas have traditionally been used in India to cure stomach ulcers.

❥ **Avoid foods that increase stomach-acid production.** These include fried foods, tea, coffee, salt, chocolate, strong spices, animal fat, and carbonated drinks. Milk also falls into this category, despite the persistent belief among some people that milk soothes the stomach.

Nutrient Recommendations

❥ **Bioflavonoids** help reduce stomach acid levels. They also counteract the production and secretion of histamine, a chemical known to stimulate the release of gastric acid. In addition, bioflavonoids help make vitamin C more effective (see the vitamin C entry on this list). Best juice sources of bioflavonoids: apricots, bell peppers, berries (blueberry, blackberry, and cranberry), broccoli, cabbage, cantaloupes, cherries, citrus fruit, grapes, parsley, plums, prunes, and tomatoes.

❥ **Vitamin A** and **carotenes** protect the mucous membranes of the stomach and intestines. Vitamin A is available in fruits and vegetables as carotenes, which are converted by the body into vitamin A as needed. Best juice sources of carotenes in general (in order of effectiveness): carrots, kale, parsley, spinach, chard, beet greens, watercress, mangoes, cantaloupes, apricots, broccoli, and romaine lettuce.

❥ **Vitamin C** promotes wound healing and protects against infections. Best juice sources of vitamin C (in order of effectiveness): kale, parsley, broccoli, Brussels sprouts, watercress, cauliflower, cabbage, strawberries, papaya, spinach, citrus fruit, turnips, mangoes, asparagus, and cantaloupes.

❥ **Vitamin E** promotes healing and aids in reducing levels of stomach acid. Best juice sources of vitamin E (in order of effectiveness): spinach, watercress, asparagus, carrots, and tomatoes.

❥ **Vitamin K** aids healing and neutralizes stomach acid. It can also help prevent bleeding. Best juice sources of vitamin K (in order of effectiveness): turnip greens, broccoli, lettuce, cabbage, spinach, watercress, asparagus, and string beans.

🌶 **Zinc** increases production of the protective substance mucin, and it may help heal ulcers. Best juice sources of zinc (in order of effectiveness): ginger root, turnips, parsley, garlic, carrots, grapes, spinach, cabbage, lettuce, cucumbers, and tangerines.

Herb Recommendations

🌶 **Aloe vera,** in a dosage of four ounces daily, helps stop ulcer bleeding and speeds the healing process. Do not use aloe bitters.

🌶 **Bilberry, calendula flower, goldenseal,** and **myrrh** all have antiulcer properties. They also inhibit the growth of *H. pylori* bacteria. Avoid goldenseal if you are pregnant, and do not use it for more than ten days at a time.

🌶 **Licorice,** in the form of deglyrrhizinated licorice (DGL), promotes healing of gastric and duodenal ulcers. DGL is available in chewable tablets from most health food stores; take between meals or twenty minutes before meals. Unlike other forms of licorice, DGL can be taken indefinitely.

Juice Ingredient Recommendations

🌶 **Alfalfa** and **wheatgrass** juices are good sources of vitamin K and blood-purifying chlorophyll. These juices prevent bleeding, aid healing, and neutralize stomach acid. Barley grass juice is another good choice.

🌶 **Cabbage** juice has been found to be very successful in treating peptic ulcers. Research has shown that drinking one quart of raw cabbage juice each day results in the healing of an ulcer within an average of three weeks. Cabbage juice contains mucinlike compounds believed by researchers to be the healing agents. Celery also contains these compounds.

🌶 **Parsley** juice is rich in beta-carotene, bioflavonoids, vitamin C, and zinc. Intake should be limited to a safe, therapeutic dose of $1/2$ to 1 cup per day. Parsley can be toxic in overdose, and should be especially avoided by pregnant women.

🌶 **Pineapple** juice contains bromelain, an enzyme that improves digestion and relieves symptoms.

🌶 **Purple grape** juice with seeds contains substances that act as anti-inflammatory agents and strengthen tissues.

Juice Recipes

PURE GREEN SPROUT DRINK

1 organic cucumber, scrubbed well

1 large handful sunflower sprouts, rinsed

1 small handful buckwheat sprouts, rinsed

1 small handful alfalfa sprouts, rinsed

Cut the cucumber in half lengthwise. Bunch up the sprouts, and push through the feed tube with the cucumber. Stir the juice, and pour into a glass. Serve at room temperature or chilled, as desired.

WHEATGRASS LIGHT

1 organic Golden or Red Delicious apple, washed

1 small handful wheatgrass, rinsed

2–3 sprigs mint, rinsed (optional)

¼ small or medium lemon, washed, or peeled if not organic

Cut the apple into sections that fit your juicer's feed tube. Bunch up the wheatgrass and mint (if using) and push them through the feed tube with the apple and lemon. Stir the juice, and pour into a glass. Serve at room temperature or chilled, as desired.

THE MORNING ENERGIZER

½ organic Red or Golden Delicious apple, washed

5 medium carrots, scrubbed well, green tops removed, ends trimmed

½ small beet with leaves and stems, scrubbed well

½ small or medium lemon, washed, or peeled if not organic

½- to 1-inch piece fresh ginger root, washed

Cut the apple into sections that will fit your juicer's feed tube. Juice the apple along with the carrots, beet, lemon, and ginger. Stir the juice, and pour into a glass. Serve at room temperature or chilled, as desired.

GRAPE EXPECTATIONS

3 plums, washed, stones removed

½ pound organic purple grapes with small stems* and seeds, washed

8 organic strawberries with caps, washed

¼ small or medium lemon, washed, or peeled if not organic

Cut the plums in half, and juice with the grapes, strawberries, and lemon. Stir the juice, and pour into a glass. Serve at room temperature or chilled, as desired.

*Large stems can dull your juicer's blade.

ANTIULCER CABBAGE EXPRESS

3–4 pounds green cabbage, washed (spring or summer cabbage is best)

1 tomato, washed or 1 orange or lemon, peeled

1 pound organic celery with leaves, washed

Cut the cabbage and tomato or fruit into sections that fit your juicer's feed tube, and juice with the celery. Stir the juice, and pour into a container. Refrigerate in the covered container, and drink throughout the day.

SWEET CALCIUM COCKTAIL

1 three-inch chunk fresh pineapple, scrubbed well or peeled if not organic

1–2 kale leaves, washed

Cut the pineapple into strips that fit your juicer's feed tube. Bunch up the kale, and push through the feed tube with the pineapple. Stir the juice, and pour into a glass. Serve at room temperature or chilled, as desired.

MAGNESIUM SPECIAL

5 medium carrots, scrubbed well, green tops removed, ends trimmed

2 stalks organic celery with leaves, washed

1/2 small beet with leaves and stems, scrubbed well

2 broccoli florets, washed

1/2 small or medium lemon, washed, or peeled if not organic

Juice the carrots, celery, beet, broccoli, and lemon. Stir the juice, and pour into a glass. Serve at room temperature or chilled, as desired.

BEAUTIFUL BONE SOLUTION

1 organic Golden or Red Delicious apple, washed

1–2 kale leaves, washed

1 handful parsley, rinsed

1 stalk organic celery, washed

1/4 small or medium lemon, washed, or peeled if not organic

1/2- to 1-inch piece fresh ginger root, washed

Cut the apple into sections that fit your juicer's feed tube. Bunch up the kale and parsley, and push through the feed tube with the apple, celery, lemon, and ginger. Stir the juice, and pour into a glass. Serve at room temperature or chilled, as desired.

POPEYE'S POWER

$\frac{1}{2}$ medium organic apple, any kind, washed

1 handful organic spinach, washed

1 small handful parsley, rinsed

4 medium carrots, scrubbed well, green tops removed, ends trimmed

1 stalk organic celery with leaves, washed

$\frac{1}{2}$ beet with leaves, scrubbed well

Cut the apple into sections that will fit your juicer's feed tube. Bunch up the spinach and parsley, and push them through the feed tube with the apple, carrots, celery, and beet. Stir the juice, and pour into a glass. Serve at room temperature or chilled, as desired.

TRIPLE C

$\frac{1}{4}$ small head green cabbage, washed

4 carrots, scrubbed well, green tops removed, and ends trimmed

4 stalks organic celery with leaves, washed

Cut the cabbage into sections that fit your juicer's feed tube. Juice the cabbage along with the carrots and celery. Stir the juice, and pour into a glass. Serve at room temperature or chilled, as desired.

STRAWBERRY-CANTALOUPE COCKTAIL

$\frac{1}{2}$ ripe organic cantaloupe with seeds, washed, or peeled if not organic

1 cup organic strawberries, washed

Cut the cantaloupe into strips that fit your juicer's feed tube. Juice the cantaloupe and strawberries; stir the juice and pour into a glass. Serve at room temperature or chilled, as desired.

DIGESTIVE TONIC

$\frac{1}{2}$ pear, washed

$\frac{1}{2}$ organic apple, any kind, washed

5 carrots, scrubbed well, green tops removed, ends trimmed

Cut the pear and apple into sections that fit your juicer's feed tube. Juice them with the carrots. Stir the juice, and pour into a glass. Serve at room temperature or chilled, as desired.

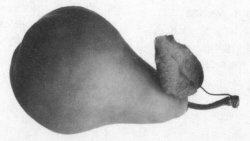

Varicose Veins and Hemorrhoids

Veins, unlike the more muscular arteries, contain valves that help keep blood flowing smoothly back to the heart. Defects in the vein walls lead to dilation of the veins and damage to the valves, which causes blood to pool in the veins. The veins then bulge, becoming widened, distended, and sometimes twisted—a condition referred to as varicose veins. This condition may be without symptoms, or it may be associated with aching tender or sore legs, feelings of heaviness, or pain in the legs (where most varicose veins form). Fluid retention, discoloration, and ulceration of the skin can develop.

If the affected veins are near the surface, they pose very little danger. However, this condition can be more serious if it involves obstruction and valve defects of the deeper veins of the legs. This type of varicose vein can lead to thrombophlebitis, an inflammation of the veins that in turn can lead to blood-clot development. Varicose veins are caused by a variety of factors, including a low-fiber diet and standing for long periods of time. This condition affects about half of all middle-aged adults.

Hemorrhoids are a type of varicose vein that occurs in the anus or rectum. Symptoms may include pain, rectal itching or bleeding, and blood in the stool. Hemorrhoids are usually caused by a low-fiber diet, constipation (*see* **Constipation**), or liver dysfunction.

Diet Recommendations

❥ **Eat a high-fiber, low-fat diet.** A high-fiber diet is the most important component in the treatment and prevention of varicose veins and hemorrhoids. At least 50 percent of your diet should consist of raw foods—fruits, vegetables, juices, sprouts, seeds, and nuts. Eating more fiber and less fat will help you maintain a healthy weight. This is another important consideration, since being overweight can contribute to varicose vein and hemorrhoid development. For more information, see Basic Guidelines for the Juice Lady's Health and Healing Diet (page 313).

❥ **Eat more ginger, garlic, and onions.** People with varicose veins have a decreased ability to break down the fibrin surrounding the affected vein. These foods help break down fibrin.

Nutrient Recommendations

❥ **Essential fatty acids (EFAs)** can be helpful in maintaining blood-vessel health. Take one tablespoon of unrefined flaxseed or hemp oil daily. For more information, see the fats and oils section in Basic Guidelines for the Juice Lady's Health and Healing Diet (page 313).

❥ **Vitamin C** and **bioflavonoids** work together to strengthen blood vessels. Best juice sources of vitamin C (in order of effectiveness): kale, parsley, broccoli, Brussels sprouts, watercress, cauliflower, cabbage, strawberries, papaya, spinach, citrus fruit, turnips, mangoes, asparagus, and cantaloupes. Best juice sources of bioflavonoids: apricots, bell peppers, berries (blueberry, blackberry, and cranberry), broccoli, cabbage, cantaloupes, cherries, citrus fruit, grapes, parsley, plums, prunes, and tomatoes.

❥ **Vitamin E** improves circulation and helps prevent the typical heavy feeling in the legs associated with varicose veins. Best juice sources of vitamin E (in order of effectiveness): spinach, watercress, asparagus, carrots, and tomatoes.

❥ **Vitamin K** is helpful for bleeding hemorrhoids. Best juice sources of vitamin K (in order of effectiveness): turnip greens, broccoli, lettuce, cabbage, spinach, watercress, asparagus, and string beans.

❥ **Zinc** is an anti-inflammatory that aids healing. Best juice sources of zinc (in order of effectiveness): ginger root, turnips, parsley, garlic, carrots, grapes, spinach, cabbage, lettuce, cucumbers, and tangerines.

Herb Recommendations

❥ **Gotu kola** helps strengthen tissue structure around frail veins and also improves blood flow.

❥ **Horse chestnut** has been used effectively for treating varicose veins as a poultice contained in compression stockings. (To learn how to use a poultice, see an herbalist.)

Juice Ingredient Recommendations

❥ **Blackberry, blueberry, cherry,** and **raspberry** juices contain anthocyanidins and proanthocyanidins, pigments that help strengthen vein walls and increase the muscular tone of the veins.

❥ **Garlic** and **ginger** juices help break down fibrin.

❥ **Parsley** juice is an important source of several nutrients, including bioflavonoids, vitamin C, and zinc. Intake should be limited to a safe, therapeutic dose of $^1/_2$ to 1 cup per day. Parsley can be toxic in overdose, and should be especially avoided by pregnant women.

 Pineapple juice contains the enzyme bromelain, which promotes fibrin breakdown. Bromelain can also help prevent the formation of the hard, lumpy skin that forms around varicose veins.

 Purple grapes are actually beneficial because of compounds in their seeds, which improve the support structure of vein walls.

Juice Recipes

CHERRY JUBILEE

1 three-inch chunk fresh pineapple, scrubbed well or peeled if not organic

½ organic Golden or Red Delicious apple, washed

6–8 organic Bing cherries, washed, pits removed

Cut the pineapple into strips, and the apple into sections, that fit your juicer's feed tube, and juice them with the cherries. Stir the juice, and pour it into a glass. Serve at room temperature or chilled, as desired.

ANTIAGING COCKTAIL

1 small bunch organic purple grapes (about 1 cup) with small stems* and seeds, washed

½ cup blueberries, blackberries, or raspberries, washed

¼ small or medium lemon, washed, or peeled if not organic

½-inch piece fresh ginger root, washed

*Large stems can dull your juicer's blade.

Juice the grapes, berries, lemon, and ginger. Stir the juice, and pour into a glass. Serve at room temperature or chilled, as desired.

THE IMMUNE BUILDER

1 organic Golden or Red Delicious apple, washed

1 turnip, scrubbed well

1 handful watercress, rinsed (optional)

5 carrots, scrubbed well, green tops removed, ends trimmed

1 large garlic clove with peel, washed

Cut the apple and turnip into sections that fit your juicer's feed tube. Bunch up the watercress (if using), and push it through the feed tube with the apple, turnip, carrots, and garlic. Stir the juice, and pour into a glass. Serve at room temperature or chilled, as desired.

THE GINGER HOPPER

½ organic Red or Golden Delicious apple, washed

5 medium carrots, scrubbed well, green tops removed, ends trimmed

½- to 1-inch piece fresh ginger root, washed

Cut the apple into sections, and juice along with the carrots and ginger. Stir the juice, and pour into a glass. Serve at room temperature or chilled, as desired.

SWEET CALCIUM COCKTAIL

1 three-inch chunk fresh pineapple, scrubbed well or peeled if not organic

1–2 kale leaves, washed

Cut the pineapple into strips that fit your juicer's feed tube. Bunch up the kale, and push through the feed tube with the pineapple. Stir the juice, and pour into a glass. Serve at room temperature or chilled, as desired.

SPRING TONIC

1 medium vine-ripened tomato, washed

1 organic cucumber, scrubbed well

8 asparagus stems, washed

½ small or medium lemon, washed, or peeled if not organic

Cut the tomato into sections that fit your juicer's feed tube. Cut the cucumber in half lengthwise. Juice the tomato, cucumber, asparagus, and lemon. Stir the juice, and pour into a glass. Serve at room temperature or chilled, as desired.

PINK PASSION POTION

1 organic Red Delicious apple, washed

½ cup fresh or frozen (thawed) cranberries, rinsed

1 bunch organic purple grapes, with seeds and small stems,* washed

⅛ small beet (no stems or leaves) for color, scrubbed well (optional)

¼ small or medium lemon, washed, or peeled if not organic

*Large stems can dull your juicer's blade.

Cut the apple into sections that fit your juicer's feed tube. Juice the apple, cranberries, grapes, beet (if using), and lemon. (To prevent the cranberries from flying out of the machine while juicing, place the cranberries in the juicer first, place an apple section on top of them, and cover with the plunger. Turn on the machine, and push the plunger to begin the juicing process.) Stir the juice, and pour into a glass. Serve at room temperature or chilled, as desired.

POPEYE'S POWER

½ medium organic apple, any kind, washed

1 handful organic spinach, washed

1 small handful parsley, rinsed

4 medium carrots, scrubbed well, green tops removed, ends trimmed

1 stalk organic celery with leaves, washed

½ beet with leaves, scrubbed well

Cut the apple into sections that will fit your juicer's feed tube. Bunch up the spinach and parsley, and push them through the feed tube with the apple, carrots, celery, and beet. Stir the juice, and pour into a glass. Serve at room temperature or chilled, as desired.

BEAUTIFUL BONE SOLUTION

1 organic Golden or Red Delicious apple, washed

1–2 kale leaves, washed

1 handful parsley, rinsed

1 stalk organic celery, washed

¼ small or medium lemon, washed, or peeled if not organic

½- to 1-inch piece fresh ginger root, washed

Cut the apple into sections that fit your juicer's feed tube. Bunch up the kale and parsley, and push through the feed tube with the apple, celery, lemon, and ginger. Stir the juice, and pour into a glass. Serve at room temperature or chilled, as desired.

MAGNESIUM SPECIAL

5 medium carrots, scrubbed well, green tops removed, ends trimmed

2 stalks organic celery with leaves, washed

½ small beet with leaves and stems, scrubbed well

2 broccoli florets, washed

½ small or medium lemon, washed, or peeled if not organic

Juice the carrots, celery, beet, broccoli, and lemon. Stir the juice, and pour into a glass. Serve at room temperature or chilled, as desired.

RASPBERRY SUNRISE

1 orange, peeled

1 cup raspberries, washed

Divide the orange into segments that fit your juicer's feed tube, and juice it with the raspberries. Stir the juice, and pour it into a glass. Serve at room temperature or chilled, as desired.

Water Retention

Water retention, also known as edema, is an abnormal accumulation of fluid in the spaces between the cells or within body cavities. Fluid is always moving in and out of cells, between cells and tissue spaces, and between the blood and the tissues. The force of blood pressure tends to push water out of the blood and into tissue spaces, and to pull water into the blood from the tissues. Normally, there is a dynamic balance between the "push and pull" forces, but when an imbalance occurs, edema is the result.

Water retention can be confined to a localized area, such as the lower legs and ankles, or generalized, affecting the whole body. Localized water retention in the lower extremities is often the result of poor venous return. This means the blood is pumped by the heart to the extremities, but the body does not do an efficient job of moving it from the extremities back to the heart.

There are many possible causes of water retention. Some are serious, such as congestive heart failure, and some are lifestyle-related, such as standing or sitting all day. A factor that contributes to edema is poor capillary structure, known as poor vascular integrity. If the walls of the capillaries are not strong and resilient, they become more permeable. This makes it easier to push water out of the blood into tissue spaces. One sign of poor vascular integrity is easy bruising (*see* **Bruises**).

Diet Recommendations

❥ **Drink plenty of water.** Although it might seem counterproductive, drinking plenty of water helps reduce water retention. The reason has to do with your body's response to water retention. As water is lost from your blood into the tissue spaces, the nonwater parts of your blood (cells, minerals, protein) become more concentrated. This signals your body to hold onto the water it has, so that your blood can maintain proper dilution. Your body does this by changing the way your kidneys filter your blood so that less water is released into the urine. Drinking plenty of water will help keep your body from concentrating urine and retaining more water.

❥ **Eat adequate protein.** Protein deficiency is a known cause of edema. Plasma osmotic pressure is one of the forces that pulls water from tissues back into the blood, and is directly related to the amount of protein in the blood. This means you should eat high-quality, low-fat protein, such as fish, skinless chicken, and combinations of grains and legumes. However, if the edema is caused by kidney problems, it is *not* advisable to increase your protein intake. If you have edema, consult with your doctor before eating more protein. The Kidney Cleanse (page 328) may be helpful.

❥ **Choose plenty of those foods and juices that support your liver.** The liver plays an important role in regulating the protein content of your blood. Foods that support liver function can be helpful in dealing with many conditions, including water retention. "Liver foods," such as beets and artichokes, can help the liver function at its best. Other "liver friends" include peas, parsnips, potatoes, pumpkin, sweet potatoes, squash, yams, beans (green and yellow), broccoli, Brussels sprouts, cabbage, carrots, cauliflower, celery, chives, cucumber, eggplant, garlic, kale, kohlrabi, okra, onion, and parsley. Bitter greens and herbs, such as mustard greens and dandelion leaves, are especially helpful in stimulating the liver. For more information, see the Liver Cleanse (page 333).

❥ **Eat and juice your vegetables.** Also eat and juice fruit, but in smaller quantities. Fruits and vegetables contain a lot of water. In addition, they contain a lot of bioflavonoids and vitamin C, substances that help improve tissue integrity and can help reduce the tendency of capillaries to leak fluid into the surrounding tissue spaces. Fruits and vegetables that have the most bioflavonoids are those that are brightly or darkly colored orange, yellow, red, purple, blue, or dark green. Berries and cherries are especially high in bioflavonoids, and blueberries are particularly good for maintaining blood-vessel integrity. Eat fruit and use fruit juice sparingly, however, to avoid consuming too much fruit sugar. Use fruit primarily as a flavoring for vegetable juices, or dilute it by half with water.

❥ **Avoid sweets.** In Chinese medicine, water retention is considered a "damp" condition. Foods that are cold, sweet, or mucus-forming contribute to this dampness, and should be avoided in excess. Foods that combine one or more of these qualities, such as ice cream—cold, sweet, and mucus-forming—are the worst for damp conditions, and should be avoided. Foods that are thought to "dry up" damp conditions are celery, lettuce, pumpkin, scallions, turnips, corn, and legumes (beans, lentils, split peas). Bitter herbs and salad greens are also helpful.

❥ **Use salt sparingly.** High levels of sodium in the body will cause the body to retain water in order to dilute the sodium. This is why low-sodium diets are often prescribed for people who have water retention problems or high blood pressure.

Nutrient Recommendations

❧ **Vitamin B$_6$ (pyridoxine)** may help ease water retention by acting against sodium retention. Best juice sources of vitamin B$_6$ (in order of effectiveness): kale, spinach, turnip greens, bell peppers, and prunes.

❧ **Vitamin E** can help maintain blood-vessel integrity, which helps to keep fluid from leaking out of the blood vessels. Best juice sources of vitamin E (in order of effectiveness): spinach, watercress, asparagus, carrots, and tomatoes.

Herb Recommendations

❧ **Burdock** and **yellow dock** stimulate liver function. Burdock is also mildly diuretic, that is, it helps remove water from the body.

❧ **Corn silk** is a good diuretic.

Juice Ingredient Recommendations

❧ **Asparagus** juice, a diuretic, helps cleanse the kidneys.

❧ **Cantaloupe (with the seeds), cucumber, lemon, parsley,** and **watermelon** juices are all diuretics. Parsley juice intake should be limited to a safe, therapeutic dose of $1/2$ to 1 cup per day. Parsley can be toxic in overdose, and should be especially avoided by pregnant women.

❧ **Dandelion leaf** juice helps fight water retention.

Juice Recipes

KIDNEY TONIC

1 organic cucumber, scrubbed well

8 asparagus stems, washed

5 medium carrots, scrubbed well, green tops removed, ends trimmed

$1/2$ small beet with leaves and stems, scrubbed well

$1/2$ small or medium lemon, washed, or peeled if not organic

Cut the cucumber in half lengthwise, and juice it with the asparagus, carrots, beet, and lemon. Stir the juice, and pour it into a glass. Serve at room temperature or chilled, as desired.

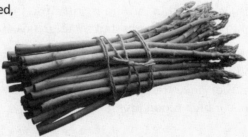

STRAWBERRY-CANTALOUPE COCKTAIL

½ ripe organic cantaloupe with seeds, washed, or peeled if not organic

1 cup organic strawberries, washed

Cut the cantaloupe into strips that fit your juicer's feed tube. Juice the cantaloupe and strawberries; stir the juice and pour into a glass. Serve at room temperature or chilled, as desired.

WATERMELON REFRESHER

1-inch slice watermelon, with seeds and well-scrubbed rind

Cut the watermelon into strips that fit your juicer's feed tube. Juice the watermelon, and pour into a glass. Serve at room temperature or chilled, as desired.

AFTERNOON REFRESHER

1 medium to large organic cucumber, scrubbed well

½ small or medium lemon, washed, or peeled if not organic

Cut the cucumber in half lengthwise, and juice with the lemon. (For an especially cooling version, let the juice splash over a few ice cubes in the juice pitcher.) Stir the juice, and pour into a glass. Serve at room temperature or chilled, as desired.

LIVER LIFE TONIC

½ organic green apple such as Granny Smith or Pippin, washed

1 handful dandelion greens, washed

5 carrots, scrubbed well, green tops removed, ends trimmed

½ small lemon, washed, or peeled if not organic

Cut the apple into wedges that will fit your juicer's feed tube. Bunch up the dandelion greens, and push through the feed tube with the apple, carrots, and lemon. Stir the juice, and pour into a glass. Serve at room temperature or chilled, as desired.

TRIPLE C

¼ small head green cabbage, washed

4 carrots, scrubbed well, green tops removed, and ends trimmed

4 stalks organic celery with leaves, washed

Cut the cabbage into sections that fit your juicer's feed tube. Juice the cabbage along with the carrots and celery. Stir the juice, and pour into a glass. Serve at room temperature or chilled, as desired.

PARSLEY PEP

1 small bunch parsley, rinsed

2 stalks organic celery with leaves, washed

2 large carrots, scrubbed well, green tops removed, ends trimmed

1/2 small or medium lemon, washed, or peeled if not organic

Bunch up the parsley, and push it through the feed tube with the celery, carrots, and lemon. Stir the juice, and pour it into a glass. Serve at room temperature or chilled, as desired.

BEAUTIFUL BONE SOLUTION

1 organic Golden or Red Delicious apple, washed

1–2 kale leaves, washed

1 handful parsley, rinsed

1 stalk organic celery, washed

1/4 small or medium lemon, washed, or peeled if not organic

1/2- to 1-inch piece fresh ginger root, washed

Cut the apple into sections that fit your juicer's feed tube. Bunch up the kale and parsley, and push through the feed tube with the apple, celery, lemon, and ginger. Stir the juice, and pour into a glass. Serve at room temperature or chilled, as desired.

TOMATO FLORENTINE

1 vine-ripened tomato, washed

1 handful organic spinach, washed

2–3 fresh basil leaves (optional)

1/2 small or medium lemon, washed, or peeled if not organic

Cut the tomato into sections that will fit your juicer's feed tube. Bunch up the spinach and basil leaves (if using), and push through the feed tube with the tomato and lemon. Stir the juice, and pour into a glass. Serve at room temperature or chilled, as desired.

THE GINGER HOPPER

1/2 organic Red or Golden Delicious apple, washed

5 medium carrots, scrubbed well, green tops removed, ends trimmed

1/2- to 1-inch piece fresh ginger root, washed

Cut the apple into sections, and juice along with the carrots and ginger. Stir the juice, and pour into a glass. Serve at room temperature or chilled, as desired.

Yeast Infections

See **Candidiasis.**

Basic Guidelines for the Juice Lady's Health and Healing Diet

Juicing can help you achieve and maintain optimal health, but it works best when used as part of an overall diet plan. In this section, I'll first explain the three most important principles of my health and healing diet. I will then provide daily servings and food recommendations for each of the major food groups before giving a sample menu based on those recommendations.

THE PRINCIPLES BEHIND THE HEALTH AND HEALING DIET

I believe that whole, fresh, low-fat foods—preferably raw foods—are the foundation of a healthy diet, while fast and prepared foods are to be avoided.

Eat a High-Fiber, Low-Fat, Whole-Foods Diet

Complex carbohydrates—vegetables, whole grains, and legumes—should compose the largest portion of your food intake, about 55 to 70 percent. This percentage can include a limited amount of the simple carbohydrates (sugars) found in fruit, but don't overdo the fruit, especially if you have a disorder that requires tight control of blood-sugar levels. Protein should make up between 15 and 20 percent of your diet, and fat should account for the remaining 15 to 25 percent. Although eating enough protein is important to overall health, there is evidence that too much protein can contribute to reduced immune function. Too much of the wrong types of fat (saturated and processed fats, such as margarine and hydrogenated oils) reduce immune-cell activity. The typical Western diet falls short on the essential fatty acids (EFAs) found in cold-water fish and in certain unrefined seed and vegetable oils (see page 316).

Avoid Fast and Prepared Foods

Most commercial foods are loaded with salt, preservatives, and additives. Too much salt causes sodium to be drawn into cells and potassium to be pulled out. That creates an imbalance in which cells are unable to absorb what they need or excrete wastes and unwanted materials efficiently. Consequently, they cease to effectively carry out vital metabolic processes. Toxic wastes build up inside the cells and sludge accumulates outside. The symptoms of this "clogging up" and slowing down at the cellular level are fatigue, poor immune function, and ultimately disease. Preservatives and additives add to this toxic load.

Drink Fresh Juice and Eat More Raw Foods

Eat more of your carbohydrates as raw fruits, vegetables, fresh juice, sprouts, seeds, and nuts if you want to enjoy high-level health. Raw foods, especially if they are organically grown, contain an abundance of nutrients in peak condition, particularly the health-promoting enzymes and phytonutrients (along with valuable vitamins and minerals). These nutrients are created through photosynthesis, a process made possible by chlorophyll—the material that makes plants green. In photosynthesis, the plant combines carbon dioxide from the air with water from the soil by using light energy from the sun. This energy is what gives raw foods their nutritional value, especially the nutrition found in raw enzymes. As I explained on page 9, enzymes are lost in cooking, and enzyme deficiencies can hinder the chemical reactions necessary for optimal health. The nutrients in raw foods haven't been degraded by sitting in a can for six months, nor have they been adulterated by food additives (some of which have themselves been associated with various health problems). And what's more, raw foods taste delicious. Nothing compares with the tangy sweetness of a red bell pepper or a ripe tart apple.

To move to a state of vibrant health and energy, nutritional experts recommend that you make 50 to 75 percent of your diet raw food. This percentage may seem staggeringly high until you consider that juicing, which is fast and easy, can make up half of that amount. Juicing enables you to quickly consume a lot of vegetables and fruits in a glass. You may not reach the 75-percent goal (I hope you will), but whatever steps you make in that direction are good.

THE DIET GUIDELINES

Below you will find a list of the food categories that make up the Juice Lady's Health and Healing Diet, which are based on the government's food-pyramid recommendations—for example, Bread, Cereal, Rice, Pasta. For all categories, I recommend organically grown food (see page 14). I have specified those foods that are recommended for this diet, and those foods that should be avoided.

Bread, Cereal, Rice, Pasta (6–11 servings per day)

For this group, a single serving is 2 slices of bread; $^1/_2$ cup dense cereal (hot or cold); 1 cup cooked pasta; $^3/_4$ cup cooked rice.

Recommended Foods: All organically grown whole grains, such as rye, millet, buckwheat, whole wheat, cornmeal, oats, brown rice; wheat germ, bran. Whole-grain pasta and noodles. Best bread choice: sprouted whole-grain bread baked at a very low temperature; these breads can be found at most health food stores and must be refrigerated at all times. Snacks: air-popped popcorn, whole-grain crackers without added sugar or preservatives, baked whole grain chips.

Foods to Avoid: White breads and crackers, refined flour pasta and noodles, white rice, refined and sugared cereals, potato chips, fried corn chips, fried potatoes, buttered/commercial popcorn, cakes, cookies, donuts, commercial muffins (high in sugar and fat).

Vegetables (a minimum of 3–5 servings per day)

For this group, a single serving is 1 cup lettuce or other leafy greens; $^1/_2$ cup cooked vegetables; 1 cup vegetable juice.

Recommended Foods: All organically grown, fresh, raw or lightly cooked vegetables. Steamed or baked potatoes, new red potatoes, sweet potatoes, yams; baked squash. All vegetable juices.

Foods to Avoid: Canned vegetables, fried vegetables, canned or bottled vegetable juices. Frozen vegetables should be used only if fresh produce is not available.

Fruits (2–4 servings per day)

For this group, a single serving is 1 medium whole fruit; $^1/_2$ cup chopped fruit; 1 cup fruit juice.

Recommended Foods: All fresh, raw, organically grown fruits and fruit juices.

Foods to Avoid: All canned fruits, and canned, bottled, or frozen juices. Frozen fruit should be used only if fresh produce is not available.

Meat, Poultry, Fish, Beans, Eggs, Nuts, and Seeds (2–3 servings per day)

For this group, a single serving is 4 ounces cooked meat, poultry, or fish; $1/2$ cup dried beans or peas; 1 egg; 2 tablespoons nut butter; $1/4$ cup nuts or seeds.

Recommended Foods: Eggs and skinless poultry (free-range and organically fed); lean meat; all fish and seafood, but especially fatty cold-water fish for their omega-3 fatty acids (see next page). All beans, lentils, and split peas, especially sprouted legumes such as bean and lentil sprouts. All soy products, such as tofu and tempeh. All nuts (almonds, walnuts, and hazelnuts are best), nut butters, seeds, and seed butters, especially sprouted seeds such as sunflower.

Foods to Avoid: Luncheon or canned meats, hot dogs, bacon, sausage, organ meat (which contains more toxins than muscle meat), fatty meat, char-broiled meat, fried chicken and red meat, poultry skin, all deep-fried products. All meat and poultry raised with hormones, antibiotics, and other drugs. Peanut butter with added oil and sugar. Nuts roasted in oil and/or salted. Refried beans with lard.

Milk, Yogurt, Cheese (2–3 servings; optional)

For this group, a single serving is 1 cup milk; 1 ounce cheese; $1/2$ cup cottage cheese; 1 cup yogurt.

Recommended Foods: Organic dairy products and dairy alternatives. Growing numbers of people are allergic to or intolerant of dairy products. Dairy also tends to be quite mucus-forming. You can also obtain calcium from such dark leafy greens as kale (very calcium rich); corn tortillas with lime added; soy products; seeds, especially sunflower and sesame; and nuts, especially almonds. For milk, you can substitute fortified soy milk (especially good for women due to the protective activity of phytoestrogens), rice milk, or almond milk. Substitute soy cheese for dairy cheese. If you choose to eat dairy products, choose low-fat milk, cheese, and plain yogurt.

Foods to Avoid: Cheese with yellow dye (choose brands that are all natural), whole milk, sweetened yogurt, ice cream, sour cream.

Fats and Oils (recommended servings not yet determined)

For this group, a single serving is 1 tablespoon butter or oil; 2 tablespoons salad dressing.

Recommended Foods: Americans eat too much saturated fat and not enough essential fatty acids (EFAs). There are a number of oils rich in EFAs, which come in two types, omega-3 and omega-6 fatty acids. Hemp oil contains a good balance of omega-3 and omega-6 fatty acids, as well as gamma-linolenic acid (GLA). Soybean oil contains omega-3s and -6s. Flaxseed oil is rich in omega-3 fatty acids. A mixture of flaxseed oil and sesame or sunflower oil will offer a balance of omega-3 and omega-6 fatty acids. Extra virgin olive oil is good for other reasons, but contains smaller amounts of omega-3; it can be mixed with hemp or flaxseed oil, in equal parts, to improve the essential fatty acid balance. You can take one to two tablespoons per day of an EFA-rich oil, such as unrefined hemp or flaxseed oil, as a supplement; mix hemp or flaxseed oil with juice, or "chase" it with juice. You may also prepare dishes with any of the oils mentioned. Purchase only pure, unrefined, organic oils (they can be found at health food stores). For delicious recipes using flaxseed oil, get a copy of the book *Flax for Life* (see Appendix A).

Some fish oils are associated with clean arteries and freedom from fatty degeneration. The health secrets of these oils involve two omega-3 fatty acids: eicosapentaenoic acid (EPA) and docosahexaenoic acid (DHA). Essential fatty acids in flaxseed, hemp, and several other oils provide the raw materials that allow our bodies to manufacture EPA and DHA. The richest sources of EPA and DHA themselves are fatty cold-water fish, such as salmon, herring, sardines, trout, halibut, cod, and mackerel. Oils from these fishes are available in supplement form.

Foods to Avoid: Margarine, shortening, and partially hydrogenated oils (they contain *trans*-fatty acids); fried and deep-fried oils and refined commercial oils contain toxic fatty acid derivatives. *Trans*-fatty acids and altered fatty acid derivatives can have adverse effects on cell membranes and brain development in infants, and can damage the cardiovascular system, liver, and immune system. Avoid any oils not specifically mentioned in the recommended foods section.

Miscellaneous

Foods that do not fall into any of the previous categories; no recommended servings.

Recommended Foods: Herbal teas, green tea, garlic, ginger, herbal seasonings.

Foods to Avoid: Coffee, soft drinks, fruit drinks, powdered drinks, alcohol, sweets, salt, anything with aspartame, preservatives, dyes, additives, fake fat. All food produced with pesticides and/or herbicides (plants) and antibiotics and/or growth hormones (animals).

A SAMPLE MENU

To see how you can put the diet guidelines to work in your everyday life, take a look at this sample menu.

Breakfast

Juice, such as The Morning Energizer (page 23) or Morning Sunrise (page 184), and/or toasted sprouted grain bread with nut butter (all-natural almond or cashew butter is the best choice) or muesli (there's a recipe in *The Healthy Gourmet,* Appendix A) or smoothie with protein powder, such as Mango Mon (page 130) or The Calcium Champ (page 223).

Midmorning Energy Snack

Juice, such as Cherry Jubilee (page 237) or The Ginger Hopper (page 32), with vegetable sticks and/or $^{1}/_{4}$ cup raw nuts or seeds

Lunch

Green leafy salad with tuna and/or Cherie's Quick Energy Soup (page 264) and sprouted grain bread

Midafternoon Energy Break

Juice, such as Santa Fe Salsa Cocktail (page 68) or Afternoon Refresher (page 75), or smoothie, such as Tropical Suprise (page 196)

Dinner

Main course salads, such as Chicken Curry Salad or Multigrain Salad Florentine (see "Two Main Course Salads" on the next page), since main course salads incorporate lots of green leafy vegetables with small amounts of either animal protein or grains and legumes, and a cup of soup or baked squash or sweet potato; or a stir-fry with lots of vegetables and chicken, meat, or seafood, and brown rice

Evening Snack

Fresh fruit or juice, such as Sweet Dreams Nightcap (page 28)

Two Main Course Salads

A main course salad makes a great dinner: fast, healthy, delicious. What you can put in a main course salad is only limited by your tastes and imagination, but should always include a variety of natural, nutrient-packed ingredients. Here's a couple of ideas to help you get started; they are adapted from my cookbook, *The Healthy Gourmet* (New York: Clarkson Potter, 1996).

MULTIGRAIN SALAD FLORENTINE

4 SERVINGS

1 cup cooked quinoa (optional)*
1 cup cooked spelt berries (optional)*
$\frac{1}{2}$ cup cooked brown rice
2 medium carrots, scrubbed and grated
1 bunch fresh spinach, washed, drained, and torn into bite-size pieces
$\frac{1}{2}$ cup chopped toasted pecans (optional)

Dressing
1 lemon, juice and zest
2–3 tablespoons extra-virgin olive oil
2 tablespoons finely chopped fresh basil, or 2 teaspoons dried
1 large garlic clove, pressed
1 teaspoon honey
Pinch cayenne pepper
Pinch sea salt (optional)

*Quinoa and spelt are two delicious grains available at health food stores. If you do not use them, increase the amount of brown rice used to 1 cup.

1. In a large salad bowl, combine the quinoa and spelt (if using), brown rice, and carrots.

2. In a small bowl, whisk together all of the dressing ingredients.

3. Pour the dressing over the grain mixture, and combine well.

4. Just before serving, toss in the spinach, mixing gently. Sprinkle with toasted pecans, if using.

CHICKEN CURRY SALAD

4 SERVINGS

2 cups cooked skinless chicken, cut into bite-sized pieces

4 cups romaine or green leaf lettuce, washed, dried, and torn into bite-sized pieces

1 cup baby field greens (or any other greens as desired), washed and dried

1 cup chopped cilantro

½ cup chopped red onion

½ cup chopped green onion

½ cup alfalfa sprouts (optional)

Lemon Curry Dressing

3 tablespoons extra-virgin olive oil

3 tablespoons fresh lemon juice

3 tablespoons reduced-fat mayonnaise

2 teaspoons honey

1–2 teaspoons curry powder

2 tablespoons chopped fresh basil, or 1–2 teaspoons dried

¼ teaspoon sea salt (optional)

1. In a small bowl, whisk together the dressing ingredients, and set aside three-quarters of the dressing. Add the chicken, and toss to coat. Chill until ready to serve.

2. In a large bowl, combine the remaining salad ingredients. Just before serving add the chicken and remaining dressing, toss to mix, and serve immediately.

The Elimination Diet

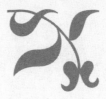

Many physicians believe that the "oral food challenge," in which potential food allergens are first eliminated from the diet and then gradually reintroduced, is the best way to identify food allergies. The Elimination Diet is designed to do just that. For the first seven days (the cleansing period), eat only the foods listed in this diet. (Read labels carefully to eliminate all other foods.) If your symptoms are related to food sensitivity, they will typically disappear by the end of the week. If they do not disappear, it is possible that a reaction to a food in the elimination diet is responsible. In that case, go to an even more restricted diet—lamb or sweet potato is usually at fault. After the elimination-diet period, you may introduce one food every two days. A detailed record should be kept as to when the food was introduced and what symptoms appeared after it was eaten. Keep in mind that some reactions are delayed up to forty-eight hours.

FOODS THAT CAN BE EATEN DURING THE ELIMINATION DIET

- **Allowed Beverage:** water

- **Allowed Cereal and Grains:** brown rice cereals, such as cream of brown rice. Bread made with rice flour. Rice cakes.

- **Allowed Condiments:** sea salt and white vinegar

- **Allowed Fats:** Willow Run margarine (found at many health food stores) and olive oil

- **Allowed Fruit and Juices:** apricots, cranberries, peaches, pears, prunes (all should be fresh, not bottled or canned)

- **Allowed Meat:** lamb

❧ **Allowed Vegetables:** sweet potatoes (boiled or baked), beets and beet greens (fresh), spinach (fresh). Vegetables can be steamed and seasoned with allowed condiments and fats.

SAMPLE ELIMINATION DIET MENU

Breakfast

Apricot, pear, or prune juice

Stewed prunes or pear sauce

Brown rice cereal
with juice substituted for milk

Rice bread, toasted

Willow Run margarine

Lunch

Pear juice

Baked sweet potato

Beet (with greens)

Broiled lamb chop

Rice cake

Peach

Dinner

Spinach salad with approved condiments

Baked sweet potato

Brown rice

Lamb roast

Pear

The Cleansing Programs

Just like a home needs a thorough "spring cleaning" occasionally, the interior of your own physical house also needs a thorough cleansing if you want to achieve optimum health. The body was made to handle an occasional toxic substance, such as spoiled food, but not the kind of abuse we give ourselves and are forced to encounter as a result of environmental toxins. We are continually tempted to eat a host of unhealthy substances, such as fried foods, high-fat snacks, refined foods, fake foods, and foods with preservatives and dyes. We are bombarded with pesticides, herbicides, chemical fertilizers, and other noxious chemicals in our air, soil, and water. All these substances serve to weaken and congest the body.

Toxic and congestive substances can overwhelm the organs of elimination and can build up within the body's tissues. Substances that are not broken down and excreted are generally stored in the intestines, gallbladder, kidneys, liver, and skin. Therefore, cleansing these organs periodically helps promote health and healing. I've learned through personal experience this can only happen through specific plans designed to promote "housecleaning" in each specific organ.

Detoxifying the body is worth the effort because the benefits are astounding. You will look more vibrant—wrinkles will diminish, skin color will improve, dark circles under the eyes will eventually disappear, and hair and nails will grow better. Best of all, you will enjoy health and vitality. You will feel more energetic, and have greater mental clarity and a higher sense of well-being. If you have ailments, you will give your body a much greater opportunity to heal them.

Organically grown, freshly made fruit and vegetable juices will help you no matter what else you do, but if your organs of elimination are congested, you won't get the best results for all your juicing efforts. It is a bit like continuing to wax a linoleum floor that has a buildup of old wax and dirt. You will never achieve the clean, shiny floor you want until you strip off the old gunk first. Just like the floor, we all need to get rid of the "old gunk" that builds up in our bodies.

What follows is the basic juice fast as a starting point for all internal cleansing, plus programs I've used personally to purify the kidneys, gallbladder, intestines, liver, and skin. (I recommend using the Kidney Cleanse before using any of the other cleansing programs; all the programs cause toxins to be released from the body, and the kidneys will have an easier time of it if they are working at full efficiency.) These programs work. I urge you to use them periodically because this is one of the most important steps you can take toward improved health and toward getting the full benefit of your juicing for health and healing program.

THE JUICE FAST

Every year my husband and I make our annual pilgrimage to The Optimum Health Institute (OHI) of San Diego. We have been going there since 1991 for the cleansing benefits of their one-week raw food and juice fasting program, what we call our "tune-up." We lose weight. Facial lines fade—we both swear the program wipes away at least five years from our faces. We always leave feeling renewed. But most importantly, we will never know the diseases that these total body cleansing weeks help us prevent.

No one has been able to explain why drinking only fresh juices for a period of several days works such a miracle, but "miracle" is the right word. Wrinkles soften, the body firms, and the skin and hair look healthier. Blood pressure and cholesterol levels come down. Aches and pains diminish. Over time, disorders begin to heal.

Whenever you are sick, the body is sending a signal. It needs rest—both from strenuous work and from foods that are toxic or difficult to digest. Juice fasting gives the digestive system a time out. It aids the immune system in clearing out dead, diseased, and damaged cells, and supports immune cells with an abundance of nutrients. Sludge that accumulates in spaces between the cells can be cleared away. There is an opportunity to reduce amounts of lipofuscin—the brown material caused by fat degeneration that is responsible for age spots. Juice fasting clears out poisons right down to the cellular level.

Juice fasting is a safe and easy way to detoxify your internal organs, tissues, and cells. Fasting has been written about for centuries, was used by the Essenes (a monastic sect active at the time of Christ), and has been a part of nearly all religious practices throughout history. Today the Orthodox Christian Church (for example, Greek or Russian) carries on the ancient tradition by practicing cycles of fasting and feasting throughout the year.

I do not recommend strict water fasts because they are too hard on the body. Too many toxins are released, and without the addition of nutrients that neutralize and bind them, you can do yourself more harm than good. The antioxidants—vitamins C and E, beta-carotene, selenium, and various enzymes and phytochemicals—are found abundantly in fresh juices. These scavengers bind harmful toxins and carry them out of the body while you fast.

Some words of caution. Children under eighteen should not follow a strict juice fast unless recommended by a health professional, although fresh fruit and vegetable juices are great supplements to a child's diet. Diabetics should seek a physician's approval before juice fasting. Anyone with hypoglycemia should avoid fruit juice and dilute carrot juice with an equal amount of purified water, and can benefit from the addition of protein powder to the juice.

Herbal Recommendations

Beneficial herbal teas include dandelion root and nettles, which help cleanse the liver and kidneys. If you purchase these herbs in bulk, steep one-half teaspoon of either herb in a pint of hot water for ten minutes, strain, and drink warm. Lemon may be added for flavor, but do not use any sweetener.

Bulking agents, such as psyllium husks, can be added to fresh juice. They act as bulk laxatives. Mix two teaspoons to a glass of juice two to three times during the day. These high-fiber agents also help to curb appetite. (For more information, see the Intestinal Cleanse, page 334.)

Juice Recommendations

Specific juices that are beneficial include:

- *Cleansing juices:* Beets (good for the liver), cabbage, wheatgrass, sprouts (any kind), lemon, carrot, celery, green bell pepper, orange, parsley, grapefruit, and apple.

- *Diuretics:* Cucumber, parsley, watermelon, cantaloupe with the seeds, lemon, kiwi fruit, asparagus.

The Juice Fast Sample Menu

The suggested menu is a guideline for the juice fast and can be modified whenever necessary to meet your individual needs. Keep the fast from one to three days.

Breakfast

THE MORNING ENERGIZER

½ organic Red or Golden Delicious apple, washed
5 medium carrots, scrubbed well, green tops removed, ends trimmed
½ small beet with leaves and stems, scrubbed well
½ small or medium lemon, washed, or peeled if not organic
½- to 1-inch piece fresh ginger root, washed

Cut the apple into sections that will fit your juicer's feed tube. Juice the apple along with the carrots, beet, lemon, and ginger. Stir the juice, and pour into a glass. Serve at room temperature or chilled, as desired.

Midmorning Break

WALDORF TWIST

1 organic Red or Golden Delicious apple, washed
3 stalks organic celery with leaves, washed
¼ small or medium lemon, washed, or peeled if not organic

Cut the apple into sections that will fit your juicer's feed tube, and juice along with the celery and lemon. Stir the juice, and pour into a glass. Serve at room temperature or chilled, as desired.

Lunch

POPEYE'S POWER

½ medium organic apple, any kind, washed
1 handful organic spinach, washed
1 small handful parsley, rinsed
4 medium carrots, scrubbed well, green tops removed, ends trimmed
1 stalk organic celery with leaves, washed
½ beet with stems and leaves, scrubbed well

Cut the apple into sections that will fit your juicer's feed tube. Bunch up the spinach and parsley, and push them through the feed tube with the apple, carrots, celery, and beet. Stir the juice, and pour into a glass. Serve at room temperature or chilled, as desired.

Happy Hour

SANTA FE SALSA COCKTAIL

1 medium vine-ripened tomato, washed
½ medium organic cucmber, scrubbed well
¼ cup cilantro, rinsed
¼ small or medium lime or lemon, washed, or peeled if not organic
Dash of hot sauce (optional)

Cut the tomato into sections that fit your juicer's feed tube. Cut the cucumber in half again lengthwise. Bunch up the cilantro, and push through the feed tube with the tomato, cucumber, and lime or lemon. Pour the juice into a glass, add the hot sauce (if using), and stir. Serve at room temperature or chilled, as desired.

Dinner

CHERIE'S QUICK ENERGY SOUP

1¼ cups fresh carrot juice (5–7 medium, or approx. 1 pound, yield about 1 cup)
1 avocado, peeled and seed removed
½ teaspoon ground cumin

Place the carrot juice, avocado, and cumin in a blender, and purée until smooth. Pour the mixture into a single soup bowl, and chill until ready to serve.

Bedtime Snack

SWEET DREAMS NIGHTCAP

2 romaine lettuce leaves, washed
1 handful parsley, rinsed
4 carrots, scrubbed well, green tops removed, ends trimmed
3 organic celery stalks with leaves, washed

Bunch up the lettuce leaves and parsley, and push through the feed tube with the carrots and celery. Stir the juice, and pour into a glass. Serve at room temperature or chilled, as desired.

Breaking the Fast

Breaking the fast properly is as important as the fast itself. If the fast is broken with bad food choices, you could do more harm than good. Make the day after a fast a strict vegan food day (no animal products), and eat the largest portion of your food raw—fresh fruits and vegetables. A suggested menu for breaking the juice fast follows.

Breakfast

Juice or smoothie: _____ (your choice)
Fruit or vegetable salad flavored with lemon juice
Herbal tea

Midmorning Snack

Juice: _____ (your choice)

Lunch

Cherie's Quick Energy Soup (see page 327)
or any vegetarian soup of your choice
Vegetable salad with lemon juice

Midafternoon Snack

Juice: _____ (your choice) or herbal tea

Dinner

Vegetable soup or steamed vegetables
Vegetable salad

Bedtime Snack

Vegetable juice: _____ (your choice) or herbal tea

THE KIDNEY CLEANSE

The kidneys perform two important functions: they remove waste from the blood by excreting urine, and they maintain proper fluid balance in the body. Poor dietary habits—eating highly refined carbohydrates, ingesting too much alcohol, eating large amounts of animal protein and fat, consuming foods (such as dairy products) that contain a lot of calcium, and eating too much salt—produce toxins that overload the kidneys, making them less effective. This reduced effciency contributes to kidney stone development and to other kidney ailments.

Symptoms of possible kidney problems include blood in the urine, burning or pain during urination, cloudy urine, a cold sensation in the lower half of the body, dark circles under the eyes, frequent urination (especially at night), foul-smelling or dark urine, incontinence, and pain in the eyes. (If you suspect kidney stones or have a urinary tract infection, see your doctor *immediately*.)

The following kidney cleanse program can reduce the toxic load on the kidneys, which allows them in turn to do their job of clearing toxins from the bloodstream. If you have a kidney disease, consult your health care provider first.

The Seven-Day Kidney Cleanse Program

❦ Drink plenty of purified water—from eight to ten glasses per day.

❦ Either daily or every other day, use an enema to gently cleanse your system (see "Enemas and Colonics" on page 334).

❦ Every day, drink one to two 8-ounce glasses of fresh juices that help to cleanse and support the kidneys. Choose from the following:
   • Asparagus, tomato, cucumber, and lemon
   • Cantaloupe with seeds
   • Carrot, celery, and parsley
   • Carrot, beet, and coconut
   • Cucumber and mint
   • Watermelon
   • Nettles, cucumber, and lemon

Cucumber, watermelon, cantaloupe, asparagus, lemon, kiwi, and parsley juices are all good diuretics.

❦ If you have a urinary tract infection, drink cranberry juice every day. (For more information, *see* **Bladder Infections;** that section includes a recipe for Cranberry-Apple Cocktail.)

❦ Drink nettles tea (see Appendix A for Arise & Shine's Kidney Life Tea and Kidney Life herbal supplements).

THE GALLBLADDER CLEANSE

The function of the gallbladder is to store and concentrate bile (which is made in the liver) until it is needed in the small intestine. The liver makes bile out of cholesterol, water, lecithin, mucin, bile acids, and other organic and inorganic substances. Bile acids are the check-and-balance of this system, designed to keep cholesterol soluble so it doesn't form stones. It is the typical Western diet of high-fat, fiber-depleted, refined foods that causes gallstones, which can cause abdominal pain, nausea, and vomiting (*see* **Gallstones**).

The cleansing program outlined here can purge the gallbladder of stones, including the "silent stones" that don't cause symptoms. I did a gallbladder flush for the first time when I was 30 because a reflexologist suggested it. I had experienced considerable pain when he worked on the reflex points on my feet that corresponded to the liver/gallbladder area. I was surprised by the purge, and I've been a believer in this program ever since.

Consult your health care professional before trying this program. Also, if you know you have gallstones, suspect that you might, are over age forty, or have not used cleansing programs before, and if you've eaten a typical Western diet most of your life, it is advisable not to try the Seven-Day Gallbladder Flush until you've used several other cleansing programs, including the Liver Cleanse (page 333) and the Intestinal Cleanse (page 332). For several weeks beforehand, you should also switch to a low-fat, high-fiber diet that is mostly vegetarian, with the occasional addition of fish or chicken. It is especially important to follow this diet during the cleansing period. If you try to flush the gallbladder while eating a high-fat, low-fiber diet, the gallbladder could release a larger stone that could block the bile duct, which would require immediate surgery. If you don't think that the Seven-Day Gallbladder Flush is for you right now, see the Beginner's Gallbladder Cleanse on page 331. The beginner's program should dissolve any stones present and bring relief for gallbladder problems.

The Seven-Day Gallbladder Flush

❧ Monday through Friday, drink at least two 8-ounce glasses of freshly made apple juice. Choose any kind of apple you wish; Golden or Red Delicious, Granny Smith, or Pippin are among my own favorites. (Just make sure they're organic!) If you have a blood-sugar disorder, such as hypoglycemia or diabetes, choose only green apples, such as Granny Smith or Pippin, and dilute the apple juice with at least four ounces of purified water or you can substitute lemon and water—the juice of one lemon in eight to ten ounces of water.

⊃ Eat a low-fat, high-fiber diet Monday through Friday. Avoid coffee, alcohol, soft drinks, junk food, sweets, red meat, dairy, and wheat.

⊃ Either daily or every other day, use an enema to gently cleanse your system (see "Enemas and Colonics" on page 334).

⊃ Drink only freshly made vegetable and fruit juices on Saturday, and eat no solid food. (See the Juice Fast sample menu on page 325.) Saturday evening before retiring, drink four ounces of gently warmed extra-virgin, cold-pressed olive oil mixed with four ounces of freshly squeezed lemon juice; shake together in a jar to combine. (This is about the worst stuff I've ever tasted, but it works.)

⊃ On Sunday morning, drink eight ounces of prune juice—you will want to be at home during this process. (Dilute the prune juice with four ounces of purified water if you have a sugar-metabolism problem.) Within a few hours, the gallbladder should purge.

⊃ What should you expect? Stones can range in size from that of orange seeds to that of dimes, or they can appear as a thick liquid if they have been softened by the juices. Colors can range from light to dark green to turquoise. (I only mention this so you won't think you are viewing something from Mars when the flush is successful.)

The Beginner's Gallbladder Cleanse

⊃ Use a lipotropic supplement formula that includes choline, methionine, betaine, folic acid, and vitamin B_{12}. The lipotropic formula helps remove fat from the liver and increases bile solubility. Also, use an herbal formula that includes dandelion root, milk thistle, artichoke leaves, turmeric, and boldo. The herbal formula also increases bile solubility (see Arise and Shine under the Liver Cleanse in Appendix A). These formulas are readily available in health food stores.

⊃ Eat more fresh vegetables and fruits.

⊃ Use a gel-forming fiber, such as psyllium husk or flaxseed, daily. Mix two teaspoons in eight ounces of fresh juice or water, two or three times a day.

⊃ Reduce your intake of saturated fats, cholesterol, sugar, and animal proteins. Completely avoid fried foods.

⊃ For one week, drink the following juices every day:
- Carrot, beet, and cucumber combined, three 8-ounce glasses.

- Carrot, celery, and endive combined, two 8-ounces glasses.

✑ Drink the juice of one lemon in eight ounces of hot water up to eight times per day.

THE INTESTINAL CLEANSE

The small intestine is made up of three segments: duodenum, jejunum, and ileum. Mineral absorption takes place in the duodenum, the first segment. Absorption of water-soluble vitamins, carbohydrates, and proteins occurs mostly in the jejunum, and the ileum, the last segment, is where fat-soluble vitamins, fat, cholesterol, and bile salts are absorbed. The large intestine (colon) also is made up of three segments: ascending, transverse, and descending. The large intestine is where the stool is formed. Although most of the water in the food is absorbed through the small intestine, more water is absorbed through the large intestine, as are electrolytes, mineral salts that help maintain the body's fluid balance.

Eating overly cooked, fried, junk, or spoiled food, or sweets like candy and ice cream; drinking coffee or alcohol; or taking drugs (prescription or recreational) can stimulate mucus secretion throughout the entire alimentary canal. This is normal, and is the body's natural way of protecting itself against the occasional encounter with bad food. But when we ingest these substances every day—and for some people, every meal and in between meals—mucus and waste build up on the intestinal wall. Pancreatic juices help to both digest food and cleanse mucus from the intestines. However, continual poor food choices lead to constant mucus secretion, and the digestive juices cannot eliminate the overload of waste.

As intestinal waste builds up, intestinal motion becomes less effective and material takes longer to pass through the digestive tract. This can contribute to constipation (*see* **Constipation**). Built-up mucus and waste also can be a breeding ground for parasites. I struggled with parasites for years, until I discovered this intestinal cleansing process. (For more information, *see* **Parasitic Infections.**) In addition, waste buildup can interfere with nutrient absorption, and can allow toxins to reenter the bloodstream.

It's not hard to see why a clean intestinal tract is so important to good health. The following three- to four-week program will reduce waste buildup in the intestines and allow for the more efficient absorption of nutrients. If you have an intestinal disease, such as Crohn's disease or diverticulitis, check with your health care provider first. (If you want to use a prepackaged intestinal cleansing kit, Arise & Shine offers a Cleanse Thyself Program; see Appendix A.)

The Intestinal Cleanse Program

❧ Drink three high-fiber shakes every day for three to four weeks. Make these shakes with psyllium husk and betonite clay (available at most health food stores or through Arise & Shine). Psyllium husk powder is a fibrous bulking agent that thickens and gels when mixed with juice or water. Betonite clay is an absorbent clay, used for centuries for internal purification. It draws out metals, drugs, toxins, waste, and mucus. To make each shake, mix one tablespoon of betonite clay with from eight to ten ounces of juice or water in a jar and shake. Add two teaspoons psyllium husk powder and shake again. Drink immediately, as psyllium husk gels quickly and the mixture becomes very thick. If using water, you can add a little fresh lemon juice or cranberry juice concentrate to this mixture to make it more palatable. Have a shake for breakfast, and for midmorning and midafternoon breaks. These shakes are very filling and you probably won't be as hungry during this cleanse, which makes it easier to lose weight, if that is a goal.

❧ Use colonics or cleansing enemas once or twice a week to remove excess waste that has accumulated. This also will help to relieve any adverse symptoms, such as headaches, fatigue, sleepiness, or aches and pains, you may experience as toxins are released (see "Enemas and Colonics" on page 334).

❧ Eat two meals a day; make the high-fiber shake and fresh juice your breakfast. The program works best if both meals are vegetarian—see the suggested menu for breaking the juice fast on page 328.

THE LIVER CLEANSE

The liver is the largest internal organ of the body and one of the most important. It performs various metabolic functions involving carbohydrate, protein, and fat usage; vitamin and mineral storage; and detoxification or excretion of chemical compounds, such as hormones, drugs, and pesticides. The liver also filters more than one liter of blood each minute and acts as a primary blood reservoir. In addition, the liver creates and secretes bile.

To a great extent, your health and vitality depend on the healthy functioning of your liver. Exposure to toxic chemicals, drugs, alcohol, or hepatitis, along with eating a typical Western diet, can lead to a sluggish or impaired liver. A liver that is even slightly sluggish can negatively affect your health. This is especially true because the liver is a prime place for the body to store poisons that can't be excreted. Highly toxic chemicals are

Enemas and Colonics

Though not a practice to rely on daily, enemas are very helpful during all cleansing programs. The colon, kidneys, lungs, and skin can become overwhelmed with the release of toxins during a cleanse, and skin eruptions, headaches, and flulike symptoms can result. Enemas assist the body in the elimination process and help minimize symptoms. Many people are not familiar with enemas today; however, their therapeutic benefits have been known for centuries.

To make a cleansing enema, add the juice of one lemon to two quarts of distilled lukewarm water. To administer the enema, lie down on your right side, draw both knees toward the abdomen, and insert the nozzle into the anus. (It's a good idea to first lubricate the nozzle with vitamin E oil or a lubricant jelly.) Take a deep breath to facilitate drawing the greatest amount of fluid into the colon. Retain the fluid for between three and four minutes during a cleansing enema, and between twelve and fifteen minutes during a retention enema. Gently massage the lower abdomen while retaining the fluid.

After taking the enema, it is a good idea to replace lost minerals by drinking an eight-ounce glass of mixed carrot and celery juice. You also need to replace your beneficial intestinal flora by taking supplements of "friendly" probiotic bacteria—*Lactobacillus acidophilus* and *Bifidobacterium infantis.* (I recommend Ultra Flora Plus DF by Metagenics; see Appendix A.)

In some cases, colonics may be used for a more thorough cleansing. Colonics are administered higher in the bowel than is possible with standard enemas, and are performed by a trained technician using specialized equipment. Talk to your health care provider before taking a colonic.

known to pass through the liver, including residues from pesticides and herbicides. And it doesn't take megadoses of unhealthy substances to weaken the livers of some people. For example, researchers have found even small amounts of alcohol can cause fat deposits in the livers of susceptible individuals.

The symptoms of a sluggish liver are numerous and varied. They include abdominal discomfort, aches and pains, brown age spots on face and hands, anal itching, bad breath, body odor, sallow or jaundiced complexion, whitish or yellow tongue coating, digestive problems (belching and flatulence), dizziness, drowsiness after eating, fatigue, frequent urination at night, migraine headaches or headaches that involve a feeling of fullness or heaviness in the head, inability to tolerate heat or cold, sleep-lessness, irritability, loss of memory or inability to concentrate, loss of sex-ual desire, lower back pain, malaise, menstrual problems, nervousness and anxiety, pain around the right shoulder blade and shoulder, puffy eyes and/or face, red nose, small red spots on the skin (either smooth or raised and hard), and sinus problems. Allergies, candidiasis, constipation, hemorrhoids, cellulite, and premenstrual syndrome are all associated with a malfunctioning liver.

Optimizing liver function focuses on cleansing, protecting, and nour-ishing the liver. The following program does just that. If you have a liver disease, consult your health care provider first.

The Seven-Day Liver Cleanse

For seven days, eat a vegan diet, which means you exclude all animal products. Avoid alcohol, tobacco, sweets, and junk food completely. Add the following foods to your daily diet plan, and use the coffee enema once or twice during the week. If you miss a day, begin again.

Carrot Salad

Place one cup of finely shredded carrots, or carrot pulp leftover from juic-ing, in a bowl. If shredding the carrots, they should be a mushy consisten-cy; use a food processor or fine grater. (It's easiest to use carrot pulp.) Combine one tablespoon extra-virgin, cold-pressed olive oil with one tablespoon fresh lemon juice. You may add more olive oil and lemon juice, but not less. I also like to add a dash of cinnamon. Whisk the olive oil and lemon juice together in a small bowl. Pour the mixture over the shredded carrots or carrot pulp, and mix well.

Vegetable Broth

This delicious broth provides important nutrients needed during the cleansing process. Eat one to two cups of the broth each day.

2–3 cups chopped fresh string beans
2–3 cups chopped zucchini
2–3 stalks chopped celery
1–3 tablespoons chopped parsley
1 tablespoon chopped garlic

Steam the string beans, zucchini, and celery over purified water until soft, but still green. Place the cooked vegetables, plus the parsley and garlic, in a blender, and purée until smooth. Add a bit of the steaming water, if needed, but the broth should be fairly thick. Season to taste with minced ginger, cayenne, vegetable seasoning, or herbs of your choice.

Fresh Beet Juice

Drink from three to eight ounces of fresh beet juice daily. Because of its strong taste, I recommend that you mix beet juice with other juices that are milder in flavor, such as carrot, cucumber, endive, lemon, or apple. Beet juice has been used for decades to cleanse and support the liver. Endive has been used traditionally to promote the secretion of bile; this is helpful for the liver and gallbladder.

Other Beneficial Juices

Juices that are beneficial for the liver include apricot, chervil, dandelion, gooseberry, papaya, radish, string bean, tomato, and wheatgrass. Many of these juices are used in the following recipes.

LIVER LIFE TONIC

½ organic green apple such as Granny Smith or Pippin, washed
1 handful dandelion greens, washed
5 carrots, scrubbed well, green tops removed, ends trimmed
½ small lemon, washed, or peeled if not organic

Cut the apple into wedges that will fit your juicer's feed tube. Bunch up the dandelion greens, and push through the feed tube with the apple, carrots, and lemon. Stir the juice, and pour into a glass. Serve at room temperature or chilled, as desired.

SINUS SOLUTION

2 medium vine-ripened tomatoes, washed
4 radishes with green tops, washed
½ small or medium lime or lemon, washed, or peeled if not organic

Cut the tomatoes into sections that fit your juicer's feed tube. Juice the tomatoes along with the radishes and lime or lemon. Stir the juice, and pour into a glass. Serve at room temperature or chilled, as desired.

JACK & THE BEAN

1 large vine-ripened tomato, washed
2 romaine lettuce leaves, washed
8 organic string beans, washed
3 Brussels sprouts, washed
½ small or medium lemon, washed, or peeled if not organic

Cut the tomato into sections that fit your juicer's feed tube. Bunch up the lettuce leaves, and push through the feed tube with the tomato, string beans, Brussels sprouts, and lemon. Stir the juice, and pour into a glass. Serve at room temperature or chilled, as desired.

WHEATGRASS LIGHT

1 organic Golden or Red Delicious apple, washed
1 small handful wheatgrass, rinsed
2–3 sprigs mint, rinsed (optional)
¼ small or medium lemon, washed, or peeled if not organic

Cut the apple into sections that fit your juicer's feed tube. Bunch up the wheatgrass and mint (if using) and push them through the feed tube with the apple and lemon. Stir the juice, and pour into a glass. Serve at room temperature or chilled, as desired.

Milk Thistle (Silymarin)

Take one capsule of the herb milk thistle after each meal. Milk thistle contains some of the most potent liver cleansing and protecting compounds known. Silymarin, which is the most-studied active ingredient in milk thistle, enhances liver function and inhibits factors that cause hepatic damage. Because of its antioxidant properties, silymarin also helps prevents free-radical damage to the liver. (A product I have used and recommend is "Liver Life" by Arise and Shine; see Appendix A.)

Coffee Retention Enema

Coffee retention enemas can help remove toxins from the liver by causing the liver to produce more bile and by stimulating bile flow. During this process, the liver can dump toxins into the bile quickly. Note that drinking coffee does not help cleanse the liver. As a beverage, coffee overstimulates the adrenal glands and is not a healthful addition to your cleansing program.

To prepare the coffee enema, add 3 heaping tablespoons of ground coffee to 1 quart of purified water in a pot made of enamel, stainless steel, or other nonreactive substance. (Use organically grown coffee, because the chemicals used to grow conventional coffee could add to the toxic load on the liver.) Let the coffee boil slowly for three minutes, then cover the pot and simmer for another seventeen minutes. Strain the grounds from the liquid, and cool the liquid to body temperature before placing in the enema bag. To administer the enema, see "Enemas and Colonics" on page 334.

It is possible for a coffee enema to cause nausea because of the toxins that are released. If this happens, drink several cups of peppermint tea, preferably from organically grown herbs. That will help dilute the toxic bile overflow and bring relief.

THE SKIN CLEANSE

The skin is the largest organ of the body. It has numerous functions, one of which is excretion. It assists the body in eliminating small amounts of water, salts, various organic compounds, toxins, and poisons. When other organs of elimination are overloaded, the skin will do everything possible to facilitate excretion. Since the skin acts as a protective barrier between the body and the millions of foreign substances in our environment, it can become overwhelmed with toxins and react with pimples, bumps, acne, redness, rashes, scales, age spots, and other unsightly conditions.

Whether your skin is dull, breaking out with pimples or bumps, is showing signs of aging, or just needs more life, a cleansing program will help it look healthier and more glowing. I recommend any of the cleansing programs in this section to improve your skin's health. Internal cleansing is very important because your skin reflects the inner state of your body. Beautiful, healthy skin begins on the inside. The following purge could help you with a "jump start" toward beautiful skin. (If you would like to try a prepackaged skin cleanse program, Mt. Shasta Herb and Health offers the Bring 'Em Back Alive Skin Purge kit; see Appendix A).

The Seven-Day Skin Purge

❧ Use juices that help to detoxify the skin (drink at least two 8-ounce glasses per day for one week):

- Cucumber, carrot, and celery

- Cucumber and lemon

- Apple, pineapple, and cucumber

- Carrot, parsnip, and green bell pepper

- Spinach and carrot

- Asparagus and tomato

❧ Either daily or every other day, use an enema to gently cleanse your system (see "Enemas and Colonics" on page 334).

❧ Drink from eight to ten 8-ounce glasses of purified water per day—for the rest of your life.

APPENDIX A

Sources of Information and Products

The first part of this appendix contains sources of general information and products that can help you improve your overall health. The second section contains sources of information and products that can help you tackle specific disorders, while the third section contains sources of products you can use in the cleansing programs.

INFORMATION AND PRODUCTS FOR OVERALL HEALTH

Flaxseed Oil Recipes

Flax for Life by Jade Butler
At health food stores, or order from Barlean's Organic Oils at (800) 445-FLAX

Health Institutes

Hippocrates Health Institute
1443 Palmdale Court
West Palm Beach FL 33411
(800) 842-2125

Optimum Health Institute of Austin
Route 1 Box 339J
Cedar Creek TX 78612
(512) 303-4817

Optimum Health Institute of San Diego
6970 Central Avenue
Lemon Grove CA 91945-2198
(800) 993-4325

Healthy Cooking

The Healthy Gourmet by Cherie Calbom (New York: Clarkson Potter, 1996)

Organic Produce—Information

Campaign for Sustainable Agriculture
12 North Church Street
Goshen NY 10924
(914) 294-0633

Environmental Working Group
Suite 600
1718 Connecticut Avenue N.W.
Washington DC 20009
(202) 667-6982

Mothers & Others for a Livable Planet
40 West 20th Street
New York NY 10011
(212) 242-0010

The Organic Food Alliance
Suite 531
2111 Wilson Boulevard
Arlington VA 22201
(703) 276-9498

Organic Foods Production of North America
P.O. Box 1078
Greenfield MA 01302

Organic Produce—Mail Order

Diamond Organics
P.O. Box 2159
Freedom CA 95019
(800) 922-2396

Walnut Acres Organic Farms
Penn Creek PA 17862
(800) 433-3998

Probiotic Supplements

Ultra Flora Plus DF by Metagenics; available through some doctors, or by
calling (800) 522-6382

INFORMATION AND PRODUCTS FOR
SPECIFIC DISORDERS

Asthma

Asthma: Clinical Pearls in Nutrition & Complementary Therapies by Kirk Hamilton. To order, call (916) 483-1085 or fax (916) 483-1431, or write 3301 Alta Arden, Suite 2, Sacramento CA 95825

Attention Deficit Disorder

Is This Your Child? by Doris Rapp (New York: William Morrow, NY 1991)
Is This Your Child's World? by Doris Rapp (New York: Bantam Books NY, 1996)

Cancer

Center for Alternative Cancer Research
412 G Street N.E.
Washington DC 20069

People Against Cancer
P.O. Box 10
Otho IA 50569
(515) 972-4444 or fax (515) 972-4415

Third Opinion by John M. Fink (Garden City Park NY: Avery Publishing Group, 1997, (800) 548-5757)

Epilepsy

The Epilepsy Diet Treatment: An Introduction to the Ketogenic Diet by John Freeman (New York: Demos Publications, 1994)

MCT cooking oil: Thin Oil (plain, olive, and butter-flavored) is available from Sound Nutrition at (800) 437-6863

Insomnia

Melatonin: Source Naturals sublingual tablets (orange- or pepermint-flavored), available at health food stores

Menopause

Wild yam: Pro-Gest from Professional Technical Services, (800) 888-6814

Parasitic Infections

Combination herbal products: WormSquirm 1 and WormSquirm 2 by Arise & Shine, (800) 688-2444

PRODUCTS FOR THE CLEANSING PROGRAMS

Kidney Cleanse

Kidney Life Tea and Kidney Life herbal supplements from Arise & Shine, (800) 688-2444

Intestinal Cleanse

Cleanse Thyself Program from Arise & Shine, (800) 688-2444. Includes betonite clay and psyllium husk powder along with herbal supplements

Liver Cleanse

Liver Life from Arise and Shine, (800) 688-2444. Includes milk thistle, artichoke leaf, dandelion root, bayberry root, bulpleurum, Oregon grape root, burdock root, black walnut hulls, wild yam root, fennel seed, stillingia root, and mandrake root

Skin Cleanse

Bring 'Em Back Alive Skin Purge from Mt. Shasta Herb and Health, (888) 343-7225. Includes a mustard bath, an herbal tea, and an herbal enema

Appendix B

Body Mass Index (BMI) Chart

There are a lot of ways to determine your ideal weight, but one of the most accurate and easiest to use is the Body Mass Index (BMI) system. BMI is calculated from height and weight; basically the more you weigh, the higher your BMI will be. Overweight is defined as having a BMI of 25.0 to 29.9 and obesity as having a BMI of 30.0 and above. To use the following chart, simply find your height, look across to find your weight, and then go to the top of the chart to find your BMI.

BODY MASS INDEX

BMI	20	21	22	23	24	25	26	27	28	29	30	31	32	33	34
HEIGHT							WEIGHT IN POUNDS								
4'10"	96	100	105	110	115	119	124	129	134	138	143	148	153	158	162
4'11"	99	104	190	114	119	124	128	133	138	143	148	153	158	163	168
5'0"	102	107	112	117	122	127	132	138	143	148	153	158	163	168	174
5'1"	106	111	116	122	127	132	138	143	148	153	158	164	169	174	180
5'2"	109	115	120	126	131	136	142	147	153	158	163	169	175	180	186
5'3"	113	118	124	130	135	141	146	152	158	164	164	169	175	180	186
5'4"	116	122	128	134	140	145	151	157	163	169	175	180	186	192	197
5'5"	120	126	132	138	144	150	156	162	168	174	180	186	192	198	204
5'6"	124	130	136	142	148	155	161	167	173	179	186	192	198	204	210
5'7"	127	134	140	147	153	159	166	172	178	185	191	198	204	211	217
5'8"	132	139	145	152	158	165	172	178	185	191	197	203	210	216	223
5'9"	135	142	149	155	162	169	176	182	189	196	203	209	216	223	230
5'10"	140	147	154	161	168	175	182	189	196	202	209	216	222	229	236
5'11"	143	150	157	164	171	179	186	193	200	208	215	222	229	236	243

BMI	20	21	22	23	24	25	26	27	28	29	30	31	32	33	34
HEIGHT						WEIGHT IN POUNDS									
6'0"	147	155	162	170	177	185	192	199	207	214	221	228	235	242	250
6'1"	151	158	166	174	181	189	196	204	211	219	227	235	242	250	257
6'2"	155	164	171	179	187	195	203	210	218	225	233	241	249	256	264
6'3"	160	168	176	184	192	200	207	216	224	232	240	248	256	264	272
6'4"	164	172	181	189	197	205	214	222	230	238	246	254	263	271	279

Clinical guidelines on the identification, evaluation and treatment of overweight and obesity in adults. National Institutes of Health; National Heart, Lung and Blood Institute (1998).

If your height or weight is not listed, you can determine your own BMI by using the following formula:

$$\frac{\text{Weight (pounds)}}{\text{Height (inches)}^2} \times 705 = \text{BMI}$$

To use this formula, just follow these steps. Let's assume, for the sake of this example, that you are 5 feet, 4 inches tall, and weigh 121 pounds.

1. First, calculate your height in inches, and square it—in other words, multiply the number by itself. In our example, your height is 64 inches. So:

    64 × 64 = 4,096

2. Now, write down your weight in pounds. In our example, your weight is 121 pounds.

3. Divide the smaller number (in this case, 121) by the larger number (4,096), rounding off your answer to the nearest hundredth:

    121 ÷ 4,096 = .03

4. Multiply your final number—.03—by 705.

    .03 × 705 = 21

    In this example, your BMI is 21.

    It is important to remember that if you are very muscular you can have a higher-than-recommended BMI and not be overweight. You should also note that if you have been overweight for many years the recommended BMI for your height may not be a realistic goal. Don't be discouraged—any weight loss is better than no loss at all.

References

All About Juice

Batmanghelidj, BF. *Your Body's Many Cries for Water.* Falls Church VA: Global Health Solutions, Inc., 1995.

Calbom, C, Chelf, VR. *Cooking for Life.* Garden City Park NY: Avery Publishing Group, 1993.

Kleiner, SM. "Defense Plants: Foods That Fight Disease," *The Physician and Sports Medicine* 25(12):89–90, December 1997.

Murray, M. *The Complete Book of Juicing.* Rocklin CA: Prima Publishing, 1992.

"Organic Tomatoes, Vitamin C and Calcium," *Nutrition Week,* 28(24):7, 19 June 1998; taken from the April 1998 issue of *Hort/Science,* 33(2):255–257.

Winston, C. "Phytochemicals: Guardians of Our Health," *Journal of the American Dietetic Association* 97(10, Suppl. 2):S199–S204, October 1997.

Wolf, AM, Wolf, AMD. "Phytochemicals: The Newest Frontier in Disease Prevention," *Hospital Medicine* 55–56, August 1998.

Wong, H, et al. "Total Antioxidant Capacity of Fruits," *Journal of Agricultural and Food Chemistry* 44:701–705, 1996.

Food Sources of Vitamins and Minerals

Grogg, JL, Gropper, SS, et al. *Advanced Nutrition and Human Metabolism.* 2nd ed. New York: West Publishing Co., 1995.

Haas, EM. *Staying Healthy With Nutrition.* Berkeley CA: Celestial Arts, 1992.

Kirschmann, GJ, Kirschmann, JD. *Nutrition Almanac.* 4th ed. New York: McGraw-Hill, 1996.

Allergies

Barnett, RA. *Tonics.* New York: Harper-Collins, 1997.

Damjanov, I. *Pathology for the Health-Related Professional.* Philadelphia: W.B. Saunders, 1996.

Heinerman, J. *Heinerman's Encyclopedia of Healing Juices.* Englewood Cliffs NJ: Prentice Hall, 1994.

Keegan, L. *Healing Nutrition.* Albany NY: Delmar Publications, 1996.

Kenton, L, Kenton, S. *Raw Energy.* London: Century Publishing, 1985.

Lust, JB. *Raw Juice Therapy.* London: Thorsons Publishers Limited, 1958.

Murray, MT. *The Healing Power of Foods.* Rocklin CA: Prima Publishing, 1993.

Murray, M, Pizzorno, J. *The Encyclopedia of Natural Medicine.* 2nd ed. Rocklin CA: Prima Publishing, 1998.

Polunin, M. *Healing Foods.* New York: DK Publishing, Inc., 1997.

Alzheimer's Disease

Behl, C, et al. "Vitamin E Protects Nerve Cells From Amyloid Protein Toxicity," *Bio-*

chemical and Biophysical Research Communications 944–950, July 1992.

Copestake, P. "Aluminum and Alzheimer's Disease—An Update," Food Chem Tox 31:670–685, 1993.

Damjanov, I. Pathology for the Health-Related Professional. Philadelphia: W.B. Saunders, 1996.

Murray, MT. The Healing Power of Foods. Rocklin CA: Prima Publishing, 1993.

Murray, M, Pizzorno, J. The Encyclopedia of Natural Medicine. 2nd ed. Rocklin CA: Prima Publishing, 1998.

Newman, PE. "Could Diet Be One of the Causal Factors of Alzheimer's Disease?" Medical Hypotheses 39:123–126, October 1992.

Riley, ME, et al. "Evaluation of a New Nutritional Supplement for Patients with Alzheimer's Disease," Journal of the American Dietetic Association 90:433–435, March 1990.

Roberts, HJ. "Allopathic specific condition review: Alzheimer's disease," Protocol Journal of Botanical Medicine 2(1):94, 1997. In: Rister, R. Japanese Herbal Medicine: The Healing Art of Kampo. Garden City Park NY: Avery Publishing Group, 1999.

Anemia

Gleerup, A, et al. "Iron Absorption From the Whole Diet: Comparison of the Effect of Two Different Distributions of Daily Calcium Intake," American Journal of Clinical Nutrition 61(1):97–104, 1995.

Haas, EM. Staying Healthy With Nutrition. Berkeley CA: Celestial Arts, 1992.

Hallberg, L, et al. "Calcium Effect of Different Amounts on Nonheme- and Heme-Iron Absorption in Humans," American Journal of Clinical Nutrition 53(1):112–119, 1991.

Hoffmann, D. The Herbal Handbook: A User's Guide to Medical Herbalism. Rochester NY: The Healing Arts Press, 1988.

Kappor, R, Mehta, U. "Iron Status and Growth of Rats Fed Different Dietary Iron Sources," Plant Foods for Human Nutrition L44(1):29–34, 1993.

Layrisse, M, Garcia-Casal, MN. "Strategies for the Prevention of Iron Deficiency Through Foods in the Household," Nutrition Reviews 55(6):233–239, 1997.

Layrisse, M, Garcia-Casal, MN, et al. "The Role of Vitamin A on the Inhibitors of Nonheme Iron Absorption: Preliminary Results," Nutritional Biochemistry 8:61–67, 1997.

Lieberman, S, Bruning, N. The Real Vitamin & Mineral Book. Garden City Park NY: Avery Publishing Group, 1990.

Lynch, SR, et al. "Inhibitory Effect of Soybean Protein-Related Moiety on Iron Absorption in Humans," American Journal of Clinical Nutrition 60(4):567–572, 1994.

Murray, M, Pizzorno, J. The Encyclopedia of Natural Medicine. Rocklin CA: Prima Publishing, 1990.

el-Shobaki, FA, Saleh, ZA. "The Effect of Some Beverage Extracts on Intestinal Iron Absorption," Zeitschrift für Ernahrungswissenchaft 29(4):264–269, 1990.

Siegenber, D, et al. "Ascorbic Acid Prevents the Dose-Dependent Inhibitory Effects of Polyphenols and Phytates on Nonheme-Iron Absorption," American Journal of Clinical Nutrition 53:537–541, 1991.

Whiting, SJ. "The Inhibitory Effect of Dietary Calcium on Iron Availability: A Cause for Concern?" Nutrition Reviews 53(3):77–80, 1995.

Anxiety and Panic Attacks

Alschuler, L. Botanical Medicine I, II, III, IV (lectures). Seattle: Bastyr University, 1998.

Benjamin, J, et al. "Inositol Treatment in Psychiatry," Psychopharmacology Bulletin 31:167–175, 1995.

Boris, M, et al. "Foods and Additives are Common Causes of the Attention Deficit Hyperactive Disorder in Children," Annals of Allergy 72:462–468, 1994.

Boulenger JP, Uhde, TW. "Caffeine Consumption and Anxiety: Preliminary Results of a Survey Comparing Patients with Anxiety Disorders with Normal Controls," *Psychopharmacology Bulletin* 18:53, 1982.

Bruce, M, et al. "Anxiogenic Affects of Caffeine in Patients with Anxiety Disorders," *Archives of General Psychiatry* 49: 867–869, 1992.

Charney, DS, et al. "Increased Anxiogenic Effects of Caffeine in Patients with Panic Disorders," *Archives of General Psychiatry* 43:233, 1985.

DePrietas, ET, et al. "Effects of Caffeine in Chronic Psychiatry Patients," *American Journal of Psychiatry* 136:1337–1338, 1979.

Gorman, JM, et al. "Hypoglycemia and Panic Attacks," *American Journal of Psychiatry* 141:101, 1984.

Grogg, JL, Gropper, SS, Hunt, SM. *Advanced Nutrition and Human Metabolism.* 2nd ed. New York: West Publishing Co., 1995.

Haas, EM. *Staying Healthy With Nutrition.* Berkeley CA: Celestial Arts, 1992.

Java, Vino, Chocolate, and Cigars (lecture). Seattle: Thorne Research Seminar, 15 November, 1997.

Kahn, RS, Westenberg, HGM. "L-5-Hydroxytryptophan in the Treatment of Anxiety Disorders," *Journal of Affective Disorders* 8:197–200, 1985.

Kirschmann, GJ, Kirschmann, JD. *Nutrition Almanac.* 4th ed. New York: McGraw-Hill, 1996.

Leznoff, A. "Preventative Challenges to Patients with Multiple Chemical Sensitivity," *Journal of Allergy and Clinical Immunology* 99(4):438–442, 1997.

Mohler, H, et al. "Nicotinamide is a Brain Constituent with Benzodiazepine Actions," *Nature* 278:563, 1979.

Rowe, KS, et al. "Synthetic Food Coloring and Behavior: a Dose Response Effect in a Double-Blind, Placebo-Controlled, Repeated-Measures Study," *Pediatrics* 125: 691–698, 1994.

Volz, HP, Kieser, M. "Kava-Kava Extract WS 1490 Versus Placebo in Anxiety Disorders—A Randomized Placebo-Controlled 25-Week Outpatient Trial," *Pharmacospsychiatry* 30:1–5, 1997.

Voocovi, PP, et al. "Nicotinic Acid Effectiveness in the Treatment of Benzadiazepine Withdrawal," *Current Therapy Research* 41:1017, 1987.

White, HL, et al. "Extracts of Ginkgo Biloba Leaves Inhibit Monoamine Oxidase," *Life Sciences* 58(16):1315–1321, 1996.

Asthma

Barnett, RA. *Tonics.* New York: HarperCollins, 1997.

Britton, J. "Dietary Magnesium, Lung Function, Wheezing, and Airway Hyperreactivity in a Random Adult Population Sample," *Lancet* 344:357–362, 1994.

Damjanov, I. *Pathology for the Health-Related Professions.* Philadelphia: W.B. Saunders, 1996.

Dry, J, Vincent, D. "Effect of Fish Oil Diet on Asthma: Results of a 1-Year Double-Blind Study," *International Archive of Allergy and Applied Immunology* 95:156–157, 1991.

Gursche, S. *Healing With Herbal Juices.* Burnaby BC, Canada: Alive Books, 1993.

Hatch, GE. "Asthma, Inhaled Oxidants and Dietary Antioxidants," *American Journal of Clinical Nutrition* 61(Suppl.): 625S–630S, 1995.

Monteleone, CA, Sherman, AR. "Nutrition and Asthma," *Archives of Internal Medicine* 157:23–34, January 1997.

Murray, M, Pizzorno, J. *The Encyclopedia of Natural Medicine.* 2nd ed. Rocklin CA: Prima Publishing, 1998.

Soutar, A. "Bronchial Reactivity and Dietary Antioxidants," *Thorax* 52:166–170, February 1997.

Troisi, RJ. "A Prospective Study of Diet and Adult-Onset Asthma," *American Respiratory and Critical Care Medicine* 151: 1401–1408, 1995.

Attention Deficit Disorders

Goldman, EL. "Ritalin Wrongly Used to Diagnose Attention Deficit," *Family Practice News* 33, 1 November 1995.

Murray, M, Pizzorno, J. *The Encyclopedia of Natural Medicine.* 2nd ed. Rocklin CA: Prima Publishing, 1998.

Rapp, D. *Is This Your Child?* New York: Quill, 1991.

Rapp, D. *Is This Your Child's World?* New York: Bantam Books, 1996.

Sever, Y, et al. "Iron Deficiency in Children with Attention Deficit Hyperactivity Disorder," *Neuropsychobiology* 35:178–180, 1997.

Stevens, LJ, et al. "Essential Fatty Acid Metabolism in Boys with Attention-Deficit Hyperactivity Disorder," *American Journal of Clinical Nutrition* 62:761–768, 1995.

Tuthill, RW. "Hair Lead Levels Related to Children's Classroom Attention-Deficit Behavior," *Archives of Environmental Health* 51(3):214–220, May/June 1996.

Bladder Infections

Alschuler, L. Botanical Medicine I, II, III, IV (lectures). Seattle: Bastyr University, 1998.

Avorn, J, et al. "Reduction of Bacteriuria and Pyuria After Ingestion of Cranberry Juice," *Journal of the American Medical Association* 271(10):751–754, 9 March 1994.

Bernstein, J, et al. "Depression of Lymphocyte Transformation Following Oral Glucose Ingestion," *American Journal of Clinical Nutrition* 30:613, 1977.

Fleet, JC. "New Support for a Folk Remedy: Cranberry Juice Reduces Bacteriuria and Pyuria in Elderly Women," *Nutrition Reviews* 52(5):168–170, May 1994.

Foxman, B, et al. "First-time Urinary Tract Infection and Sexual Behavior," *Epidemiology* 6(2):162–168, March 1995.

Gaby, A. Therapeutic Nutrition I, II (lectures). Seattle: Bastyr University, 1998.

Girodon, F, Lombard, M, et al. "Effect of Micronutrient Supplementation on Infection in Institutionalized Elderly Subjects: A Controlled Trial," *Annals of Nutrition and Metabolism* 41(2):98–107, 1997.

Goldhar, J. "Anti-*Escherichia coli* Adhesion Activity of Cranberry and Blueberry Juices," *Advances in Experimental Medicine and Biology* 15:179–183, 1996.

Grimble, RF, "Effects of Antioxidative Vitamins on Immune Function with Clinical Applications," *International Journal for Vitamin and Nutrition Research* 67(5):312–320, 1997.

"Inhibitory Activity of Cranberry Juice on Adherence of Type 1 and Type P Fimbriated *Escherichia coli* to Eucaryotic Cells," *Antimicrobial Agents and Chemotherapy* 33(1): 92–98, January 1989.

Levy, R, Shriker, O, et al. "Vitamin C for the Treatment of Recurrent Furunculosis in Patients with Impaired Neutrophil Functions," *Journal of Infectious Disease* 173(6):1502–1505, June 1996.

Lundberg, JO, Carlsson, S, et al. "Urinary Nitrite: More Than a Marker of Infection," *Urology* 50(2):189–191, August 1997.

Naganawa, R, Suzuki, A, et al. "Inhibition of Microbial Growth by Ajoene, a Sulfur-Containing Compound Derived From Garlic," *Applied and Environmental Microbiology* 62(11):4238–4242, November 1996.

Pitchford, P. *Healing With Whole Foods: Oriental Traditions and Modern Nutrition.* Berkeley CA: North Atlantic Books, 1993.

Rees, LP, et al. "A Quantitative Assessment of the Antimicrobial Activity of Garlic," *World Journal of Microbiology and Biotechnology* 9:303–307, 1993.

Sanchez, A, et al. "Role of Sugars in Human Neutrophilic Phagocytosis," *American Journal of Clinical Nutrition* 26(11): 1180–1184, November 1973.

Bruises

Beckham, N. *Family Guide to Natural Therapies.* New Canaan CT: Keats Publishing, 1996.

Haas, EM. *Staying Healthy With Nutrition.* Berkeley CA: Celestial Arts, 1992.

Hoffmann, D. *The Herbal Handbook: A User's Guide to Medical Herbalism.* Rochester NY: Healing Arts Press, 1988.

Hoffmann, D. *The New Holistic Herbal.* 3rd ed. Rockport MA: Element Books, Inc., 1992.

Moore, M. *Medicinal Plants of the Pacific West.* Santa Fe NM: Red Crane Books, 1993.

Murray, MT. *Encyclopedia of Nutritional Supplements.* Rocklin CA: Prima Publishing, 1996.

Pitchford, P. *Healing With Whole Foods: Oriental Traditions and Modern Nutrition.* Berkeley CA: North Atlantic Books, 1993.

Thomas, CL. *Taber's Cyclopedic Medical Dictionary.* 17th ed. Philadelphia: F.A. Davis Co., 1993.

Bursitis and Tendinitis

Arora, R, Kapoor, N et al. "Anti-inflammatory Studies on *Curcuma longa* (Turmeric)," *Indian Journal of Medicial Research* 59:1289–1295, 1971.

Millen, A, Wilson CWM. "The Metabolism of Ascorbic Acid in Rheumatoid Arthritis," *Proc Nutri Sci* 35:8A–9A, 1976.

Panganamala, RV, Cronwell, DG. "The Effects of Vitamin E on Arachidonic Acid Metabolism," *Annals of the New York Academy of Sciences* 393:376–391, 1982.

Pizzorno, J, Murray, MT. *Encyclopedia of Natural Medicine.* 2nd ed. Rocklin CA: Prima Publishing, 1998.

Taussig, S. "The Mechanism of the Physiological Action of Bromelain," *Medical Hypotheseis* 6:9–14, 1980.

Weil, A. *Vitamins and Minerals.* New York: Ivy Books, 1997.

Yoshimoto, T, Furukawa, M, et al. "Flavonoids: Potent Inhibitors of Arachidonate 5-Lipoxygonase," *Biochemistry and Biophysical Research Communications* 116: 612–618, 1983.

Cancer

Belman, S. "Onion and Garlic Oil Inhibit Tumor Growth," *Carcinogenesis* 4(8):1063–1065, 1983.

Bendich, A. "Vitamin C and Immune Response," *Food Technology* 41:112–114, 1987.

Cameron, E, Pauling, L. *Proceedings of the National Academy of Sciences* 73(10): 3685–3689 (October 1976). In: Lieberman, S, Bruning, N. *The Real Vitamin and Mineral Book.* Garden City Park NY: Avery Publishing Group, 1997.

Craig, WJ. "Phytochemicals: Guardians of Our Health," *Journal of the American Dietetic Association* 97(10 Suppl2):S199–S204, October 1997.

Dowd, P, et al. "Single-Nutrient Effects of Immunologic Functions," *Journal of the American Medical Association* 245:53–58, 1981.

Gerster, H. "Anticarcinogenic Effect of the Common Carotenoids," *International Journal for Vitamin and Nutrition Research* 63:93–121, 1993,

Hoffer, A, Pauling, L. *Journal of Orthomolecular Medicine* 5(3):143–154 (1990). In: Lieberman, S, Bruning, N. *The Real Vitamin and Mineral Book.* Garden City Park NY: Avery Publishing Group, 1997.

Kuhnau, J. "The Flavonoids: A Class of Semi-Essential Food Components: Their Role in Human Nutrition," *World Review of Nutrition and Diet* 24:117–191, 1976.

Lai, CN, et al. "Chlorophyll: The Active Factor in Wheat Sprout Extract Inhibiting the Metabolic Activation of Carcinogens in Vitro," *Nutrition and Cancer* 1(3):19–21, 1978. In: Wigmore, A. *The Wheatgrass Book.* Garden City Park NY: Avery Publishing Group, 1985.

Lai, CN, et al. "Anti-mutagenic Activities of Common Vegetables and Their Chlorophyll Content," *Mutation Research* 77: 245–250, 1980. In: Kenton, L, Kenton, S. *Raw Energy.* London: Century Publishing, 1985.

Pizzorno, J. *Total Wellness*. Rocklin CA: Prima Publishing, 1996.

Semba, RD. "Vitamin A, Immunity and Infection," *Clinical Infectious Diseases* 19: 489–499, 1994.

Steinmetz, K, Potter, JD. "Vegetables, Fruit and Cancer, I: Epidemiology," *Cancer Causes Control* 2:325–357, 1991.

Steinmetz, K, Potter, JD. "Vegetables, Fruit and Cancer, II: Mechanisms," *Cancer Causes Control* 2:427–442, 1991.

Talska, G, et al. "Genetically Based n-Acetyltransferase Metabolic Polymorphism and Low-Level Environmental Exposure in Carcinogens," *Nature* 369: 154–156, 1994. In: Murray, M, Pizzorno, J. *Encyclopedia of Natural Medicine*. 2nd ed. Rocklin CA: Prima Publishing, 1998.

Watson, RR, et al. "Selenium and Vitamins A, E, and C: Nutrients with Cancer Prevention Properties," *Journal of the American Dietetic Association* 86(4): 505–510, 1986.

Weil, A. *Vitamins and Minerals*. New York: Ivy Books, 1997.

Candidiasis

Babu, U, Failla, ML. "Respiratory Burst and Candidacidal Activity of Peritoneal Macrophages are Impaired in Copper-Deficient Rats," *Journal of Nutrition* 120(12): 1692–1699, December 1990.

Boyne, R, Arthur, JR. "The Response of Selenium-Dependent Mice to *Candida albicans* Infection," *Journal of Nutrition* 116: 816–822, May 1986.

The Burton Goldberg Group (J. Strohecker, exec ed). *Alternative Medicine: The Definitive Guide*. Puyallup WA: Future Medicine Publishing, 1994, pp. 587–593.

"*Candida albicans* and Foods Containing Yeast." Seattle: Bastyr University Nutrition Clinic, 1998. Photocopy.

De Schepper, L. "Candida." 1986, pp. 28–32.

Drutz, DJ. "*Lactobacillus* Prophylaxis for *Candida* Vaginitis," comment in: *Annals of Internal Medicine* 116(5):419–420, March 1992.

Edman, J, et al. "Zinc Status in Women with Recurrent Vulvovaginal Candidiasis," *American Journal of Obstetrics and Gynecology* 155:1082–1085, 1986.

Gaia Multimedia, Inc. *Condition: Vaginitis/leukorrhea. Body System: Reproductive System*. Produced by the Alchemical Medicine Research and Teaching Association. Interactive Body/Mind Information System (IBIS), Version 1.2, 1994.

Hilton, E, et al. "Ingestion of Yogurt Containing *Lactobacillus Acidophilus* as Prophylaxis for Candidal Vaginitis," *Annals of Internal Medicine* 116(5):353–357, March 1992.

Horrowitz, BJ, et al. "Sugar Chromatography Studies in Recurrent Candida Vulvovaginitis," *The Journal of Reproductive Medicine* 29(7):441–443, July 1984.

Kennedy, MJ, et al. "Mechanisms of Association of *Candida albicans* With Intestinal Mucosa," *Journal of Medical Microbiology* 24(4):333–341, December 1987.

MacDonald, TM, et al. "The Risks of Symptomatic Vaginal Candidiasis After Oral Antibiotic Therapy," *Quarterly Journal of Medicine* 86(7):419–424, July 1993.

Olkowski, AA, et al. "Effects of Diets of High Sulphur Content and Varied Concentrations of Copper, Molybdenum, and Thiamin on In Vitro Phagocytic and Candidacidal Activity of Neutrophils in Sheep," *Research in Veterinary Science* 48(1):82–86, January 1990.

Pizzorno, JE, Murray, MT. *The Textbook of Natural Medicine*. Seattle:Bastyr University Publications, 1992, IV:Candid-1-6.

Reed, BD, et al. "The Association Between Dietary Intake and Reported History of *Candida* Vulvovaginitis," *The Family Practice* 29(5):509–515, 1989.

Rochilitz, S. *Allergies and Candida With the Physicist's Rapid Solution*. 2nd ed. Setauket NY: Human Ecology Balancing Sciences, Inc., 1989, pp. 69–91.

Canker Sores

Balch, J Balch, P. *Prescription for Nutritional Healing*. Garden City Park NY: Avery Publishing Group, 1990.

Hay, KD, et al. "The Use of an Elimination Diet in the Treatment of Recurrent Aphthous Ulceration of the Oral Cavity," *Oral Surgery* 57:504–507, 1984.

Murray, MT. *Encyclopedia of Nutritional Supplements*. Rocklin CA: Prima Publishing, 1996.

Wray, D, et al. "Recurrent Aphthae Treatment With Vitamin B_{12}, Folic Acid, and Iron," *British Medical Journal* 2:490–493, 1975.

Cardiovascular Disease

Anderson, JW, et al. "Oat Bran Cereal Lowers Serum Total and LDL Cholesterol in Hypercholesterolemic Men," *American Journal of Clinical Nutrition* 52:495–499, 1990.

Anderson, JW, et al. "Meta Analysis of the Effects of Soy Protein Intake on Serum Lipids," *New England Journal of Medicine* 333:276–282, 1995.

Aronov, DM, et al. "Clinical Trial of Wax-Matrix Sustained Release Niacin in a Russian Population with Hypercholesteremia," *Archives of Family Medicine* 5:567–575, 1996.

Ascherio, A, et al. "Trans Fatty Acids Intake and Risk of Myocardial Infarction," *Circulation* 89:94–101, 1994.

Berkow, R (ed). *The Merck Manual*. 16th ed. Rahway NJ: Merck Research Laboratories, 1992.

Bianchi, C, et al. "Alcohol Consumption and the Risk of Acute Myocardial Infarction in Women," *Journal of Epidemiology and Community Health* 47:308–311, 1993.

Block, G, Langseth, L. "Antioxidant Vitamins and Disease Prevention," *Food Technology* 80–84, July 1994.

Breithaupt-Grogler, K, et al. "Protective Effect of Chronic Garlic Intake on Elastic Properties of Aorta in the Elderly," *Circulation* 96:2649–2655, 1997.

Camargo, CA, et al. "Prospective Study of Moderate Alcohol Consumption and Risk of Peripheral Arterial Disease in U.S. Male Physicians," *Circulation* 95:577–580, 1997.

Cappuccio, FP, MacGregor, GA. "Does Potassium Supplementation Lower Blood Pressure? A Meta-Analysis of Published Trials," *Journal of Hypertension* 9:465–473, 1991.

Carbonneau, MA, et al. "Supplementation with Wine Phenolic Compounds Increases the Antioxidant Capacity of Plasma and Vitamin E of Low-Density Lipoprotein Without Changing the Lipoprotein Copper Ion Oxidability: Possible Explanation by Phenolic Location," *European Journal of Clinical Nutrition* 51: 682–690, 1997.

Cerda, JJ, et al. "The Effects of Grapefruit Pectin on Patients at Risk for Coronary Heart Disease Without Altering Diet or Lifestyle," *Clinical Cardiology* 11:589–594, 1988.

Chisholm, A, et al. "Effect on Lipoprotein Profile of Replacing Butter with Margarine in a Low Fat Diet: Randomized Study with Hypercholesteremic Subjects," *British Medical Journal* 312:931–934, 1996.

Cotran, RS, et al. *Robbins Pathologic Basis of Disease*. 5th ed. Philadelphia: W.B. Saunders Company, 1994.

Crestanello, JA, et al. "Elucidation of a Tripartite Mechanism Underlying the Improvement in Cardiac Tolerance to Ischemia by Coenzyme Q_{10} Pretreatment," *Journal of Thoractic and Cardiovascular Surgery* 111:443–450, 1996.

Croft, KD, et al. "Oxidative Susceptibility of Low-Density Lipoproteins—Influence of Regular Alcohol Use," *Alcoholism and Clinical Experimental Research* 20:980–984, 1996.

Davini, P, et al. "Controlled Study on L-Carnitine Therapeutic Efficacy in Post-Infarction," *Drugs Under Experimental Clinical Research* 18:355–365, 1992.

Frankel, EN, et al. "Inhibition of Oxidation of Human Low-Density Lipoprotein by Phenolic Substances in Red Wine," *Lancet* 341:454–457, 1993.

Gatto, LM, et al. "Ascorbic Acid Induces a Favourable Lipoprotein Profile in Women," *Journal of the American College of Nutrition* 15:154–158, 1996.

Geleijnse, JM, et al. "Dietary Electrolyte Intake and Blood Pressure in Older Subjects: The Rotterdam Study," *Journal of Hypertension* 14:737–741, 1996.

Gey, KF. "Cardiovascular Disease and Vitamins. Concurrent Correction of Suboptimal Plasma Antioxidant Levels May, as Important Part of Optimal Nutrition, Help to Prevent Early Stages of Cardiovascular Disease and Cancer, Respectively," *Bibliotheca Nutritio et Dieta* 52:75–91, 1995.

Gillman, MW, et al. "Protective Effect of Fruits and Vegetables on Development of Stroke in Men," *Journal of the American Medical Association* 273:1113–1117, 1995.

Graham, IM, et al. "Plasma Homocysteine as a Risk Factor for Vascular Disease. The European Concerted Action Project," *Journal of the American Medical Association* 277:1775–1781, 1997.

Imai, K, Nakachi, K. "Cross Sectional Study of Effects of Drinking Green Tea on Cardiovascular and Liver Diseases," *British Medical Journal* 310:693–696, 1995.

Jenkins, DJ, et al. "Effect of Diet High in Vegetables, Fruit, and Nuts on Serum Lipids," *Metabolism* 46:530–537, 1997.

Kurowska, EM, et al. "Effects of Substituting Dietary Soybean Protein and Oil for Milk Protein an Fat in Subjects with Hypercholesteremia," *Clinical and Investigative Medicine* 20:162–170, 1997.

Lark, SM. *Women's Health Companion.* Berkeley CA: Celestial Arts, 1995.

McCarron, DA. "Role of Adequate Dietary Calcium Intake in the Prevention and Management of Salt-Sensitive Hypertension," *American Journal of Clinical Nutrition* 65:712S–716S, 1997.

Miura, S, et al. "Effects of Various Natural Antioxidants on the Copper Ion Mediated Oxidative Modification of Low Density Lipoprotein," *Biological and Pharmaceutical Bulletin* 18:1–4, 1995.

Mizushima, S, et al. "Fish Intake and Cardiovascular Risk Among Middle-Aged Japanese in Japan and Brazil," *Journal of Cardiovascular Risk* 4:191–199, 1997.

Mori, TA, et al. "Interactions Between Dietary Fat, Fish and Fish Oils and Their Effects on Platelet Function in Men at Risk of Cardiovascular Disease," *Arteriosclerosis, Thrombosis, and Vascular Biology* 17:279–286, 1997.

Morrison, III, et al. "Serum Folate and Risk of Fatal Coronary Heart Disease," *Journal of the American Medical Association* 275:1893–1896, 1996.

Murray, MT. *The Complete Book of Juicing.* Rocklin CA: Prima Publishing, 1992.

Murray, MT. *The Healing Power of Herbs.* 2nd ed. Rocklin CA: Prima Publishing, 1995.

Murray, MT, Pizzorno, J. *The Encyclopedia of Natural Medicine.* 2nd ed. Rocklin CA: Prima Publishing, 1998.

Ness, AR, Powles, JW. "Fruits and Vegetables, and Cardiovascular Disease: A Review," *International Journal of Epidemiology* 26:1–13, 1997.

Ness, AR, et al. "Vitamin C Status and Blood Pressure," *Journal of Hypertension* 14:503–508, 1996.

Oliver, MF. "It Is More Important to Increase the Intake of Unsaturated Fats than to Decrease the Intake of Saturated Fats: Evidence from Clinical Trials Relating to Ischemic Heart Disease," *American Journal of Clinical Nutrition* 66:980S–986S, 1997.

Olson, BH, et al. "Psyllium Enriched Cereals Lower Blood Total Cholesterol and LDL Cholesterol but Not HDL Cholesterol in Hypercholesterolemic Adults: Results of Meta-Analysis," *Journal of Nutrition* 127:1973–1980, 1997.

Orekhov, AN, Tertov, VV. "In Vitro Effect

of Garlic Powder Extract on Lipid Content in Normal and Atherosclerotic Human Aortic Cells," *Lipids* 32:1055–1060, 1997.

Ornish, D, et al. "Can Lifestyle Changes Reverse Coronary Heart Disease? The Lifestyle Heart Trial," *Lancet* 336:129–133, 1990.

Palmer, JR, et al. "Coffee Consumption and Myocardial Infarction in Women," *American Journal of Epidemiology* 141: 724–731, 1995.

Pucciarelli, G, et al. "The Clinical and Hemodynamic Effects of Propionyl-L-Carnitine in the Treatment of Congestive Heart Failure," *Clinica Terapeutica* 141: 379–384, 1992.

Rifier, VA, Khachadurian, AK. "Effects of Vitamin C and E Supplementation on the Copper Mediated Oxidation of HDL and on HDL Mediated Cholesterol Efflux," *Atherosclerosis* 127:19–26, 1996.

Robbers, J, et al. *Pharmacognosy and Pharmacobiotechnology.* Baltimore: Williams & Wilkins, 1996.

Robertson, D, et al. "Tolerance to the Humoral and Hemodynamic Effects of Caffeine in Man," *Journal of Clinical Investigation* 67:1111–1117, 1981.

Robertson, J, et al. "The Effect of Raw Carrots on Serum Lipids and Colon Function," *American Journal of Clinical Nutrition* 32:1889–1892, 1979.

Robinson, K, et al. "Low Circulating Folate and Vitamin B_6 Concentrations: Risk Factors for Stroke, Peripheral Vascular Disease, and Coronary Artery Disease, European COMAC Group," *Circulation* 97:437–443, 1998.

Salonen, JT, et al. "Effects of Antioxidant Supplementation on Platelet Function: A Randomized Pair-Matched Placebo Controlled Double Blind Trial in Men with Low Antioxidant Status," *American Journal of Clinical Nutrition* 53:1222–1229, 1991.

Santos, MJ, et al. "Influence of Dietary Supplementation with Fish on Plasma Fatty Acid Composition in Coronary Heart Disease Patients," *Annals of Nutrition and Metabolism* 39:52–62, 1995.

Schneider, J, et al. "Alcohol Lipid Metabolism and Coronary Heart Disease," *Herz* 21:217–226, 1996.

Skrabal, F, et al. "Low Sodium/High Potassium Diet for Prevention of Hypertension: Probable Mechanisms of Action," *Lancet* 2:895–900, 1981.

Soja, AM, Mortensen, SA. "Treatment of Chronic Cardiac Insufficiency With Coenzyme Q_{10}, Results of Meta-Analysis in Controlled Clinical Trials," *Ugeskr Laeger* 159:7302–7308, 1997.

Takamatsu, S, et al. "Effects on Health of Dietary Supplementation with 100 mg d-Alpha Tocopheryl Acetate Daily for 6 Years," *Journal of International Medical Research* 23:342–357, 1995.

Tavani, A, et al. "Beta Carotene Intake and Risk of Nonfatal Acute Myocardial Infarction in Women," *European Journal of Epidemiology* 13:631–637, 1997.

Troisi, R, et al. "Trans Fatty Acid Intake in Relation to Serum Lipid Concentrations in Adult Men," *American Journal of Clinical Nutrition* 56:1019–1024, 1992.

Weber, C, et al. "The Coenzyme Q_{10} Content of the Average Danish Diet," *International Journal for Vitamin and Nutrition Research* 67:123–129, 1997.

Werbach, M. *Healing With Food.* New York: HarperCollins Publishers, 1993.

Willett, WC, et al. "Intake of Trans Fatty Acids and Risk of Coronary Heart Disease Among Women," *Lancet* 341:581–585, 1993.

Wise, KJ, et al. "Interactions Between Dietary Calcium and Caffeine Consumption on Calcium Metabolism in Hypertensive Humans," *American Journal of Hypertension* 9:223–229, 1996.

Carpal Tunnel Syndrome

Bernstein, AL, Dinesen, JS. "Brief Communication: Effect of Pharmacologic Doses of Vitamin B_6 on Carpal Tunnel Syndrome, Electroencephalographic Results in Pain," *Journal of the American College of Nutrition* 12(1):73–76, February 1993.

Folkers K, Ellis J. "Successful Therapy with Vitamin B_6 and Vitamin B_2 of the Carpal Tunnel Syndrome and Need for Determination of the RDA's for Vitamin B_6 and B_2 Disease States," *Annals of the New York Academy of Sciences* 585:295–301, 1990.

Fuhr, JE, et al. "Vitamin B_6 Levels in Patients with Carpal Tunnel Syndrome," *Archives of Surgery* 124:1329–1330, 1989.

Gaby, A, Wright, J. *Nutritional Therapy In Medical Practice.* Seattle: Gaby/Wright Seminars, 1996, p. 18.

Gaia Multimedia, Inc. *Carpal Tunnel Syndrome.* Produced by the Alchemical Medicine Research and Teaching Association. Interactive Body/Mind Information System (IBIS), Version 1.2, 1994.

Gould, JS, Wissinger, HA. "Carpal Tunnel Syndrome in Pregnancy," *Southern Medical Journal* 71:144, 1978.

Haas, EM. *Staying Healthy With Nutrition.* Berkeley CA: Celestial Arts, 1992, p. 22.

Ombregt, L, et al. *A System of Orthopedic Medicine.* London: WB Saunders, Co., 1995, pp. 393–399.

Pizzorno, J, Murray, M. *Textbook of Natural Medicine.* Seattle: Bastyr University Publications, 1992, VI:CTS-1-2.

Roe, D. *Drug-Induced Nutritional Deficiencies.* Westport CT: AVI, 1976, pp. 166–167.

Werbach, M. *Nutritional Influences on Illness.* New Canaan CT: Keats Publishing, 1988, pp. 192–193.

Chronic Fatigue Syndrome

Barnes, CL, et al. "Chronic Fatigue Syndrome: What are the Facts?" *The Journal of Practical Nursing* 24–31, September 1993.

The Burton Goldberg Group (J. Strohecker, exec ed). *Alternative Medicine: The Definitive Guide.* Puyallup WA: Future Medicine Publishing, 1994, pp. 616–624.

Carter, RE. "Chronic Intestinal Candidiasis as a Possible Etiological Factor in the Chronic Fatigue Syndrome," *Medical Hypotheses* June 44(6):507–515, 1995.

Cox, IM, Campbell, MJ, et al. "Red Blood Cell Magnesium and Chronic Fatigue Syndrome," *Lancet* 337:757–760, 1991.

Douglass, J. "Nutrition, Nonthermally-Prepared Food and Nature's Message to Man," *Journal of the International Academy of Preventative Medicine* VII(2). July 1982. In: Kenton, L, Kenton, S. *Raw Energy.* London: Century Publishing Co. Ltd., 1984.

Haas, EM. *Staying Healthy With Nutrition.* Berkeley CA: Celestial Arts, 1992.

Hoffmann, D. *The Herbal Handbook: A User's Guide to Medical Herbalism.* Rochester NY: Healing Arts Press, 1988.

Hoffmann, D. *The New Holistic Herbal.* 3rd ed. Rockport MA: Element Books, Inc., 1992.

Jacobson, W, et al. "Serum Folate and Chronic Fatigue Syndrome," *Neuropsychobiology* 35(1):16–23, 1997.

Murray, M, Pizzorno, J. *The Encyclopedia of Natural Medicine.* Rocklin CA: Prima Publishing, 1990.

Pitchford, P. *Healing With Whole Foods: Oriental Traditions and Modern Nutrition.* Berkeley CA: North Atlantic Books, 1993.

Pizzorno, J, Murray, MT. *The Textbook of Natural Medicine.* Seattle: Bastyr University Publications, 1992, Mono Ch-1.

Pliophys, AV, Pliophys, S. "Amantadine and L-Carnitine Treatment of Chronic Fatigue Syndrome," *Lancet* 337:757–760, 1991.

Pliophys, AV, Pliophys, S. "Serum Levels of Carnitine in Chronic Fatigue Syndrome: Clinical Correlates," *Neuropsychobiology* 32(3):132–138, 1995.

Pompei, R, Pani, A, et al. "Antiviral Activity of Glycyrrhizic Acid," *Experientia* 36(3):304–305, 1980.

Straus, SE, Dale, DK, et al. "Allergy and the Chronic Fatigue Syndrome," *Journal of Allergy and Clinical Immunology* 81(5): 791–795, 1988.

Colds

Abbas, AK, Lichtman, et al. *Cellular and Molecular Immunology.* Philadelphia: WB Saunders Co., 1994, pp. 328, 396.

Balch, J Balch, P. *Prescription for Nutritional Healing.* 2nd ed. Garden City Park NY: Avery Publishing Group, 1997, pg. 209.

Baurn, MK, et al. "HIV-1 Infection in Women is Associated With Severe Nutritional Deficiencies," *Journal of Acquired Immune Deficiency Syndromes and Human Retrovirology* 16(4):272–278, 1997.

Cowgill, UM. "The Distribution of Selenium and Mortality Owing to Acquired Immune Deficiency Syndrome in the Continental US," *Biological Trace Element Research* 56(1):43–61, 1997.

Garland, MI, Hagneyer, KO. "The Role of Zinc Lozenges in Treatment of the Common Cold," *Annals of Pharmacotherapy* 32(1):63–69, 1998.

Glasziou, PP, MacKerras, DEM. "Vitamin A Supplementation in Infectious Diseases: A Meta Analysis," *British Medical Journal* 306:366–370, 1993.

Haas, E. *Staying Healthy With Nutrition: The Complete Guide to Diet and Nutritional Medicine.* Berkeley CA: Celestial Arts Publishing, 1992, pp. 96, 213.

Hemil, AH. "Vitamin C and Common Cold Incidence: A Review of Studies with Subjects Under Heavy Physical Stress," *International Journal of Sports Medicine* 17(5):379–383, 1996.

Hemil, AH. "Vitamin C, the Placebo Effect, and the Common Cold: A Case Study of How Preconceptions Influence the Analysis of Results," *Journal of Clinical Epidemiology* 49(10):1079–1084, October 1996.

Hemil, AH. "Vitamin C Intake and Susceptibility to the Common Cold," *British Journal of Nutrition* 77(1):59–72, 1997.

Hunt, C, et al. "The Clinical Effects of Vitamin C Supplementation in Elderly Hospitalized Patients with Acute Respiratory Infections," *International Journal for Vitamin and Nutrition Research* 64(3):212–219, 1994.

Kiremidjian-Schumacher, L, et al. "Supplementation With Selenium and Human Immune Cell Functions II: Effect on Cytotoxic Lymphocytes and Natural Killer Cells," *Biological Trace Element Research* 41(1–2):115–127, 1994.

Makowska-Zwierz, W, et al. "The Effect of Vitamin E on Granulocyte Function in Patients With Recurrent Infections," *Archivm Immunologiae et Therapiae Experimentalis (Warz)* 39(1–2):109–115, 1991.

Mossad, SB, et al. "Zinc Gluconate Lozenges for Treating the Common Cold: A Randomized Double-Blind, Placebo-Controlled Study," *Annals of Internal Medicine* 125(2):81–88, 1996.

Murray, MT. *The Complete Book of Juicing.* Rocklin CA: Prima Publishing, 1992, pp. 71, 136, 157, 209–210, 214.

Murray, MT. *The Healing Power of Herbs.* 2nd ed. Rocklin CA: Prima Publishing, 1992, pp. 102, 124, 355.

Murray, MT, Pizzorno, J. *The Encyclopedia of Natural Medicine.* 2nd ed. Rocklin CA: Prima Publishing, 1998, pp. 148–157, 371–376.

Novick, SG, et al. "Zinc Induced Suppression of Inflammation in the Respiratory Tract, Caused by Infection with Human Rhinovirus and Other Irritants," *Medical Hypotheses* 49(4):347–357, 1997.

Peretz, A. "Lymphocyte Response is Enhanced by Supplementation of Elderly Subjects with Selenium-Enriched Yeast," *American Journal of Clinical Nutrition* 53(5): 1323–1328, 1991.

Price, S, Price, L. *Aromatherapy for Health Professionals.* New York: Churchill Livingstone, 1995, pp. 249, 253.

See, DM, et al. "In Vitro Effects of Echinacea and Ginseng on Natural Killer and Antibody-Dependent Cell Cytotoxicity in Healthy Subjects and Chronic Fatigue Syndrome or Acquired Immunodeficiency Syndrome Patients," *Immunopharmacology* 35(3):229–235, 1997.

Werbach, M. *Healing With Food.* New York: Collins Publishers, 1993, pp. 77, 201.

Colitis

Bartels, M, et al. "What Is the Role of Nutrition in Ulcerative Colitis? A Contribution to the Current Status of Diet Therapy in Treatment of Inflammatory Bowel Disease," *Langenbecks Arch fur Chirurgie* 380 (1):4–11, 1995.

Belluzzi, A, et al. "Effect of an Enteric-Coated Fish-Oil Preparation on Relapses in Crohn's Disease," *The New England Journal of Medicine* 34:1557–1560, 13 June 1996.

Burke, A, et al. "Nutrition and Ulcerative Colitis," *Baillieres Clinical Gastroenterology* 11(1):153–174, March 1997.

"Dietary and Other Risk Factors of Ulcerative Colitis: A Case-Controlled Study in Japan," *Journal of Clinical Gastroenterology* 19(2):166–171, September 1994.

Heaton, K., et al. "Treatment of Crohn's Disease With an Unrefined-Carbohydrate, Fibre-Rich Diet," *British Medical Journal* 2:764–766, September 1979.

Hoffmann, D. *The New Holistic Herbal.* Rockport MA: Element, Inc. 1990.

Hyde, AC. "An Herbal Practitioner's Approach to Irritable Bowel Syndrome," *The European Journal of Herbal Medicine* 1(2): 44–47, Summer 1994.

Jarrett, M, et al. "Comparison of Diet Composition in Women With and Without Functional Bowel Disorder," *Gastroenterology Nursing* 16(6):253–258, June 1994.

Jones, V, et al. "Crohn's Disease: Maintenance of Remission by Diet," *Lancet* 1:177–180, July 1985.

Meier, R. "Chronic Inflammatory Bowel Disease and Nutrition," *Schweizerische Medizinische Wochenschrift Supplement* 79:14S–24S, 1996.

Murray, M, Pizzorno, J. *Encyclopedia of Natural Medicine.* Rocklin CA: Prima Publishing, 1990.

Peck, P. "Glutamine Should be Figured Into IBD Formulation," *Family Practice News* 22, 1 June 1994.

Raif, S, et al. "Pre-illness Dietary Factors in Inflammatory Bowel Diseae," *Gut* 40(6):754–760, June 1997.

Reichert, R. "Treatment of Ulcerative Colitis with Boswellia Serrata," *Quarterly Review of Natural Medicine* 175–176, Fall 1997.

Rhodes, JM. "Unifying Hypothesis for Inflammatory Bowel Disease and Associated Colon Cancer: Sticking the Pieces Together With Sugar," *Lancet* 346:40–44, 6 January 1996.

Sandler, RS. "Epidemiology of Irritable Bowel Syndrome in the United States," *Gastroenterology* 99(2):409–415, August 1990.

Shoda, R, et al. "Epidemiologic Analysis of Crohn's Disease in Japan: Increased Dietary Intake of n-6 Polyunsaturated Fatty Acids and Animal Protein Relates to the Increased Incidence of Crohn's Disease in Japan," *American Journal of Clinical Nutrition* 63:741–745, 1996.

Sonnerville, K, et al. "Delayed Release Peppermint Oil Capsules (Colpermin) for the Spastic Colon Syndrome: A Pharmacokinetic Study," *British Journal of Clinical Pharmacology* 18:638–640, 1984. In: Murray, M, Pizzorno, J. *The Encyclopedia of Natural Medicine.* Rocklin CA: Prima Publishing, 1990, p. 399.

Thornton, J, et al. "Diet and Crohn's Disease: Characteristics of the Pre-illness Diet," *British Medical Journal* September 2:762–764, 1979.

Tragnone, A, et al. "Dietary Habits as Risk Factors for Inflammatory Bowel Disease," *European Journal of Gastroenterology* 7(1): 47–51, January 1995.

Vernia, P, et al. "Lactose Malabsorption and Irritable Bowel Syndrome. Effect of a Long-Term Lactose-Free Diet," *Italian Journal of Gastroenterology* 27(3):117–121, April 1995.

Walker, AR. "Diet and Bowel Diseases—Past History and Future Prospects," *South*

African Medical Journal 68(3):148–152, 3 August 1985.

Constipation

Badiali, D, et al. "Effect of Wheat Bran in the Treatment of Chronic, Nonorganic Constipation: A Double-Blind Controlled Trial," *Digestive Diseases and Sciences* 40(2):349–356, February 1995.

"Help for When You're Constipated," *Family Practice Recertification* 17(4):54, April 1995.

Lupton, JR, et al. "Barley Bran Flour Accelerates Gastrointestinal Transit Time," *Journal of American Dietetic Association* 93:881–885, 1993.

Cravings

Barnett, RA. *Tonics.* New York: HarperCollins, 1997.

Blundall, JE, et al. "Mechanisms of Appetite Control and Their Abnormalities in Obese Patients," *Hormone Research* 39: 72–76, 1993.

Burton, BT, Foster, WR. *Human Nutrition.* New York: McGraw-Hill Book Co., 1998.

Carper, J. Food: Your *Miracle Medicine.* New York: HarperCollins, 1993.

Christensen, L, Somers, S. "Comparison of Nutrient Intake Among Depressed and Nondepressed Individuals," *International Journal of Eating Disorders* 20:105–109, July 1996.

Dye, L, Blundell, JE. "Menstrual Cycle and Appetite Control: Implications for Weight Regulation," *Human Reproduction* 12:1142–1151, June 1997.

Haas, EM. *Staying Healthy With Nutrition.* Berkeley CA: Celestial Arts, 1992.

Heller, RF. "Hyperinsulinemic Obesity and Carbohydrate Addiction: The Missing Link is the Carbohydrate Frequency Factor," *Medical Hypotheses* 42:307–312, May 1994.

Hunt, D. *No More Cravings.* New York: Warner Books, 1987.

Kenton, L, Kenton, S. *Raw Energy.* London: Century Publishing, 1985.

Mercer, ME. "Food Cravings, Endogenous Opiad Peptides, and Food Intake: A Review," *Appetite* 29:3225–3252, December 1997.

Monte, T. *World Medicine: The East West Guide to Healing Your Body.* New York: Jeremy P. Tarcher, 1993, p. 216.

Sayegh, R, et al. "The Effect of a Carbohydrate-Rich Beverage on Mood, Appetite, and Cognitive Function in Women with Premenstrual Syndrome," *Obstetrics and Gynecology* 86:520–528, October 1995.

Wallach, JD, Lan, M. *Rare Earth's Forbidden Cures.* Bonita CA: Double Happiness Publishing Co., 1994.

Depression

Alpert, JE, Fava, M. "Nutrition and Depression: the Role of Folate," *Nutrition Reviews* 55:145–149, 1997.

Anada, RF, et al. "Depression and the Dynamics of Smoking. A National Perspective," *Journal of the American Medical Association* 264:1583–1584, 1990.

Balch, JF, Balch, PA. *Prescription for Nutritional Healing.* Garden City Park NY: Avery Publishing Group, 1990.

Bell, JR, et al. "Brief Communication. Vitamin B_1, B_2, and B_6 Augmentation of Tricyclic Antidepressant Treatment in Geriatric Depression with Cognitive Dysfunction," *Journal of the American College of Nutrition* 11:159–163, 1992.

Bell, JR, et al. "Symptom and Personality Profiles of Young Adults From College Student Population with Self-Reported Illness from Foods and Chemicals," *Journal of the American College of Nutrition* 12: 693–702, 1993.

Birmaher, B, et al. "Cellular Immunity in Depressed, Conduct Disorder, and Normal Adolescents: Role of Adverse Life Events," *Journal of the American Academy of Child and Adolescent Psychiatry* 33:671–678, 1994.

Bottiglieri, T. "Folate, Vitamin B_{12}, and Neuropsychiatric Disorders," *Nutrition Review* 54:382–390, 1996.

Bucco, G. "Fading the Winter Blues," *Herbs for Health* 34–37, 1998.

Christensen, L, Somers, S. "Adequacy of the Dietary Intake of Depressed Individuals," *Journal of the American College of Nutrition* 13:597–600, 1994.

Ellenbogen, MA, et al. "Mood Response to Acute Tryptophan Depletion in Healthy Volunteers: Sex Differences and Temporal Stability," *Neuropsychopharmacology* 15: 465–474, 1996.

Hibben, JR, Salem, N. "Dietary Polyunsaturated Fatty Acids and Depression: When Cholesterol Does Not Satisfy," *Journal of the American College of Nutrition* 62:1–9, 1995.

Irwin, M, et al. "Depression and Reduced Natural Killer Cytoxicity: a Longitudinal Study of Depressed Patients and Control Subjects," *Psychological Medicine* 22:1045–1050, 1992.

Maes, M. "A Review of the Acute Phase Response in Major Depression," *Reviews in the Neurosciences* 4:407–416, 1993.

Murray, M, Pizzorno, J. *Encyclopedia of Natural Medicine.* 2nd ed. Rocklin CA: Prima Publishing, 1998.

Van Straten, M. *Healing Foods.* New York: Barnes & Noble, 1997.

Werbach, MR. *Nutritional Influences on Illness.* New Canaan CT: Keats, 1990.

Young, SN. "Use of Tryptophan in Combination With Other Antidepressant Treatments: A Review," *Journal of Psychiatry and Neuroscience* 16:241–246, 1991.

Diabetes Mellitus

Alschuler, L. Botanical Medicine I, II, III, IV (lectures). Seattle: Bastyr University, 1998.

Borkman, M, et al. "The Relation Between Insulin Sensitivity and the Fatty-Acid Composition of Skeletal-Muscle Phospholipids," *The New England Journal of Medicine* 328:238, 1993. In: Rudin, D, Felix, C. *Omega-3 Oils.* Garden City Park NY: Avery Publishing Group, 1996, pp. 63–64.

Cunningham, JJ. "Micronutrients as Nutriceutical Interventions in Diabetes Mellitus," *Journal of the American College of Nutrition* 17:7–10, 1998.

Gaby, A. Therapeutic Nutrition I, II (lectures). Seattle: Bastyr University, 1998.

Geil, PB, Anderson, JW. "Nutrition and Health Implications of Dry Beans: Review," *Journal of the American College of Nutrition* 13:549–558, 1994.

Grogg, JL, Gropper, SS, Hunt, SM. *Advanced Nutrition and Human Metabolism.* 2nd ed. New York: West Publishing Co., 1995.

Haas, EM. *Staying Healthy With Nutrition.* Berkeley CA: Celestial Arts, 1992.

Heinerman, J. *Heinerman's Encyclopedia of Healing Juices.* Englewood Cliffs NJ: Prentice Hall, 1994.

Jovanovic-Peterson, L, Peterson, CM. "Review of Gestational Diabetes Mellitus and Low-Calorie Diet and Physical Exercise as Therapy," *Diabetes/Metabolism Reviews* 12: 287–308, 1996.

Jovanovic-Peterson, L, Peterson, CM. "Vitamin and Mineral Deficiencies Which May Predispose to Glucose Intolerance of Pregnancy," *Journal of the American College of Nutrition* 15:14–20, 1996.

Kenton, L, Kenton, S. *Raw Energy.* London: Century Publishing, 1985.

Kirschmann, GJ, Kirschmann, JD. *Nutrition Almanac.* 4th ed. New York: McGraw-Hill, 1996.

Mann, JI. "The Role of Nutritional Modifications in the Prevention of Macrovascular Complications of Diabetes," *Diabetes* 46(2):S125–S130, 1997.

McCarron, DA, et al. "Nutritional Management of Cardiovascular Risk Factors: A Randomized Clinical Trial," *Archives of Internal Medicine* 157:169–177, 1997.

Mertz, W. "A Balanced Approach to Nutrition for Health: The Need for Biologically Essential Minerals and Vitamins (see comments)," *Journal of American Dietetic Association* 94:1259–1262, 1994.

Mooradian, AD, et al. "Selected Vitamins and Minerals in Diabetes," *Diabetes Care* 17:464–479, 1994.

"Nutrition Recommendations and Principles for People with Diabetes Mellitus," *Journal of American Dietetic Association* 504–506, 1994.

Toeller, M. "Diet and Diabetes," *Diabetes/Metabolism Reviews* 9:93–108, 1993.

Diverticulitis and Diverticulosis

Balch, JF, Balch, PA. *Prescription for Nutritional Healing.* Garden City Park NY: Avery Publishing Group, 1990.

Burton, BT. *Human Nutrition.* New York: McGraw-Hill, 1988.

Dean, R, et al. "Preventing Diverticulosis," *The Canadian Nurse* 86:35–36, September 1990.

Malbey, R. *The New Age Herbalist.* New York: McMillian Publishing Co., 1988.

O'Keefe, S. "Nutrition and Gastrointestinal Disease," *Scandinavian Journal of Gastroenterology Supplement* 220:52–58, 1996.

Pitchford, P. *Healing With Whole Foods: Oriental Traditions and Modern Nutrition.* Berkeley CA: North Atlantic Books, 1993.

Silverman, HM. "Therapeutic Fiber: Its Role in Disease Treatment and Prevention," *The Journal of Practical Nursing* 40:18–26, June 1990.

Weiss, RF. *Herbal Medicine.* Beaconsfield, England: Beaconsfield Publishers LTD, 1988.

Eczema (Atopic Dermatitis)

Anderson, JA. "Milk, Eggs and Peanuts: Food Allergies in Children," *American Family Physician* 56(5):1365–1374, October 1997.

Bindslev-Jensen, C, et al. "Atopic Dermatitis," *Ugeeskr-Laeger* 159(42):6199–6204, October 1997.

Borrek, S, et al. "Gamma-Linolenic Acid-Rich Borage Seed Oil Capsules in Children with Atopic Dermatitis. A Placebo Controlled Double Blind Study," *Klinisch Padiatrie* 209(3):100–104, May 1997.

Businco, L, et al. "Breast Milk from Mothers of Children with Newly Developed Atopic Eczema has Low Levels of Long Chain Polyunsaturated Fatty Acids," *Journal of Allergy and Clinical Immunology* 91(6):1134–1139, June 1993.

Cotterill, JA. "Psychophysiological Aspects of Eczema," *Seminars in Dermatology* 3:216–219, 9 September 1990.

Di-Gioacchino, M, et al. "Allergic Contact Dermatitus to Nickel: Modification of Receptor Expression on Peripheral Lymphocytes of Woman After Oral Provocation Tests," *Giornale Italiano di Medicina del Lavoro ed Ergonomia* 19(1):56–58, January-March 1997.

Dotterud, LK. "Role of Food in Atopic Eczema," *Tidsskrift Norske Laegeforening* 116(28):3335–3340, November 1996.

Eberlein-Konig, B, et al. "Change of Skin Roughness Due to Lowering Air Humidity in Climate Chamber," *Acta Dermatologica Venerologica* 76(6):447–449, November 1996.

Flyvholm, MA, et al. "Nickel Content of Food and Estimation of Dietary Intake," *Zitschrift für Lebensum Unters Forsch* 179(6):427–431, December 1984.

Gmoshinskii, IV, et al. "Disordered Permeability of the Gastrointestinal Tract Barrier for Macromolecules and the Possibilities for Its Experimental Dietetic Correction," *Fiziolohichnyi Zhurnal I M Sechenova* 79(6):115–127, June 1993.

Host'ynek, JJ. "Gold: An Allergen of Growing Significance," *Food and Chemical Toxicology* 35(8):839–844, August 1997.

Leung, DY. "Atopic Dermatitis: Immunobiology and Treatment with Immune Modulators," *Clinical and Experimental Immunology* 7(1):25–30, 10 January 1997.

Majamaa, H, et al. "Intestinal Inflammation in Children with Atopic Eczema; Fae-

162

Juice Lady's Guide to Juicing for Health

cal Eosinophil Cationic Protein and Tumor Necrosis Factor-Alpha as Non-Inva-
sive Indicators of Food Allergy," *Clinical
and Experimental Allergy* 26(2):181–187,
February 1996.

Majamaa, H, et al. "Probiotics: A Novel
Approach in the Management of Food Allergy," *Journal of Allergy and Clinical Immunology* 99(2):179–185, February 1997.

"Metabolic Pathways of Essential Fatty
Acids," *Protocol Jour Bot Med* 1(1):18–19,
Summer 1995.

Morse, PF, et al. "Meta Analysis of Placebo Controlled Studies of the Efficacy of
Epogam in the Treatment of Atopic
Eczema. Relationship Between Plasma Essential Fatty Acid Changes and Clinical
Response," *British Journal of Dermatology*
121(1):75–90, July 1989.

Murray, M, Buetler. *Understanding Fats and
Oils: Your Guide to Healing with Essentail
Fatty Acids.* Encinitas CA: Progressive
Health Publishing, 1996.

Murray, M, Pizzorno, J. *The Encyclopedia of
Natural Medicine.* 2nd ed. Rocklin CA: Prima Publishing, 1998.

Ockenfels, HM, et al. "Contact Allergy in
Patients With Periorbital Eczema: An
Analysis of Allergens. Data Recorded by
the Information Network of the Department of Dermatology," *Dermatology* 195
(2):119–124, 1997.

Ring, J, et al. "Atopic Eczema, Langerhans
Cells and Allergy," *International Archives of
Allergy and Applied Immunology* 94(1–4):
194–201, 1991.

Wollenberg, A, et al. "Immunomorpho-
logical and Ultrastructoral Characteriza-
tion of Langerhans Cells and a Novel, Inflammatory Dendritic Epidermal Cell
(IDEC) Population in Lesional Skin of
Atopic Eczema," *Journal of Investigative
Dermatology* 106(3):446–453, March 1996.

Wright, S, Sanders, TA. "Adipose Tissue
Essential Fatty Acid Composition in Patients with Atopic Eczema," *European Journal of Clinical Nutrition* 45(10):501–505, October 1991.

Epilepsy and Seizures

Burhanoglin, M. "Hypozincemia in Febrile Convulsions," *European Journal of Pediatrics* 155:498–501, 1996.

Bykowski, M. "Unhealthy Liquids May
Promote Obesity," *Family Practice News* 61,
1 March 1997.

Gobbi, G., et al. "Celiac Disease, Epilepsy
and Cerebral Calcifications," *Lancet* 340:
439–442, 22 August 1992.

Kiviranta, T, Airaksinen, EM. "Low Sodium Levels in Serum Are Associated with
Subsequent Febrile Seizures," *Acta Pediatrics* 84:1372–1374, 1995.

Krahn, LE. "Use of Caffeine in Medically
Refractory Seizure Patients," *Neuropsychi-
atry, Neuropsychology and Behavioral Neurology* 7(2):136, 1994.

Maltz, G. "Ketogenic Diet Can Control
Seizures in Epileptic Children," *Family
Practice News* 23, 15 December 1994.

Murray, M. *The Encyclopedia of Nutritional
Supplements.* Rocklin CA: Prima Publishing, 1996.

Nakagawa, E., et al. "Efficacy of Pyridox-
al Phosphate in Treating an Adult With Intractable Status Epileptics," *Neurology*
48:1468–1469, May 1997.

Prasad, AN, et al. "Alternative Epilepsy
Therapies: The Ketogenic Diet, Im-
munoglobulins, and Steroids," *Epilepsia*
37(Suppl. 1):S81–S95, 1996.

Ramaekers, V, et al. "Selenium Deficiency
Triggering Intractable Seizures," *Neurological Pediatrics* 25:216–223, 1994.

Torbi, D. et al. "Free Radical Generation in
the Brain Precedes Hyperbaric Oxygen-
Induced Convulsions," *Free Radical Biology in Medicine* 13:101–106, 1992.

Eye Disorders

Ahirot-Westerlund, B, Norrby, A. "Cataracts, Vitamin E and Selenomethionine,"
Acta Ophthalmologica Scandinavica 237–
238, April 1988.

Awasthi, S, et al. "Curcumin Protects
Against 4-Hydroxy-2-Trans-Nonenal-In-

duced Cataract Formation in Rat Lenses," *American Journal of Clinical Nutrition* 64:761–766, 1996.

Bunce, GE. "Nutrition and Eye Disease of the Elderly," *Journal of Nutritional Biochemistry* 5:66–76, February 1994.

Harding, J. "Cigarettes and Cataract: Cadmium or a Lack of Vitamin C," *British Journal of Ophthalmology* 70:199–201, 1995.

Karakucuk, S, et al. "Selenium Concentrations in Serum, Lens, and Aqueous Humor of Patients with Senile Cataracts," *Acta Ophthalmologica Scandinavica* 73:323–332, 1995.

Mares-Perlman, J, et al. "Diet and Nuclear Lens Opacities," *American Journal of Epidemiology* 141(4):322–334, 1995.

Potter, AR. "Reducing Vitamin A Deficiency: Could Save the Eyesight and Lives of Countless Children," *British Medical Journal* 314:317–318, 1 February 1997.

Schalch, W. "Carotenoids in the Retina— A Review of Their Possible Role in Preventing or Limiting Damage Caused by Light and Oxygen," In: *Free Radicals and Aging.* Basel, Switzerland: Birkhauser Verlag, 1992, pp. 280–298.

Tavani, A, et al. "Food and Nutrient Intake and Risk of Cataract," *Annals of Epidemiology* 6:41–46, 1996.

Taylor, A. "Effects of Nutrition on Cataract and Macular Degeneration (Beyond Nutrition: New Views on the Function and Health Effects of Vitamins)," *New York Academy of Sciences*, 10:9–12 February 1992;10.

Taylor, A, et al. "Relations Among Aging, Antioxidant Status, and Cataract," *American Journal of Clinical Nutrition* 62(Suppl.):1439S–1447S, 1995.

White, AC, et al. "Glutathione Deficiency in Human Disease," *Journal of Nutritional Biochemistry* 5:218–226, May 1994.

Fibrocystic Breast Disease

Berkow, R (ed). *The Merck Manual.* 16th ed. Rahway NJ: Merck Research Laboratories, 1992.

Boyd, NF, et al. "Effect of a Low Fat, High Carbohydrate Diet on Symptoms of Cyclical Mastopathy," *Lancet* 2(8603):128–132, 1988.

DeCherney, AH, Pernoll, MI (eds). *Current Obstetrics and Gynaecology Diagnosis and Treatment.* East Norwalk CT: Appleton and Lange, 1994, pp. 1118–1119.

Estes, NC. "Mastodynia Due to Fibrocystic Disease of the Breast Controlled with Thyroid Hormone," *American Journal of Surgery* 142(6):764–766, 1981.

Haas, F. *Staying Healthy With Nutrition: The Complete Guide to Diet and Nutritional Medicine.* Berkeley CA: Celestial Arts Publishing, 1992, pp. 67-69, 94-98, 101-102.

Hoffmann, D. *The New Holistic Herbal.* Rockport MA: Element, Inc., 1990, p. 61.

Hoffmann, D. *Therapeutic Herbalism. A Correspondence Course in Phytotherapy.* 2-175-2-176.

Hudson, T. *Gynaecology and Naturopathic Medicine.* 3rd ed. TR Publications, 1994, ch. 7.

Lark, SM. *The Woman's Health Companion.* Berkeley CA: Celestial Arts Publishing, 1995, pp. 113–117, 191.

London, RS, et al. "The Effect of Alpha-Tocopherol on Premenstrual Symptomatology: A Double-Blind Study," *Journal of the American College of Nutrition* 2(2):115–122, 1983.

Martinez, I, et al. "Thyroid Hormones in Fibrocystic Breast Disease," *European Journal of Endocrinology* 132(6):673–676, 1995.

Meyer, EC, et al. "Vitamin E and Benign Breast Disease," *Surgery* 107(5):549–551, 1990.

Murray, MT. *The Complete Book of Juicing.* Rocklin CA: Prima Publishing, 1992, pp. 71–72, 123–124, 136, 142–143, 149, 192, 215.

Murray, MT. *The Healing Power of Herbs.* Rev. 2nd ed. Rocklin CA: Prima Publishing, 1995, pp. 173-183.

Nagata, C, Kabuto, M, Kurisu, Y, Shimizu, H. "Decreased Serum Estradiol Concentration Associated With High Dietary Intake of Soy Products in Premenopausal Japanese Women," *Nutrition and Cancer* 29(3):228–233, 1997.

Ody, P. *The Complete Medicinal Herbal.* London: Dorling Kindersley Limited, 1993, p. 85.

Pizzorno, JE, Murray, MT. *The Textbook of Natural Medicine.* Seattle:Bastyr University Publications, 1993, VI:FibCys-1-6.

Rhoades, R, Pflanzer, R. *Human Physiology.* 3rd ed. Philadelphia: Saunders College Publishing, 1996, p. 385.

Rothman, KJ, et al. "Teratogenicity of High Vitamin A Intake," *New England Journal of Medicine* 333:1369–1373, 1995.

Russell, LC. "Caffeine Restriction as Initial Treatment for Breast Pain," *Nurse Practitioner* 14(2):36–37, 40, 1989.

Sandaram, GS, et al. "Serum Hormones and Lipoproteins in Benign Breast Disease," *Cancer Research* 14(9 Pt2):3814–3816, 1981.

Stoll, BA. "Macronutrient Supplements May Reduce Breast Cancer Risk: How, When, and Which," *European Journal of Clinical Nutrition* 51(9):573–577, 1997.

Werbach, M. *Healing With Food.* New York: HarperCollins Publishers, 1993, pp.41–45.

Werbach, M, Murray, MT. *Botanical Influences on Illness: A Sourcebook of Clinical Research.* Third Line Press, 1994, p. 33.

Zych, F, et al. "Fibrocystic Disease of the Breast and Pituitary-Thyroid Axis Function," *Pol Merkuriusz Lek* 1(4):227–228, 1996.

Fibromyalgia

Eisinger, J, et al. "Studies of Transketolase in Chronic Pain," *Journal of Advancement in Medicine* 5(2):105–113, Summer 1992.

Murray, M. *Encyclopedia of Nutritional Supplements.* Rocklin CA: Prima Publishing, 1996.

Romano, T, Stiller, JW. "Magnesium Deficiency and Fibromyalgia Syndrome," *The Journal of Nutritional Medicine* 4:165–167, 1994.

St. Amand, RP. "Exploring the Fibromyalgia Connection," *The Vulvar Pain Newsletter* 1, 4–6, Fall 1996.

Gallstones

Gustafson, U, et al. "The Effect of Vitamin C in High Doses on Plasma and Biliary Lipid Composition in Patients with Cholesterol Gallstones: Prolongation of the Nucleation Time," *European Journal of Clinical Investigation* 27:387–391, 1997.

Heaton, KW, et al. "An Explanation for Gallstones in Normal-Weight Women: Slow Intestinal Transit," *Lancet* 341:8–10, 2 January 1993.

Klawansky, S, Chalmers, TC. "Fat Content of Very Low Calorie Diets and Gallstone Formation," *Journal of the American Medical Association* 268(7):873, 19 August 1992.

Ortega, R, et al. "Differences in Diet and Food Habits Between Patients with Gallstones and Controls," *The Journal of the American College of Nutrition* 16(1):88–95, 1997.

Tandon, RK, et al. "Dietary Habits of Gallstone Patients in Northern India: A Case Control Study," *Journal of Clinical Gastroenterology* 22(1):23–27, 1996.

Gout

Balch, J, Balch, P. *Prescription for Nutritional Healing.* Garden City Park NY: Avery Publishing Group, 1990.

Blau, LW. "Cherry Diet Control for Gout and Arthritis," *Texas Report on Biology and Medicine* 8:309–312, 1950.

Emmerson, BT. "Effect of Oral Fructose on Urate Production," *Annals of the Rheumatic Diseases* 33:276, 1974.

Escott-Stump, S. *Nutrition and Diagnosis-Related Care.* Philadelphia: W.B. Saunders, 1988.

Krause, M, Mahan, L. *Food, Nutrition and Diet Therapy.* Philadelphia: W.B. Saunders, 1984.

Shils, M, Young, V. *Modern Nutrition in Health and Disease.* Philadelphia: Lea & Feibiger, 1988.

Herpes

Balch J., Balch, P. *Prescription for Nutritional Healing.* Garden City Park NY: Avery Publishing Group, 1990.

Chandra, RK. "Nutrition and Immunity—Basic Considerations. Part I," *Contemporary Nutrition* 11:11, 1986.

Griffith, R, et al. "Relations of Arginine-Lysine Antagonism to Herpes Simplex Growth in Tissue Culture," *Chemotherapy* 27:209–213, 1981.

Murray, M. *Encyclopedia of Nutritional Supplements.* Rocklin CA: Prima Publishing, 1996.

Rhodes, J. "Human Interferon Action: Reciprocal Regulation by Reinoic Acid and Beta-Carotene," *Journal National Cancer Institute* 70:833–837, 1983.

Terezhalmy, GT, et al. "The Use of Water Soluble Bioflavonoid-Ascorbic Acid Complex in the Treatment of Recurrent Herpes Labialis. Oral Surgery. Oral Medicine," *Oral Pathology* 45:56–62, 1978.

High Blood Pressure (Hypertension)

Abe, Y, Umemura, S, Sugimoto, K, et al. "Effect of Green Tea Rich in Gamma-Aminobutyric Acid on Blood Pressure of Dahl Salt-Sensitive Rats," *American Journal of Hypertension* 8:74–79, 1995. In: Mitscher, L, Dolby, V. *The Green Tea Book.* Garden City Park NY: Avery Publishing Group, 1998.

Appel, LJ, et al. "A Clinical Trial of the Effects of Dietary Patterns on Blood Pressure," *The New England Journal of Medicine* 36:1117–1124, 17 April 1997.

Borok, G. "Nutritional Aspects of Hypertension," *South African Medical Journal* 76:125–126, 5 August 1989.

Gordon, L. "Exercise and Salt Restriction May be Enough for Mildy High BP," *Medical Tribune* 8, 21 December 1995.

Henry, JP, Stephens-Larson, P. "Reduction of Chronic Psychosocial Hypertension in Mice by Decaffeinated Tea," *Hypertension* 6(3):437–444, 1984. In: Mitscher, L, Dolby, V. *The Green Tea Book.* Garden City Park NY: Avery Publishing Group, 1998.

Lardinois, CK. "Nutritional Factors and Hypertension," *Archives of Family Medicine* 4:707–713, August 1995.

"Magnesium Lowers Blood Pressure," *Nutrition Week* 7, 24 May 1996.

Osborne, CG, et al. "Evidence for the Relationship of Calcium to Blood Pressure," *Nutrition Reviews* 54(12):365–381, December 1996.

Pauletto, P, et al. "Blood Pressure, Serum Lipids, and Fatty Acids in Populations on a Lake-Fish Diet or a Vegetarian Diet in Tanzania," *Lipids* 31:S309–S312, 1996 (Suppl.).

Solzback, U, et al. "Vitamin C Improves Endothelial Dysfunction of Epicardial Coronary Arteries in Hypertensive Patients," *Circulation* 96(5):1513–1519, 2 September 1997.

Stensvold, I, Tverdal, A, Solvoll, K, et al. "Tea Consumption. Relationship to Cholesterol, Blood Pressure, and Coronary and Total Mortality," *Preventive Medicine* 21:546–553, 1992. In: Mitscher, L, Dolby, V. *The Green Tea Book.* Garden City Park NY: Avery Publishing Group, 1998.

Superka, HR, et al. "Effects of Cessation of Caffeinated-Coffee Consumption on Ambulatory and Resting Blood Pressure in Men," *American Journal of Cardiology* 73: 780–784, 15 April 1994.

Hypoglycemia

Anderson, RA. "Nutritional Factors Influencing the Glucose/Insulin System: Chromium," *Journal of the American College of Nutrition* 16(5):404–410, October 1997.

Gaia Multimedia, Inc. *Condition: Hypoglycemia. Body System: Endocrine System.* Produced by the Alchemical Medicine Research and Teaching Association. Interactive Body/Mind Information System (IBIS), Version 1.2, 1994.

Haas, EM. *Staying Healthy With Nutrition.* Berkeley CA: Celestial Arts, 1992.

Hoffmann, D. *The Herbal Handbook: A User's Guide to Medical Herbalism.* Rochester NY: Healing Arts Press, 1988.

Pitchford, P. *Healing With Whole Foods: Oriental Traditions and Modern Nutrition.* Berkeley CA: North Atlantic Books, 1993.

Pizzorno, JE, Murray, MT. *The Textbook of Natural Medicine.* Seattle: Bastyr University Publications, 1992, VI:Hypo 1-7.

Rutherford, WJ. "Hypoglycemia and Endurance Exercise: Dietary Considerations," *Nutrition and Health* 6(4):173–181, 1990.

Werbach, MR. *Nutritional Influences on Illness.* New Canaan CT: Keats Publishing, Inc., 1987.

Indigestion

Al-Yahya, MA, Rafatullah, S, et al. "Gastroprotective Activity of Ginger *Zingiber officinale* Rosc. in the Albino Rats," *American Journal of Chinese Medicine* 17(1–2): 51–56, 1989.

Aroroa, A, Sharma, MP. "Use of Banana in Non-ulcer Dyspepsia," *Lancet* 355, March 1990.

Colbin, A. *Food and Healing.* New York: Ballantine Books, 1986.

Elta, GH, Behler, EM, et al. "Comparison of Coffee Intake and Coffee-Induced Symptoms in Patients with Duodenal Ulcer, Nonulcer Dyspepsia, and Normal Controls," *American Journal of Gastroenterology* 85(10):1339–1342, 1990.

Gaia Multimedia, Inc. *Interactive Body/ Mind Information System.* http://www.teleport. com/~ibis/ (1994).

Haas, EM. *Staying Healthy With Nutrition.* Berkeley CA: Celestial Arts, 1992.

Hoffmann, D. *The Herbal Handbook: A User's Guide to Medical Herbalism.* Rochester NY: Healing Arts Press, 1988.

Mahan, KL, Escott-Stump, S. *Krause's Food, Nutrition, and Diet Therapy.* 9th ed. Philadelphia: W.B. Saunders Co., 1996.

Matthews, G. "Gut Fermentation," *Journal of the Royal Society of Medicine* 85:304–305, May 1992.

Mullan, A, et al. "Food and Nutrient Intakes and Eating Patterns in Functional and Organic Dyspepsia," *European Journal of Clinical Nutrition* 48(2):97–105, February 1994.

Murray, M, Pizzorno, J. *Encyclopedia of Natural Medicine.* Rocklin CA: Prima Publishing, 1990.

Pitchford, P. *Healing With Whole Foods: Oriental Traditions and Modern Nutrition.* Berkeley CA: North Atlantic Books, 1993.

Pizzorno, J, Murray, M. *The Textbook of Natural Medicine.* Seattle: Bastyr University Publications, 1992, V:Bromel-1-4.

Warden, RA, et al. "Vitamin A Deficiency Exacerbates Methotrexate-Induced Jejunal Injury in Rat," *Journal of Nutrition* 127(5):770–776, May 1997.

Inflammation

Alschuler, L. Botanical Medicine I, II, III, IV (lectures). Seattle: Bastyr University, 1998.

Bistrian, BR, et al. "Cytokines, Muscle Proteolysis, and the Catabolic Response to Infection and Inflammation," *Proceedings of the Society for Experimental Biology and Medicine* 200:220–223, 1992.

Denko, CW, et al. "Inflammation in Relation to Dietary Intake of Zinc and Copper," *International Journal of Tissue Reactions* 3:73–76, 1981.

Fleck, A. "Clinical and Nutritional Aspects of Changes in Acute-Phase Proteins During Inflammation," *Proceedings of the Nutrition Society* 48:347–354, 1989.

Gaby, A. Therapeutic Nutrition I, II (lectures). Seattle: Bastyr University, 1998.

Grimble, R. "Inflammation, Cytokines and Nutrition," *European Journal of Clinical Nutrition* 45:413–417, 1991.

Grimble, RF. "Nutritional Antioxidants and the Modulation of Inflammation: Theory and Practice," *New Horizons* 2:175–185, 1994.

Grogg, JL, Gropper, SS, Hunt, SM. *Advanced Nutrition and Human Metabolism.* 2nd ed. New York: West Publishing Co., 1995.

Haas, EM. *Staying Healthy With Nutrition.* Berkeley CA: Celestial Arts, 1992.

Kirschmann, GJ, Kirschmann, JD. *Nutrition Almanac.* 4th ed. New York: McGraw-Hill, 1996.

Milanino, R, Velo, GP. "Multiple Actions of Copper in Control of Inflammation: Studies in Copper-Deficient Rats," *Agents Actions Supplement* 8:209–230, 1981.

Roubenoff, R, Roubenoff, RA, et al. "Abnormal Vitamin B_6 Status in Rheumatoid Cachexia. Association with Spontaneous Tumor Necrosis Factor Alpha Production and Markers of Inflammation," *Arthritis and Rheumatism* 38:105–109, 1995.

Tate, G, Mandell, BF, et al. "Suppression of Acute and Chronic Inflammation by Dietary Gamma Linolenic Acid," *Journal of Rheumatology* 16:729-734, 1989.

Terano, T, et al. "Eicosapentaenoic Acid as a Modulator of Inflammation. Effect on Prostaglandin and Leukotriene Synthesis," *Biochemical Pharmacology* 35:779–785, 1986.

Wan, JM, et al. "Nutrition, Immune Function, and Inflammation: An Overview," *Proceedings of the Nutrition Society* 48: 315–335, 1989.

Influenza

Calbom, C. *The Healthy Gourmet.* New York: Clarkson Potter, 1996, p. 121.

Chandra, RK, McBean, LD. "Zinc and Immunity," *Nutrition* 10(1), 1994.

Halpern, GM, Trapp, CI. "Nutrition and Immunity: Where Are We Standing," *Allergy and Immunopathology* 21(3):122–126, 1993.

Nakayama, M, Suzuki, K, Toda, M, et al. "Inhibition of the Infectivity of Influenza Virus by Tea Polyphenols," *Antiviral Research* 21:289–299, 1993.

Nakayama, M, Toda, M, Okubo, S, et al. "Inhibition of the Infectivity of Influenza Virus by Black Tea Extract," *Kansenshogaku Zasshi—Journal of the Japanese Association for Infectious Diseases* 68(7): 824–829, 1994. In: Mitscher, L, Dolby, V. *The Green Tea Book.* Garden City Park NY: Avery Publishing Group, 1998.

Scaglione, F, et al. "Efficacy and Safety of the Standardized Ginseng Extract G 115 for Potentiating Vaccination Against Common Cold and/or Influenza Syndrome," *Drugs in Experimental and Clinical Research* 22(2):65–72, 1996.

Shrauzer, GN. "Selenium and the Immune Response," *The Nutrition Report* 10(3):17, 24, March 1992.

Sunkind, R. "Immunologic Mechanisms and The Role of Nutrition." In: *Principles and Practice of Environmental Medicine.* New York: Plenum Medical Book Company, 1992, pp. 159–172.

Insomnia and Jet Lag

Berry, EM, Levy, M. "Foods and Their Effects on Sleep Patterns," *International Clinical Nutrition Review* 7:76–78, April 1987.

Brown, DJ. "Valerian Root: Non-Addictive Alternative for Insomnia and Anxiety," *Quarterly Review of Natural Medicine* 221–224, Fall 1994.

The Burton Goldberg Group (J. Strohecker, exec ed). *Alternative Medicine: The Definitive Guide.* Puyallup WA: Future Medicine Publishing, 1994, pp. 838–847.

Comperatore, CA, et al. "Melatonin Efficacy in Aviation Missions Requiring Rapid Deployment and Night Operations," *Aviation, Space, and Environmental Medicine* 67(6):520–524, June 1996.

Foster, S. "A Good Night's Sleep," *Supplement to the Herb Companion* 73–74, June/July 1995.

"Halcion vs. Valerian in the Treatment of Insomnia," *American Journal of Natural Medicine* 2:7–9, May 1995.

Murray, MT. *Encyclopedia of Nutritional Supplements.* Rocklin CA: Prima Publishing, 1996.

Phillips, F, Crisp, AH, et al. "Isocaloric Diet Changes and Electroencephalographic Sleep," *Lancet* 723–725, 18 October 1975.

Pitchford, P. *Healing With Whole Foods: Oriental Traditions and Modern Nutrition.* Berkeley CA: North Atlantic Books, 1993.

Porter, JM, Home, JA. "Bed-Time Food Supplements and Sleep: Effects of Different Carbohydrate Levels," *Electroencephalography and Clinical Neurophysiology* 51:426–433, 1981.

Menopause

Bullock, C. "Soybeans: An Estrogen Replacement Alternative," *Family Practice News* 11, 6 April 1995.

Gleason, S. "Menopause: It's Not a Disease. Natural Approaches to a Change of Life," *Good Medicine* 8–10, Spring 1994.

Hunt, CD, et al. "Metabolic Responses of Postmenopausal Women to Supplemental Dietary Boron and Aluminum During Usual and Low Magnesium Intake: Boron, Calcium, and Magnesium Absorption and Retention and Blood Mineral Concentrations," *American Journal of Clinical Nutrition* 65:803–813, 1997.

Murray, M. "Essential Fatty Acid Supplementation." In: Murray, MT. *Encyclopedia of Nutritional Supplements.* Rocklin CA: Prima Publishing, 1996.

Torgerson, DJ, et al. "Alcohol Consumption May Influence Onset of the Menopause," *British Medical Journal* 315–318, 19 July 1997.

Wahlqvist, ML. "Phytoestrogens: Emerging Multifaceted Plant Compounds," *Medical Journal of Australia* 167:119–120, 4 August 1997.

Menstrual Disorders

Bagga, D, Ashley, JM, et al. "Effects of a Very Low Fat, High Fiber Diet on Serum Hormones and Menstrual Function: Implications for Breast Cancer Prevention," *Cancer* 76(3):2491–2496, 15 December 1995.

Campbell, EM, Peterkin, D, et al. "Premenstrual Symptoms in General Practice Patients: Prevalence and Treatment," *Journal of Reproductive Medicine* 42(10):637–646, October 1997.

Chan, WY, Hill, JC. "Determination of Menstrual Prostaglandin Levels in Non-Dysmenorrheic Subjects," *Prostaglandins* 15(2):365–375, February 1978.

Deutch, B. "Menstrual Pain in Danish Women Correlated with Low Omega-3 Polyunsaturated Fatty Acid Intake," *European Journal of Clinical Nutrition* 49(7): 508–516, July 1995.

Downing, I, Hutchon, DJR, et al. "Uptake of [3H]-Arachidonic Acid by Human Endometrium: Differences Between Normal and Menorrhagic Tissue," *Prostaglandins* 26:55–69, 1983.

Ermans, SJ. "Menarche and Beyond: Do Eating and Exercise Make a Difference?" *Pediatric Annals* 26(2 Supplement):S137–S141, February 1997.

Fowler, GC, Hasselquist, MB, et al. "Menstrual Irregularities: A Focused Evaluation," *Patient Care* 155–164, 15 April 1994.

Gladstar, R. *Herbal Healing for Women.* New York: Fireside, 1993.

Hoffmann, D. *The New Holistic Herbal.* Rockport MA: Element, Inc., 1990.

Kjerulff, KH, Erickson, BA, et al. "Chronic Gynecological Conditions Reported by US Women: Findings from the National Health Interview Survey, 1984 to 1992," *American Journal of Public Health* 86(2): 195–199, February 1996.

Lewis, SJ, Heaton, KW, et al. "Lower Serum Oestrogen Concentrations Associated With Faster Intestinal Transit," *British Journal of Cancer* 76(3):395–400, 1997.

Murray, MT. *The Complete Book of Juicing.* Rocklin CA: Prima Publishing, 1992, p. 462.

Murray, M, Pizzorno, J. *The Encyclopedia of Natural Medicine.* Rocklin CA: Prima Publishing, 1990.

Penland, JG, Johnson, PE. "Dietary Calcium and Manganese Effects on Menstrual Cycle Symptoms," *American Journal of Obstetrics and Gynecology* 168(5):1417–1423, May 1993.

Taussig, S, Batkin, R. "Bromelain: The Enzyme Complex of Pineapple (*Ananas comosus*) and its Clinical Application: An Update," *Journal of Ethnopharmacology.* 22:191–203, 1988. Cited in Murray, *The Complete Book of Juicing*, pp. 40–41.

Migraine

Atkinson, M. "Migraine Headaches: Some Clinical Observations on the Vascular Mechanisms and Its Control," *Annals of Internal Medicine* 21:990–997, 1944.

Bic, Z, et al. "In Search of the Ideal Treatment for Migraine Headache," *Medical Hypotheses* 50:1–7, 1998.

Colbin, A. *Food and Healing.* New York: Ballantine Books, 1986, pp. 264–266.

Gaia Multimedia, Inc. *Condition: Headache, Vascular, Body System, Nervous System.* Produced by the Alchemical Medicine Research and Teaching Association. Interactive Body/Mind Information System, Version 1.2, 1994.

Grenfell, RF. "Treatment of Migraine with Nicotinic Acid," *American Practioner* 3(9): 542–544, May 1949.

Haas, EM. *Staying Healthy With Nutrition.* Berkeley CA: Celestial Arts, 1992.

Hanington, E. "Diet and Migraine," *Journal of Human Nutrition* 34:175–180, 1980.

Hoffmann, D. *The New Holistic Herbal.* 3rd ed. Rockport MA: Element Books, 1992.

Hughes, EC, et al. "Migraine: A Diagnostic Test for Etiology of Food Sensitivity by a Nutritionally Supported Fast and Confirmed by Long-Term Report," *Annals of Allergy* 55(1):28–32, July 1985.

Johnson, BS, et al. "Efficacy of Feverfew: a Prophylactic Treatment of Migraine," *British Medical Journal* 291:569–574, August 1985.

Mansfield, IE, et al. "Food Allergy and Adult Migraine: Double-Blind and Medi-

ator Confirmation of an Allergic Etiology," *Annals of Allergy* 55(2):126–129, August 1985.

Marcus, DA, et al. "A Double-Blind Provocative Study of Chocolate as a Trigger of Headache," *Cephalalgia* 17(8):855–862, December 1997.

Mauskop, A, et al. "Deficiency in Serum Ionized Magnesium But Not Total Magnesium in Patients With Migraines. Possible Role of Ica2+/IMg2+ Ratio," *Headaches* 33(3):135–138, March 1993.

Mauskop, A, et al. "Intravenous Magnesium Sulfate Rapidly Alleviates Headaches of Various Types," *Headache* 36(3): 154–160, March 1996.

McCaren, T, et al. "Amelioration of Severe Migraine by Fish Oil," *American Journal of Clinical Nutrition* 41(4):874, April 1985.

Murray, M, Pizzorno, J. *Encyclopedia of Natural Medicine.* Rocklin CA: Prima Publishing, 1990.

Peatfield, RC. "Relationship Between Food, Wine, and Beer-Precipitated Migrainous Headaches," *Headache* June 35(6):355–357, 1995.

Pitchford, P. *Healing With Whole Foods: Oriental Traditions and Modern Nutrition.* Berkeley, CA: North Atlantic Books, 1993.

Werbach, MR. *Nutritional Influences on Illness.* New Canaan CT: Keats Publishing, 1987.

Multiple Sclerosis

Agranoff, B, Goldberg, D. "Diet and the Geographical Distribution of Multiple Sclerosis," *Lancet* 2:1061, 1974.

Alter, M. "Multiple Sclerosis and Nutrition," *Archives of Neurology* 31:262–272, 1974.

Bates, D, Fawcett, P, et al. "Polyunsaturated Fatty Acids in Treatment of Acute Remitting Multiple Sclerosis," *British Medical Journal* 2:1390–1391, 1978.

Elian, M, Dean, G. "Multiple Sclerosis Among the United Kingdom-Born Children of Immigrants From the West Indies," *Journal of Neurological Neurosurgery and Psychiatry* 50:327–332, 1987.

Hayes, CE, Cantorna, MT, et al. "Vitamin D and Multiple Sclerosis," *Proceedings of the Society of Experimental Biology and Medicine* 216(1):21–27, 1997.

Hutter, CD, Laing, P. "Multiple Sclerosis: Sunlight, Diet, Immunology and Aetiology," *Medical Hypotheses* 46(2):67–74, 1996.

Lauer, K. "The Risk of Multiple Sclerosis in the USA in Relation to Sociographic Features: A Factor-Analytic Study," *Journal of Clinical Epidemiology* 47(1):43–48, 1994.

Lauer, K. "Environmental Associations With the Risk of Multiple Sclerosis: The Contribution of Ecological Studies," *Acta Neurological Scandinavica Supplement* 161: 77–88, 1995.

Manley, P. "Diet in Multiple Sclerosis," *Practitioner* 238(1538):358–363, 1994.

Messina, VK, Burke, KI. "Position of the ADA: Vegetarian Diets," *Journal of the American Dietetic Association* 97(11): 1317–1321, 1997.

Miller, J, et al. "Double-blind Trial of Linoleate Supplementation of the Diet in Multiple Sclerosis," *British Medical Journal* 765–768, 1973.

Rosner, LJ, Ross, S. *Multiple Sclerosis: New Hope and Practical Advice for People with MS and Their Families.* Updated ed. New York: Fireside, 1992.

Swank, RL. "Multiple Sclerosis: A Fat-Oil Relationship," *Nutrition* 7(5):368–376, 1991.

Swank, RL, Dugan, BB. *The Multiple Sclerosis Diet Book.* Garden City NY: Doubleday, 1987.

Swank, RL, Dugan, BB. "Effect of Low Saturated Fat Diet in Early and Late Cases of Multiple Sclerosis," *Lancet* 336(8706): 37–39, 1990.

Swank, RL, Grimsgaard, A. "Multiple Sclerosis: The Lipid Relationship," *American Journal of Clinical Nutrition* 48:1387, 1988.

Weil, A. *Eight Weeks to Optimum Health.* New York: Alfred A. Knopf, 1997, pp. 47–52, 84. This book contains a very inspiring story of a woman's recovery from MS disability on pp. 146–148.

Osteoarthritis

Felson, DT. "Weight and Osteoarthritis," *American Journal of Clinical Nutrition* 63 (Suppl):430S–432S, 1996.

Flynn, M, et al. "The Effect of Folate and Cobalamin on Osteoarthritic Hands," *Journal of the American College of Nutrition* 13(4):351–356, 1994.

Maltz, G. "Get to the Joint: Exercise Benefits Osteoarthritis Patients," *Family Practice News* 20, 15 February 1995.

Murray, M, Pizzorno, J. *Encyclopedia of Natural Medicine.* 2nd ed. Rocklin CA: Prima Publishing, 1998.

Pizzorno, JE. "Natural Medicine Approach to Treating Osteoarthritis," *Alternative and Complementary Therapies* 93–95, January/February 1995.

Srivastava, KC, Mustafa, T. "Ginger (*Zingiber officinale*) in Rheumatism and Muscoloskeletal Disorders," *Medical Hypothesis* 39:342–348, 1992.

"Vitamin D Deficits Affect Osteoarthritis," *Nutrition Report* 14(7):54, September-October 1996.

Osteoporosis

Bellantoni, MF. "Osteoporosis Prevention and Treatment," *American Family Practice* 54(3):986–992, 1 September 1996.

Hasling, C, et al. "Calcium Metabolism in Postmenopausal Osteoporotic Women is Determined by Dietary Calcium and Coffee Intake," *Journal of Nutrition* 112: 1119–1126, 1992.

Hollenback, KA, et al. "Cigarette Smoking and Bone Mineral Density in Older Men and Women," *American Journal of Public Health* 83(9):1265–1270, September 1993.

Kidd, PM. "An Integrative Lifestyle: Nutritional Survey for Lowering Osteoporosis Risk," *Townsend Letter for Doctors* 400–405, May 1992.

Murray, M, Pizzorno, J. *Encyclopedia of Natural Medicine*. Rocklin CA: Prima Publishing, 1990.

"Osteoporosis: Not Just a Woman's Disease," *Journal of Nuclear Medicine* 37 (10):N17, 1996.

Riggs, BL, Melton, LJ. "The Prevention and Treatment of Osteoporosis," *The New England Journal of Medicine* 327(9):620-627, 27 August 1992.

Swezey, RL. "Exercise for Osteoporosis— Is Walking Enough?" *Spine* 21:2809-2813, 1996.

Szule, P, Delams, PD. "Is There a Role for Vitamin K Deficiency in Osteoporosis?" *Challenge of Modern Medicine* 24(4):303–307, 1995.

Vikhanski, L. "Magnesium May Slow Bone Loss," *Medical Tribune* 1, 23 July 1993.

Overweight/Obesity

"Appetite and High-Fat Food," *Nutrition Week* 27(12):7, 29 March 1997.

"Aspartame and Dieting," *Nutrition Week* 27(23):7, 13 June 1997.

Grant, KE, et al. "Chromium and Exercise Training: Effect on Obese Women," *Medicine and Science in Sports and Exercise* 29(8):992–998, 1997.

Jancin, B. "Whole Grain May Reduce Obesity, Hyperinsulinemia," *Family Practice News* 8, 15 May 1998.

"More than Half of Adults Classified as Overweight," *Nutrition Week* 28(22):2, 5 June 1998.

Murray, M, Pizzorno, J. *Encyclopedia of Natural Medicine*. 2nd ed. Rocklin CA: Prima Publishing, 1998.

"Obesity in Children," *Nutrition Week* (16): 7, 25 April 1997.

"Pantothenic Acid and Weight Loss," *The Nutrition Report* 61, September 1995.

Rossner, S, et al. "Weight Reduction with

Dietary Fiber Supplements: Results of Two Double-Blind Studies," *Acta Medica Scandinavia* 22:83–88, 1987.

Singh, RB, et al. "Association of Low Plasma Concentration of Antioxidant Vitamins, Magnesium, and Zinc With High Body Fat Percent Measured by Bioelectrical Impedance Analysis in Indian Men," *Magnesium Research* 11(1):3–10, 1998.

Whitaker, RC. "Predicting Obesity in Young Adulthood From Childhood and Parental Obesity," *The New England Journal of Medicine*, 337(13):869–873, 25 September 1997.

Parasitic Infections

The Burton Goldberg Group (J. Strohecker, exec ed). *Alternative Medicine: The Definitive Guide*. Puyallup WA: Future Medicine Publishing, 1994.

Gittleman, AL. *Natural Healing for Parasites*. New York: Healing Wisdom Publications, 1995.

Murray, M. *Encyclopedia of Natural Medicine*. Rocklin CA: Prima Publishing, 1990, 55-56.

Murray, M. *Encyclopedia of Nutritional Supplements*. Rocklin CA: Prima Publishing, 1996, pp. 404–405.

Nesheim, MC. "Human Nutrition Needs and Parasite Infection," *Parasitology* 107:S7–S18, 1993.

"Results of Testing for Intestinal Parasites by State Diagnostic Laboratories, United States, 1987," *Morbidity and Mortality Weekly Report* 40(SS-4);25–30, 1992.

Prostate Enlargement, Benign

Buck, AC. "Phytotherapy for the Prostate," *British Journal of Urology* 78:325–336, 1996.

Bush, LM, et al. "Zinc and the Prostate." Presented at the Annual Meeting of the American Medical Association, 1974.

Gerber, PC. "Alternative Medicine: All Eyes on NIH's Office of Alternative Medicine," *Physician Management* 30–42, March 1994.

Murray, M Pizzorno, J. *Encyclopedia of Natural Medicine.* 2nd ed. Rocklin CA: Prima Publishing, 1998.

Walker, N. *Raw Vegetable Juices.* Phoenix: Norwalk Press Publishers, 1947.

Psoriasis

Murray, MT. *The Healing Power of Herbs.* Rocklin CA: Prima Publishing, 1992.

Murray, MT. *The Healing Power of Foods.* Rocklin CA: Prima Publishing, 1993.

Murray, M, Pizzorno, J. *The Encyclopedia of Natural Medicine.* 2nd ed. Rocklin CA: Prima Publishing, 1998.

Naldi, F. "Dietary Factors and the Risk of Psoriasis: Results of an Italian Case-Controlled Study," *British Journal of Dermatology* 134:101–106, January 1996.

Rackett, SC. "Diet and Dermatology," *Journal of the American Academy of Dermatology* 29:447-459, September 1993.

Swain, R, et al. "Vitamins as Therapy in the 1990s," *Journal of American Board of Family Practice* 8:206, May/June 1995.

Respiratory Disorders

The Burton Goldberg Group (J. Strohecker, exec ed). *Alternative Medicine: The Definitive Guide.* Puyallup WA: Future Medicine Publishing, 1994, pp. 81, 816, 820–823.

De-Sole, G, et al. "Vitamin A Deficiency in Southern Ethiopia," *American Journal of Clinical Nutrition* 45(4):780–784, April 1987.

Gaia Multimedia, Inc. *Condition: Bronchitis, Pneumonia, Sinusitis. Body System: Respiratory System.* Produced by the Alchemical Medicine Research and Teaching Association. Interactive Body/Mind Information System (IBIS), Version 1.2, 1994.

Haas, EM. *Staying Healthy With Nutrition.* Berkeley CA: Celestial Arts, 1992.

Hoffmann, D. *The New Holistic Herbal.* Rockport MA: Element Books, Inc., 1992.

McCaleb, R, "Boosting Immunity with Herbs." *The Herb Research Foundation: Herb Information Greenpaper,* http://www.healthy.net/ library/articles/ passwater/ gabor.htm.

Mossad, SB, et al. "Zinc Gluconate Lozenges for Treating the Common Cold: A Randomized, Double-Blind, Placebo-Controlled Study," *Annals of Internal Medicine* 125:81–88, 1996.

Pedersen, M. *Nutritional Herbology: A Reference Guide to Herbs.* Warsaw IN: Wendell W. Whitman, Co., 1994.

Pitchford, P. *Healing With Whole Foods: Oriental Traditions and Modern Nutrition.* Berkeley CA: North Atlantic Books, 1993.

Pizzorno, JE, Murray, MT. *The Textbook of Natural Medicine.* Seattle: Bastyr University Publications, 1992, IV:ImmSupl 1-6, VI:Pneu 1-3, SinuBal.

Ryan, RE. "A Double-Blind Clinical Evaluation of Bromelains in the Treatment of Acute Sinusitis," *Headache* 7:13–27, 1967.

Schwartz, J, Weiss, S. "Dietary Factors and Their Relation to Respiratory Symptoms," *American Journal of Epidemiology* 132(1): 67–76, July 1990.

Tockman, MS, et al. "Milk Drinking and Possible Reduction of the Respiratory Epithelium," *Journal of Chronic Diseases* 39 (3):207–209, 1986.

West, CE, et al. "Epithelial Damaging Virus Infections Affect Vitamin A Status in Chickens," *Journal of Nutrition* 122(2): 333–339, February 1992.

Rheumatoid Arthritis

Blau, LW. "Cherry Diet Control for Gout and Arthritis," *Texas Report on Biology and Medicine* 8:309–312, 1950.

Darlington, LG. "Diet Therapy for Arthritis," *Nutrition and Rheumatic Diseases/ Rheumatic Disease Clinics of North America* 17(2):273–285, May 1991.

Darlington, LG, Ramsey, NW. "Clinical Review of Dietary Therapy for Rheumatoid Arthritis," *British Journal of Rheumatology* 32:507–514, 1993.

Palmblad, J, et al. "Antirheumatic Effects of Fasting," *Nutrition and Rheumatic Dis-*

ease/*Rheumatic Disease Clinics of North America* 17(2):351–362, May 1991.

Srivasiava, KC, Mustafa, T. "Ginger (*Zingiber officinale*) in Rheumatism and Musculoskeletal Disorder," *Medical Hypothesis* 39:342–348, 1992.

Volker, D, Garg, M. "Dietary N-3 Fatty Acid Supplementation in Rheumatoid Arthritis—Mechanisms, Clinical Outcomes, Controversies, and Future Directions," *Journal of Clinical Biochemical Nutrition* 20:83-97, 1996.

Zurier, RB, et al. "Gamma-Linolenic Acid Treatment of Rheumatoid Arthritis: A Randomized Placebo-Controlled Trial," *Arthritis and Rheumatism* 39(11):1808–1817, November 1996.

Stress

Andrade, FH, et al. "Effects of Selenium Deficiency on Diaphragmatic Function After Resistive Loading," *Acta Physiologica Scandinavica* 162:141–148, 1998.

Bagchi, D, et al. "Stress, Diet and Alcohol-Induced Oxidative Subsalicylate," *Journal of Applied Toxicology* 18:2–13, 1998.

Balch, JF, Balch, PA. *Prescription for Nutritional Healing.* Garden City Park NY: Avery Publishing Group, 1990, pp. 151–153.

Barnes, V, et al. "Stress, Stress Reduction and Hypertension in African Americans: An Updated Review," *Journal of the National Medical Association* 89:464–476, 1997.

Carsia, RV, McIlroy, PJ. "Dietary Protein Restriction Stress in the Domestic Turkey (*Meleagris gallopavo*) Induces Hypofunction and Remodeling of Adrenal Steroidogenic Tissue," *General and Comparative Endocrinology* 109:140–153, 1998.

Dess, NK, Choe, S, et al. "The Interaction of Diet and Stress in Rats: High-Energy Food and Sucrose Treatment," *Journal of Experimental Psychology: Animal Behavior Processes* 24:60–71, 1998.

Frame, LT, Hart, RW, et al. "Calorie Restriction as a Mechanism Mediating Resistance to Environmental Disease," *Environ-mental Health Perspectives* 106(Suppl 1):313–324, 1998.

Groff, JL, Gropper, SS, et al. *Advanced Nutrition and Human Metabolism.* 2nd ed. San Francisco: West, 1995.

Haas, EM. *Staying Healthy With Nutrition.* Berkeley CA: Celestial Arts, 1992.

Heath, JA, Dufty, AM. "Body Condition and the Adrenal Stress Response in Captive American Kestrel Juveniles," *Physiological Zoology* 71:67–73, 1998.

Hobbs, C. *Stress & Natural Healing.* Loveland CO: Interweave Press, 1997.

Konig, D, et al. "Rationale for a Specific Diet From the Viewpoint of Sports Medicine and Sports Orthopedics: Relation to Stress Reaction and Regeneration," *Orthopade* 26:942–950, 1997.

Larsen, CT, Pierson, FW, et al. "Effect of Dietary Selenium on the Response of Stressed and Unstressed Chickens to *Escherichia coli* Challenge and Antigen," *Biological Trace Element Research* 58:169–176, 1997.

Margen, S (ed). *University of California at Berkeley: The Wellness Encyclopedia of Food and Nutrition.* New York: Rebus, 1992.

Murray, M, Pizzorno, J. *Encyclopedia of Natural Medicine.* 2nd ed. Rocklin CA: Prima Publishing, 1998, pp. 379-400.

Schneider, RH, et al. "Lower Lipid Peroxide Levels in Practitioners of the Transcendental Meditation Program," *Psychosomatic Medicine* 60:38–41, 1998.

Seelig, MS. "Consequences of Magnesium Deficiency on the Enhancement of Stress Reaction. Preventative and Therapeutic Implications—A Review," *Journal of the American College of Nutrition* 13:429–446, 1994.

Skantze, HB, et al. "Psychosocial Stress Causes Endothelial Injury in Cynmolgus Monkeys Via Veta 1-Adrenoceptor Activation," *Atherosclerosis* 136:153–161, 1998.

Takahashi, K, Ohta, M, et al. "Influences of Dietary Methionine and Cysteine on Metabolic Responses to Immunological

Stress by *Escerichia coli* Lipopolysaccharide Injection and Mitogenic Response in Broiler Chickens," *British Journal of Nutrition* 78:815–821, 1997.

Toates, F. *Stress: Conceptual and Biological Aspects.* New York: John Wiley & Sons, 1995, p. 31.

VanStraten, M. *Healing Foods.* New York: Barnes & Noble, 1997, pp. 52–54.

Watkins, GG. "Music Therapy: Proposed Physiological Mechanisms and Clinical Implications," *Clin Nurse Spec* 11:43–50, 1997.

Werbach, MR. *Nutritional Influences on Illness.* New Canaan CT: Keats, 1990, pp. 155–163.

Yi, I, Stephan, FK. "The Effects of Food Deprivation, Nutritive and Non-Nutritive Feeding and Wheel Running on Gastric Stress Ulcers in Rats," *Physiology and Behavior* 63:219–225, 1998.

Tuberculosis

Balch, JF, Balch, PA. *Prescription for Nutritional Healing.* Garden City Park NY: Avery Publishing Group, 1990.

The Burton Goldberg Group (J. Strohecker, exec ed). *Alternative Medicine: The Definitive Guide.* Puyallup WA: Future Medicine Publishing, 1994.

Heinerman, J. *Encyclopedia of Healing Juices.* Englewood Cliffs NJ. Prentice Hall, 1994.

"TB Surges: Diet Link Still Unclear," *Nutrition Week* 17:6–7, 1 May 1992.

Ulcers

Albert-Puleo, M. "Physiological Effects of Cabbage with Reference to Its Potential as a Dietary Cancer-Inhibitor and Its Use in Ancient Medicine," *Journal of Ethopharmacology* 9(2):261–272, December 1983.

Aldori, WH, et al. "Prospective Study of Diet and the Risk of Duodenal Ulcer in Men," *American Journal of Epidemiology* 145:42–50, 1997.

Balch, JF, Balch, PA. *Prescription for Nutri-*

tional Healing. Garden City Park NY: Avery Publishing Group, 1990.

Cheney, G, et al. "Anti-Peptic Ulcer Dietary Factor (Vitamin "U") in the Treatment of Peptic Ulcers," *Journal of the American Dietetic Association* 25:668–672, 1950.

Murray, M, Pizzorno, J. *Encyclopedia of Natural Medicine.* 2nd ed. Rocklin CA: Prima Publishing, 1998.

Rao, NM. "Protease Inhibitors From Ripened and Unripened Bananas," *Biochemistry International* 24:13–22, 1991.

Rector, PL. *Healthy Living.* Carmel Valley CA: Healthy Living Publications, 1997.

Tovey, FI. "Diet and Duodenal Ulcer," *Journal of Gastroenterology and Hepatology* 9:177–185, 1994.

Wilson, JC. "Phytochemicals: Guardians of Our Health," *Journal of the American Dietetic Association* 97:S199–S204, 1997.

Varicose Veins and Hemorrhoids

Balch, JF, Balch, PA. *Prescription for Nutritional Healing.* Garden City Park NY: Avery Publishing Group, 1990.

Gabor, M. "The Pharmacologic Effects of Flavonoids on Blood Vessels," *Angologica* 9:355–374, 1972.

Heinerman, J. *Heinerman's Encyclopedia of Healing Juices.* Englewood Cliffs NJ: Prentice Hall, 1994.

Murray, M, Pizzorno, J. *Encyclopedia of Natural Medicine.* 2nd ed. Rocklin CA: Prima Publishing, 1998.

Rose, S. "What Causes Varicose Veins," *Lancet* 1:32, 1986.

Taussig, S. "The Mechanism of the Physiological Action of Bromelain," *Medical Hypotheses* 6:99–104, 1980.

Water Retention

Alschuler, L. Botanical Medicine I, II, III, IV (lectures). Seattle: Bastyr University, 1998.

Bertuglia, S, Malandrino, S, et al. "Effect of *Vaccinium myrillus* Anthocyanosides on

Ischemia Reperfusion Injury in Hamster Cheek Pouch Microcirculation," *Pharmacological Research* 31:183–187, 1995.

Bouskela, E, Donyo, KA. "Effects of Oral Administration of Purified Micronized Flavonoid Fraction on Increased Microvascular Permeability Induced by Various Agents and on Ischemia/Reperfusion in Diabetic Hamsters," *International Journal of Microcirculation Clinical Experiments* 15:293–300, 1995.

Bouskela, E, Svensjo, E, et al. "Oxidant-Induced Increase in Vascular Permeability is Inhibited by Oral Adminstration of S-5682 (Daflon 500 mg) and Alpha-tocopherol," *International Journal of Microcirculation Clinical Experiments* 17:18–20, 1997.

Edelstein, B. *The Woman Doctor's Guide Medical Guide for Women.* New York: William Morrow, Co., 1982.

Ihme, N, Kiesewetter, H, et al. "Leg Oedema Protection from a Buckwheat Herb Tea in Patients with Chronic Venous Insufficiency: a Single-Centre, Randomised, Double-Blind, Placebo-Controlled Clinical Trial," *European Journal of Clinical Pharmacology* 50:443–447, 1996.

Kamimur, M. "Physiology and Clinical Use of Vitamin E (author's trans.)," *Hokkaido Igaku Zasshi* 52:185–188, 1977.

"Liver Foods." Seattle: Bastyr University Nutrition Clinic, 1998. Photocopy.

McGuire, EA, Young, VR. "Nutritional Edema in a Rat Model of Protein Deficiency," *Journal of Nutrition* 116: 1209–1224, 1986.

Mian, E, et al. "Anthocyanides and the Walls of Microvessels: Further Aspects of the Mechanism of Action of Their Protective Effect in Syndromes Due to Abnormal Capillary Fragility," *Minerva Medicine* 68: 565–581, 1977.

Qiao, Y, et al. "Effects of Vitamin E on Vascular Integrity in Cholesterol-fed Guinea Pigs," *Ateriosclerosis and Thrombosis* 13:1885–1892, 1993.

Rudakova, IS, Chernukh, AM. "Changes in the State of the Microvascular Bed and in the Extent of Transcapillary Exchange by Preparations with P-Vitamin Activity," *Bibl Anat* 10:273–277, 1969.

Index